Neoliberalism, Austerity, and the Moral Economies of Young People's Health and Well-being

Peter Kelly • Jo Pike
Editors

Neoliberalism, Austerity, and the Moral Economies of Young People's Health and Well-being

palgrave
macmillan

Editors
Peter Kelly
School of Education
RMIT University
Bundoora, Victoria, Australia

Jo Pike
Leeds Beckett University,
Leeds, United Kingdom

Neoliberalism, Austerity, and the Moral Economies of Young People's Health and Well-being
ISBN 978-1-137-58265-2   ISBN 978-1-137-58266-9   (eBook)
DOI 10.1057/978-1-137-58266-9

Library of Congress Control Number: 2016955531

This Palgrave Macmillan imprint is published by Springer Nature
The registered company is Macmillan Publishers Ltd. London
The registered company address is: The Campus, 4 Crinan Street, London, N1 9XW, United Kingdom

Contents

List of Figures

List of Tables

Is Neo-Liberal Capitalism Eating Itself or Its Young?

Peter Kelly and Jo Pike

Sell Everything! Save Yourselves!

As we finalise the introduction to what we think is an important, and timely, examination of the relationships between a globalising neo-Liberal capitalism, a post-2008–2009 Global Financial Crisis (GFC) environment of recession and austerity, and the moral economies of young people's health and well-being, it appears that neo-Liberal, globalised capitalism might be about to eat itself, again. And if not itself, then it will continue, it seems, to devour its young.

At the start of 2016, in an investment note to clients, the Royal Bank of Scotland (RBS) warned that this would be a 'cataclysmic year' in

P. Kelly (✉)
RMIT University, Melbourne, VIC, Australia

J. Pike
Leeds Beckett University, Leeds, West Yorkshire, UK

© The Editor(s) (if applicable) and The Author(s) 2017
P. Kelly, J. Pike (eds.), *Neoliberalism, Austerity, and the Moral Economies of Young People's Health and Well-being*,
DOI 10.1057/978-1-137-58266-9_1

1

which 'stock markets could fall by up to 20 % and oil could slump to $16 a barrel'. Faced with cataclysm, RBS advised investors, with their own self-interests in mind, to 'sell everything except high quality bonds. This is about return of capital, not return on capital. In a crowded hall, exit doors are small'. The RBS drew strong similarities to the conditions leading up to the 2008–2009 GFC in which 'the collapse of the Lehman Brothers investment bank led to the global financial crisis. This time China could be the crisis point' (Fletcher 2016).

At the same time, and as they do each year in early January, the world's plutocrats, technocrats and largely compliant politicians gathered in the Swiss ski resort of Davos for what has come to be called the World Economic Forum (WEF). The planet's political and financial elites meet in Davos on an annual basis to discuss our common fates, or more accurately the conditions that are capable of producing and sustaining their privileges. Commentary on Davos is extensive and is often critical of the ways in which the global 0.01 % and their representatives and protectors meet in a 'public' way each year to work at maintaining processes, practices and relationships that produce and maintain this privilege in a world of profound and often deadly inequality, conflict and crisis. The challenge is not to find this sort of critique. Rather, our interest at this time is to find and put into play critique that suits the purposes we have in mind.

Aditya Chakrabortty is the senior economics commentator for *The Guardian* (UK) newspaper. Since 2008–2009 he has constructed a long CV of stories that have critically examined the GFC, the Great Recession, the UK and European Union (EU) austerity policies and the array of social, cultural and political consequences of neo-Liberal capitalism's illusory (delusional) attempts to manage its multiple, self-inflicted crises (Gray 2014). As the WEF convened at Davos, Chakrabortty (2016) wrote an article which suggested that *We've been conned by the rich predators of Davos*. The predatory metaphor seems particularly apt here.

Much of Chakrabortty's (2016) account references a report released to coincide with Davos by the global charitable organisation Oxfam on global wealth inequalities, inequalities that have widened significantly in the wake of the GFC. As Fig. 1 powerfully illustrates, the research undertaken by Oxfam (2016) claims that increasing global inequality 'has created a world where 62 people own as much as the poorest half

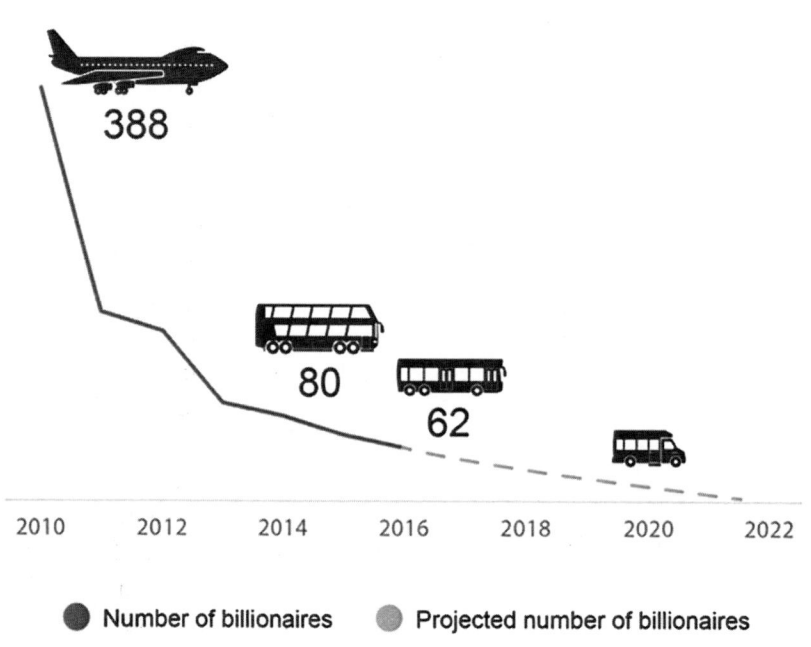

Billionaires who own the same wealth as half the world
And what transport they would fit on

388

80

62

2010   2012   2014   2016   2018   2020   2022

● Number of billionaires   ● Projected number of billionaires

Fig. 1 Number of billionaires who own as much as the poorest 50 % of the world's population. *Source*: Oxfam 2016

of the world's population'. According to Oxfam this 'number has fallen dramatically from 388 as recently as 2010 to 80 last year'. Mobilising the rhetoric of the global protest movements that emerged in the wake of the GFC (e.g. Occupy, the Spanish *Indignados* and Greek Indignant Citizens movements), Oxfam (2016) observed that

> An Economy for the 1 %, shows that the wealth of the poorest half of the world's population—that's 3.6 billion people—has fallen by a trillion dollars since 2010. This 38 per cent drop has occurred despite the global population increasing by around 400 million people during that period. Meanwhile the wealth of the richest 62 has increased by more than half a trillion dollars to $1.76tr. Just nine of the '62' are women.

Oxfam (2016) identifies a number of trends, processes and practices that have driven this escalating inequality in the period since the GFC, a period marked in spheres of human activity other than wealth accumulation, by the increasing and continuing mass unemployment of young people in economies around the world (named as *the Great Recession* in the EU and Organisation for Economic Co-operation and Development [OECD] economies), and austerity programmes that promise to forestall sovereign debt crises, in which the most vulnerable and disadvantaged carry the greatest burden. For Oxfam (2016) one of the key trends here is

> the falling share of national income going to workers in almost all developed and most developing countries and a widening gap between pay at the top and the bottom of the income scale. This particularly affects women, who make up the majority of low paid workers around the world.

In this context, Oxfam (2016) called for governments to 'make sure work delivers an acceptable standard of living for those at the bottom as well as for those at the top'. This can be achieved by 'moving minimum wage rates towards a living wage and tackling the pay gap between men and women'. Oxfam (2016) also suggested that at the privileged 0.1 % end of the spectrum, the 'already wealthy have benefited from a rate of return on capital via interest payments, dividends, etc., that has been consistently higher than the rate of economic growth'. This manifest privilege

> has been compounded by the use of tax havens which are perhaps the most glaring example set out in the report of how the rules of the economic game have been rewritten in a manner that has supercharged the ability of the rich and powerful to entrench their wealth.

The role of governments here, argued Oxfam (2016), should include developing policies and programmes to 'recover the missing billions lost to tax havens', and to commit to use these recovered billions 'to invest in healthcare, schools and other vital public services that make such a big difference to the lives of the poorest people'.[1]

---

[1] At the time of writing, pressure has increased on national governments to tackle the issue of tax havens as a result of the leaked 'Panama papers'. For a discussion of how this affects democracy,

As Chakrabortty (2016) observes, Oxfam's 'grotesque index' indicates that in terms of how many of us imagine globalised neo-Liberal capitalism should work, then things have not been right for a number of years: 'in the five years since the world recession, the very richest have grown inexorably wealthier'. Further, as Chakrabortty (2016) suggests: 'every worker on a pay freeze and every family seeing their benefits cut knows' that this massive increase in the wealth of the very few has not occurred because economies are booming, or are experiencing growth rates that result in wealth increases across the board. Rather, claims Chakrabortty (2016), it is 'because we are living in a period of *trickle-up* economics, in which the middle- and working-classes have handed over money to those right at the very top'.

For Chakrabortty (2016), reports such as Oxfam's, and much of the critique from both the left and the right about growing inequality, largely miss the point if they focus too heavily on the use of tax havens to avoid paying tax, or the situation in which the likes of Google, Apple and Amazon are able to negotiate with finance ministers in various jurisdictions about how much corporate tax that they deem it appropriate to pay (a luxury denied wage and salary earners who are subject to legislated pay-as-you-go tax scales/regimes). As bad as these tax practices and regimes may seem if we are concerned with the consequences of increased inequality, Chakrabortty (2016) insists that the story of growing inequality in the period since the GFC is one that is much more profoundly characterised by the roles of central banks around the world in printing massive amounts of money in the name of Quantitative Easing (QE). Around the globe, trillions of dollars have been pumped by central banks, not into public work programmes, infrastructure projects, bridging technologies into a post-carbon future, health infrastructure, or investments in education, training and employment initiatives that might promise some hope, some cause for optimism among the world's tens of millions of unemployed, underemployed and precariously employed young people, but into the inflation of asset prices. Assets are, by definition, held by the wealthy. Here, Chakrabortty (2016) references various sources

---

see Chakarabotty's article 'The 1 % hide their money offshore—then use it to corrupt our democracy' in *The Guardian* 10 April 2016.

which indicate, among other things, that in the period 2009–2012 the Bank of England's £375 billion QE programme had inflated the value of shares and bonds by £600 billion, and that 40 % of these gains had gone to increase the wealth of the top 5 % of UK households (Elliott 2012). In the same period, according to Emmanuel Saez, a UC Berkeley Professor of Economics, and the Director, Center for Equitable Growth, the wealthiest 1 % of US households took 91 cents of each dollar in new wealth generated, while the 99 % had to share the remaining 9 cents (Saez 2015). In the end, it is little 'wonder', according to Chakrabortty (2016), that Stanley Druckenmiller, the billionaire hedge fund manager, has labelled QE 'The biggest redistribution of wealth from the middle-class and the poor to the rich ever' (see, also, Frank 2013).

John Gray is a prolific author, a former Professor of Politics at Oxford and anti-humanist political philosopher who is deeply sceptical about the faith that many of us invest in the possibilities of human progress. Gray's (2014) *The Silence of Animals: On Progress and Other Myths* gives expression to this scepticism by suggesting that this faith is an illusion and that the idea of human progress is mythic, a secular fiction we tell ourselves as we seek a meaningfulness to human existence. In *The Silence of Animals*, he tells a troubling story of human history that continues to be marked by violence, wars, crises, totalitarianisms, 'actually existing' free markets, democracies and individualisms, and a recent faith in the possibility of human perfectibility promised through the practice of reason. His telling of this history, updated for the particular globalising challenges and crises of the early twenty-first century, embraces Marx's observation that *History repeats itself. First as tragedy, then as farce.*

For many of the young people around the globe who are the central concern for many of the contributors to this collection, the *tragedy* and the *farce* of neo-Liberal capitalism's 'eternal return' to crisis continue to be keenly felt.[2] And the work undertaken and collected here seeks to make

---

2 *The greatest weight.* What if some day or night a demon were to steal after you into your loneliest loneliness and say to you: 'This life as you now live it and have lived it, you will have to live once more and innumerable times more; and there will be nothing new in it, but every pain and every joy and every thought and sigh and everything unutterably small or great in your life will have to return to you, all in the same succession and sequence—even this spider and this moonlight between the trees, and even this moment and I myself. The eternal hourglass of existence is turned upside down again and again, and you with it, speck of dust!'

some sense to the consequences for young people of these crises under the banner of *neo-Liberalism, austerity and the moral economies of young people's health and well-being.*

Austerity and Young People's Health and Well-Being

This collection has emerged from an ongoing series of conversations that we have been involved in for a number of years, and a one-day conference held at the University of Leeds, UK, in April 2015. Much of these conversations and discussions has been framed by a sense that we need new or reinvigorated languages, new or reinvigorated vocabularies, for engaging with the long-running and increasing forms of inequalities that are just briefly hinted at in our suggestion that globalised, neo-Liberal capitalism is lurching from crisis to crisis, and in the process devouring the presents, and the futures, of hundreds of millions of young people around the world.

A central concern in reimagining some of these issues and concerns has been to think about the ways in which these increasing inequalities often have profound consequences for large populations of young people, consequences that are not just related to marginalisation from education, training and work, or to obstacles to their 'active participation' in the 'civic life' of their communities, or to their 'transitions' or their sense of 'belonging'. One way we have imagined doing this is to critically engage with the World Health Organization's (WHO 1946) very mainstream, now orthodox, understanding of health and well-being, which argues that: *Health is a state of complete physical, mental and social well-being and not merely the absence of disease or infirmity.*

The widespread, often powerful, deployment and development of this definition, such that we can call it an orthodoxy, has enabled an array of cultural, social and economic 'determinants' to be incorporated

---

Would you not throw yourself down and gnash your teeth and curse the demon who spoke thus? Or how well disposed would you have to become to yourself and to life *to crave nothing more fervently* than this ultimate eternal confirmation and seal?

From Nietzsche's *The Gay Science*, s.341, Walter Kaufmann translation. Available at http://www.theperspectivesofnietzsche.com/nietzsche/nrecur.html

into community, academic, business and policy discussions about the physical, mental and social health and well-being of different populations (young and old, who are made knowable in terms of their social class, gender, ethnic and religious background, or their geographic location).

We have suggested in a number of places (Kelly 2013, 2016; Kelly and Kamp 2015; Pike and Kelly 2014) that in this, the second decade of the twenty-first century, many young people in the OECD/EU economies, and in the developing economies of Asia, Africa and Central and South America, continue to be carrying a particularly heavy burden for many of the downstream effects of the GFC. The echoing effects of the Great Recession in Europe and the USA, for example, and the emergence of sovereign debt crises and significant austerity programmes in many EU/OECD economies represent a largely successful framing of responses to the downstream effects of the GFC as being principally about State debt levels. In this discourse, those who depend most on State-provided services, payments and programmes are the ones carrying the greatest burden of government austerity measures. It is in this sense that today's young people and young adults, and the generations who will follow and grow up in the unfolding aftermath of the GFC, will carry a particularly heavy burden in terms of changed education and employment circumstances and opportunities, consequences for physical and mental health and well-being, consumption, housing, relationship and parenting aspirations, and a sense of self in relation to the possibilities for participation in the liberal democracies (Kelly 2016).

In the EU, for example, over 4.45 million young people (under 25) were unemployed in the EU-28 area in December 2015 (an unemployment rate of 19.7 % [22.0 % in the euro area]—a rate almost twice as high as the adult unemployment rate of 10.0 %). Variations in these rates across the EU are extreme. For example, the lowest rates of youth unemployment were in Germany (7.0 %), Denmark (10.3 %) and the Czech Republic (10.9 %). The highest rates were in Greece (48.6 % in October 2015), Spain (46.0 %), Croatia (44.1 % in the fourth quarter 2015) and Italy (37.9 %) (Eurostat 2015). In addition, in 2014, 16.6 % of Europeans between 18 and 24 are classified, problematically, as neither in employment nor in education or training (NEET) (Eurostat 2016).

As many have suggested, these sorts of aggregate figures do not reveal the ways in which different groups and communities and different localities are differently impacted, how different labour markets offer more or less opportunities for particular populations of young people, or what combinations of social class, gender, ethnicity and geography shape the exclusion and marginalisation of young people from education, from work, from housing, from consumption and from the possibilities of family relationships. These gross and regionally segmented unemployment figures also do not tell us much about the types of work, the sorts of jobs that are available to many people, young and old. In *The Self as Enterprise* (Kelly 2013), we argued that work can be 'better than sex', or 'toil and drudgery', and can say much about the sorts of choices that the 'self as enterprise' can or cannot make, and how these choices echo through much of a life. Further, in many OECD and EU economies, governments have, for the last few decades, been shifting the burden for the cost of higher education to students. In this context, high levels of youth unemployment and precarious employment, student debt accompanying increased costs for higher education, housing costs that lock many out of home ownership and the challenges for young people's physical and mental health and well-being are reshaping young people's sense of self and of their chances for meaningful participation in relationships and settings that traditionally identified someone as an adult, as a citizen (Kelly 2016). In addition, hundreds of millions of children and young people around the globe face the prospect of growing up with greater levels of risk and uncertainty brought about by political instability, conflict, climate change, and technological and cultural change (Kelly and Kamp 2015).

Reflecting many of these concerns, some researchers have sought to engage with the ways in which locally produced cultures of childhood and youth are shaped by global forces, highlighting the absence of considerations of childhood and youth from discussions related to the GFC (Morrow 2009). This lack of attention to children and young people is also evident in the health-related disciplines where the widely acknowledged view that 'austerity kills' (Stuckler and Basu 2013) is a central tenet of research examining widening gaps in health inequalities, decreased investment in health-care systems and health promotion, and the impact of precarity and unemployment on mental and emotional health, food insecurity and the life choices, and chances and courses of individuals and communities. Young people, and particular populations of young people, are especially vulnerable and exposed to the sorts of crises and challenges we identify here.

Neo-Liberal Capitalism

The problem of capitalism is, in a discursive sense, a problem of 'knowing capitalism' (Thrift 2005). This is a problem that has a long history: a history of competing ways of knowing, competing purposes for knowing and competing consequences for knowing in particular ways. Thomas Piketty's (2014) *Capital in the Twenty-First Century* is probably the most widely known (if not read) recent contribution to this heritage: a contribution concerned with widening inequalities, and the ways in which the difference between returns on capital and rates of economic growth is driving the increasing global inequality that is all too evident at the start of the twenty-first century.

The problem of knowing capitalism is not one that we want to pretend to solve here, though we have engaged with the problem in greater detail elsewhere (see Kelly 2013). But knowing capitalism, in some way, is important to this collection in terms of the pervasive sense of the 'eternal return' of the crises of capitalism, our naming of capitalism as being neo-Liberal, and because we want to examine the 'moral economies' of young people's health and well-being. Our colleagues address some of these concerns in more or less detail in the chapters that follow, but at the moment we want to briefly draw on Nigel Thrift's (2005) *Knowing Capitalism* to sketch a methodological orientation or disposition to engaging the complexities, ambiguities, contradictions and paradoxes of knowing capitalism at the start of the twenty-first century—whether we call it neo-Liberal or not. The work here draws on the work done elsewhere (Kelly 2013, pp.18–20) where we referenced Thrift's (2005, p.3) position in relation to what he considers a sometimes non-reflexive, automatic response to the problem of capitalism: 'Surely capitalism is a system of oppression whose only purpose is to grind out mass commodities? And surely its Dionysian side is just one more symptom of its wrong-headedness?' Thrift's (2005, p.3) intent is to develop a much more ambivalent, even pragmatic, position to the problem of capitalism: a position that acknowledges that capitalism can be oppressive, exploitative and 'hard graft' for many. But, he suggests, it can also be 'fun': 'People get stuff from it—and not just more commodities'. In this view, capitalism 'has a kind of crazy vitality. It doesn't just line its pockets. It also appeals to gut feelings. It gets involved in all kinds of extravagant symbioses'. It is productive. It is performative. It 'adds into the world as well as subtracts'. And it reshapes the world in its own image so that it becomes difficult, even impossible, for many, to imagine something other than capitalism: a sensibility that continues to pose immense challenges for any critique of capitalism; a sensibility that produces, or fails to produce, the *crisis of ideas* that Stuart Hall and his colleagues reference in the *Kilburn Manifesto* (more on this shortly).

As Thrift indicates (2005, pp.10–11), for many commentators and critics this ambiguity is an unpopular, even wrong-headed, position, and one that attracts judgements for displaying a lack of a political stomach for the difficult task of holding capitalism to account for an array of consequences, effects and practices that should, rightly, be the object of critique and action. The problem here, in part, is what it is that we make knowable in the knowing of capitalism. What are the targets, the objects of critique? What mode of critique is appropriate for these objects? What ethos or disposition is productive in framing this critique?

Thrift (2005, p.3), for example, imagines capitalism as a 'set of networks which, though they may link in many ways, form not a total system but rather a project that is permanently "under construction"'. As a project that is permanently under construction, capitalism is also a project that is continually failing, continually escaping the ordering processes and practices of organisations, managers, consultants, commentators and academics. It is, also, a project that continually energises the production of newer, more sophisticated ordering devices and practices. As Thrift (2005, pp.1–3) argues, capitalism is always characterised by innovation, inventiveness, routine, repetition, the new, the old, the uncertain, the tried and true. Capitalism, in this sense, is 'only relatively stable and relatively predictable'; is characterised by 'all kinds of gaps and hesitations, excesses and remainders'; 'contains multiple spaces of oppression and lockdown, but it also contains little spaces of joy and generosity which cannot be locked out'; is 'enchanted'; is 'closer to the imaginary of the medieval world of dark superstitions and religious bliss than we fondly choose to believe'. Particularly, as Thrift suggests, if we are to imagine that managers of capitalist organisations are also uncertain, unsure and in the dark about 'what they are doing for quite a lot of the time'.

In a globalising world, capitalism may be the main game in town, but the game is not over, has no time limits (there appears to be no end to history), and its rules, regulations, outcomes, consequences, tools and players continue to evolve in complex, uncertain and only sometimes predictable ways. The global, regional and local economic, political and social consequences of the GFC, still echoing and unfolding in dramatic, if uneven, ways, in different contexts, are powerful manifestations of this chaos, of these crises, uncertainties and contingencies.

From this standpoint, Thrift (2005, pp.2–5) argues that any analysis of this game should be framed by a number of methodological rules. These rules, for Thrift, enable capitalism to be made known in particular ways. Knowing, in this sense, would mean adopting a particular disposition towards a *history of the present* that would seek to acknowledge in our present 'vast numbers of unresolved issues, differences of interpretation and general confusions'. This present is indeed contingent. The past, present and future are shaped by a cascading series of possibilities, *what ifs*, *if onlys* and a particular lack of any grand (intelligent) design. These ways of knowing would try to capture a sense of the performative nature of capitalism, a performativity marked by experiment, success, adaptation, complex change, crisis and the permanent possibility of failure, and of consequences that are/were not able to be imagined or planned for in any of the frameworks or models that fallible actors (human, machine, virtual) could design, develop and deploy.

So why call capitalism neo-Liberal? And not, for example, 'flexible', 'post-industrial' or 'biogenetic'. The answer here could tap into any number of academic traditions and histories. We could, as a number of our contributors do, reference the work of Michel Foucault (1983, 1985, 1986, 1991), and the governmentality literature that has drawn on and developed Foucault's legacy to imagine neo-Liberalism as an art of government, a mentality of rule. Here, neo-Liberalism is much more than economic theory, or political discourse, or public policy. In this sense, neo-Liberalism signals the emergence, development and deployment of a range of *political rationalities* and *governmental technologies* (Rose and Miller 1992) that seek to make the 'real' knowable and governable through the behaviours and dispositions of autonomous, rational, choice-making, risk aware, prudent and enterprising individuals. Individuals find a home in, and remake, the relationships between the State, Civil Society and the Economy: relationships that have been profoundly remade, though in different ways and with different consequences, in an array of national settings around the globe since the late 1970s (see Kelly 2013; Pike and Kelly 2014).

Other contributors take different routes into the neo-Liberal. As a consequence, it is not our intent to develop or impose an *orthodox* reading of neo-Liberalism, or neo-Liberal capitalism. A significant inspiration for this approach is in the ways in which the late Stuart Hall, the late Doreen Massey and Michael Rustin (2013a), and their fellow contributors, take up the challenge of rethinking the neo-Liberal ascendency *after* the GFC. In their Introduction to *After neoliberalism? The Kilburn manifesto*, Hall, Massey and Rustin (2013b) suggest that for all of neo-Liberal capitalism's 'successes' in remaking the world, and our sense of what it is to be a person, many of the overdeveloped OECD economies currently find themselves in deep trouble, and young people are carrying a particularly heavy burden for their trouble. As Hall et al. (2013b, pp.16–17), suggest

> This phase of free-market capitalism has now entered a serious economic crisis from which it cannot easily engineer an exit. But the shape of the crisis remains 'economic'. There are so far no major political fractures, no unsettlings of ideological hegemony, no ruptures in popular discourse. The disastrous effects of the crisis are clearly evident; but there is little understanding of how everyday troubles connect to wider structures. There is no serious crisis of ideas.

In much of the work done by themselves and their collaborators in the *Manifesto,* Hall et al. (2013b, pp.8–9) try to capture and analyse a sense of the moment, of our present, of young people's present. A present that is marked by recession, sovereign debt crises, austerity and the language of 'strivers and skivers' and 'lifters and leaners'—as seemingly unproblematic ways of describing self-evident realities in human experience, circumstances and orientations to the conduct of a life. For Hall and the others, the 'present economic crisis is a moment of potential rupture'. As they suggest, the 'current neoliberal settlement has … entailed the re-working of the common-sense assumptions of the earlier, social democratic settlement'. Drawing on an extensive, long-running thread in Hall's work, they suggest that every 'social settlement, in order to establish itself, is crucially founded on embedding as common sense a whole bundle of beliefs'. This common sense bundles together, however, provisionally, 'ideas beyond question, assumptions so deep that the very fact that they are assumptions is only rarely brought to light'. The bundle of beliefs we name as neo-Liberalism 'revolves around the supposed naturalness of "the market", the primacy of the competitive individual, the superiority of the private over the public'.

Yet, as they suggest, this 'outcome was not inevitable. Conflicts between social settlements and the crafting of hegemonies are the product of contending social forces' (Hall et al. 2013b, p.8). What is more, neo-Liberal views of individualised autonomy, choice, responsibility and the market are, at the same time, 'naturalised' and contested in the current settlement:

> Opening public areas for potential profit-making is accepted because it appears to be 'just economic common sense'. The ethos of the 'free market' is taken to licence an increasing disregard for moral standards, and even for the law itself. (Hall et al. 2013b, p.8)

These moral dilemmas and concerns are evidenced in suggestions that the dominance of market logics in all areas of life has 'cultivated an ethos of corruption and evasiveness'. Some examples are as follows:

> Banks, once beacons of probity, rig interest rates, mis-sell products, launder drug money, flout international embargoes, hide away fortunes in safe havens. … Graduates stacking supermarket shelves are told they don't need to be paid because they are 'getting work experience'. Commercialisation

permeates everywhere, trumps everything. Once the imperatives of a "market culture" become entrenched, anything goes. Such is the power of the hegemonic common sense. (Hall et al. 2013b, pp.14–15)

It is in this 'moment' of crisis, of possible ruptures, of a call for new thinking *after neo-Liberalism*, that this collection is situated.

The Moral Economies of Young People's Health and Well-Being

A particular concern for this collection is the concept of *moral economy/moral economies*, and what this concept offers for thinking about the choices that are imagined, are made, or not made, by a range of individuals, organisations, businesses and agencies in relation to young people's health and well-being in the context of austerity and a crisis of/for neo-Liberalism. This interest, to a large degree, develops the work we undertook in *The Moral Geographies of Children, Young People and Food: Beyond Jamie's School Dinners* (Pike and Kelly 2014).[3] There we used the concept of *moral geographies* to identify and engage with the elements of choice that relate to what it is that we *should* feed ourselves, our families, our children. We suggested that these questions of choice and what we should imagine as food extended also to the various, often complex and ambiguous, processes and practices of food production, processing, transportation and preparation. As well as to the array of personal and cultural practices that structure often idealised, always morally inflected, ideas about children, parenting and food, the family meal, the issues of young people's nutrition, health and well-being, public health 'crises' such as obesity, and the array of possible responses and interventions in relation to these issues, these crises. We were interested in the cultural, economic, social, political and spatial dimensions of these choices, the things that contribute to the shaping and the making of these choices, the normative and non-normative forces and positions that contribute to the naming and framing of what it is that we should choose to do, how we should

---

[3] This section draws on Pike and Kelly 2014, pp.1–9.

choose to prepare, present and consume our food, where and when these practices and processes should occur, who should be present, and what relations of authority are implicated in the choosing and the doing.

Citing Roger Lee and David Smith's (2011, p.2) argument in *Geographies and Moralities: International Perspectives on Development, Justice and Peace* that far from being universal and unchanging, ethics and morals 'are, in short, social constructs', we suggested that a current interest in the idea of the *moral* in a number of social science disciplines connected to a long tradition that included Nietzsche's (2003) *The Genealogy of Morals*; Weber's (2002) *The Protestant Ethic and the 'Spirit' of Capitalism*, and Foucault's (1986) *The Care of the Self*.

Lee and Smith (2011) suggest that a concern with *moral geographies* has mirrored, since the 1980s, a broad concern with the uneven, unequal development of particular places and spaces in an increasingly globalised world (see, e.g., Harvey 1996; Proctor and Smith 1999; Sack 1993, 2003; Smith 1997, 2000). Lee and Smith (2011, p.2) make a case for recognising that 'there are "moralities of geography" as well as "geographies of morality"'. We suggested that this recognition not only pointed to some of the spatial dimensions of our concern with the moral judgements associated with young people and food but, also, pointed to the 'normativity of the practice of geography, and of geographers' (Lee and Smith 2011, p.2). Lee and Smith (2011, p.1) indicate that in these moments of recognition, when 'we raise issues of spatial inequality and its social, economic and political consequences', then the normative dimensions of spatial relations, and geography's concerns with these, become apparent. What also becomes apparent in these moments, and movements, is the 'more critical issue of normative ethics: to what extent are uneven development and social inequality just?' (Lee and Smith 2011, p.1). As they indicate, the 'resolution of such questions are both reflected in, and constitutive of, the moral values of particular people in particular places'.

In our earlier work, we highlighted Lee and Smith's discussion about the complex relations between processes of development, the places and spaces shaped by these processes, and issues of justice that can be attached to these processes. In the first instance, Lee and Smith (2011, p.7) argue that if 'moralities are inescapable, distinctions like those between positive and normative thought start to look distinctly chaotic'. This chaos and complexity is made real, for Lee and Smith, in the theoretical, epistemological and methodological choices that geographers and social scientists make, and the social, economic, cultural and political practices and processes that shape the projects and work and objects of study that we become concerned with. Lee and Smith (2011, p.7) further suggest that moralities are 'profoundly geographical products of uneven development of social relations among people and between people and nature'. These differences and distinctions, and the 'tensions that are created through them, together constitute the very source of moralities'. These sorts of relations, distinctions and differentiations raise, for Lee and Smith (2011, p.8), questions about the complexity, ambiguity and character of these very relations and differentiations—in general, and in more particular contexts. There is, they suggest

> an important issue here of the extent and nature of over-determination in understanding the complex and mutually formative relationships between the 'economic' and 'culture', for example, or between the ethical and the social.

Finally, the ways in which in a variety of academic, community and political/policy discussions concerns related to social justice have been transformed into 'matters of social exclusion' indicates, for Lee and Smith (2011, p.8), the putting into play of 'an unquestioned norm (the condition from which exclusion is sustained), rather than a contested process which may be judged by certain criteria to be just or unjust'. As they suggest, the more or less successful displacement of a discourse of social justice by a discourse of social exclusion, particularly in the neo-Liberal democracies 'serves to sustain and enhance existing inequalities of power around what are represented as unproblematic norms'. In this sense, the logics of markets come to shape other (all) forms of being, and the response to manifest inequalities comes to be shaped by concerns with choice, participation, responsibility, inclusion and exclusion, and not with justice.

Building on our work on moral geographies, we have found Andrew Sayer's (2000, 2004a, b) discussions of moral economies to be generative for framing the work of this collection (see also Dogan 2010, Max Planck Institute 2016). For Sayer (2004b), 'moral economy' is a concept, originally introduced by E P Thompson (1971) in a discussion of food riots in the 'premodern' English economy of the eighteenth century, that, in a much wider sense than first imagined by Thompson, suggests a

> kind of inquiry focussing on how economic activities of all kinds are influenced and structured by moral dispositions, values and norms, and how in turn these are reinforced, shaped, compromised or overridden by economic pressures.

It is in this sense, Sayer (2004b) argues that 'moral' and 'economy' are 'best defined broadly'. The 'moral' here includes an interest in

> lay norms (informal and formal), conventions, values, dispositions and commitments regarding what is just and what constitutes good behaviour in relation to others, and implies certain broader conceptions of the good or well-being.

In this way, *contra* E.P. Thompson, Sayer (2004a, p.2) suggests that it can be useful to argue that '*all* economies—not merely pre- or non-capitalist ones—are moral economies'. In doing so, he recognises that

> Of course, just what counts as moral, as opposed to immoral, behaviour is contestable; some forms of moral economy, for example, that of the patriarchal household, might be deemed immoral, or as domination disguised as benevolence and fairness.

In his work on moral economies, Sayer (2004a, p.2) explores the 'ways in which markets and associated economic phenomena both depend on and influence moral/ethical sentiments, norms and behaviours and have ethical implications'. Importantly, given our interests in the array of choices made and not made about young people, their education, training and work, their health and well-being in a post-GFC period of ongoing crises for neo-Liberal capitalism, this broad view of the *moral* creates a space not only for assessing moral aspects of economic practices, and economic influences on morality, but also for the assessment of how economic organisation affects human well-being. (Sayers 2004b, p. 1)

In the chapters that follow, these broad conceptual and empirical concerns will be developed in ways that give a more particular, social, cultural, economic, political and geographical flavour to the ways in which the health and well-being, the life chances, life choices and life courses of hundreds of millions of young people around the world are currently being shaped and remade in the moral economies of neo-Liberalism and austerity.

Part I: After Neo-Liberalism? Rethinking Choices, Responsibilities and Young People's Futures

In Part I of this collection, our contributors, in a variety of ways, engage with the challenges set out in the *Kilburn Manifesto* to trouble, to unsettle, to make problematic, to contribute to a crisis of ideas about neo-Liberalism, austerity and the moral economies of young people's health and well-being. In different ways, the authors of chapters in this section engage with some key concepts and key ideas, with categories and new vocabularies that promise to contribute to different ways of thinking about the challenges and opportunities that continue to profoundly shape young people's life chances, life choices and life courses. These vocabularies are productive, generative and sometimes provocative. They aim to open up discussion, rather than replace a neo-Liberal orthodoxy with new orthodoxies.

Peter Kelly in Chap. 1 opens up spaces in which children and young people's marginalisation can be rethought in ways that are productive for Youth Studies at the start of the twenty-first century. In his chapter, he questions whether concepts such as *structure* and *agency*, which comprise part of the orthodoxy of Youth Studies, are well able to capture the character and experience of young people's marginalisation in a post-GFC world in which neo-Liberal, biogenetic capitalism changes the 'nature' of what it is to be an 'agent' (human and non-human). Drawing on Foucault's concept of apparatus and Braidotti's post-humanism, he asks whether structure and agency are still appropriate terms, appropriate concepts. What sorts of thinking, doing, being should sociologies of youth be concerned with? What relationships, practices, functions and consequences, what organisms, substances and apparatuses can be made present, manifestly absent, absent as Other in the doing of this work? Who or what might have that thing called agency in the twenty-first century, biogenetic, digital capitalism in which human exceptionalism looks increasingly problematic and provisional? In raising these questions, Peter argues that the promise of remaking the world cannot be invested in the autonomous, choice-making, individualised human agent/subject, and that 'structure's and 'agency' need to be reassembled in ways that are fit for what it is to be a truly networked organism.

In Chap. 2, Luke Howie and Perri Campbell take us into the world of Katniss Everdeen and *The Hunger Games* to suggest that in a post-GFC world pop culture has played a significant role in questioning neo-Liberal common sense. For Luke and Perri, *The Hunger Games* novels and films can be read as *moments that imagine the future in other terms* and are, in this sense, possible catalysts for change. But this reading requires 'diligent viewing' and a 'little imagination'. Their diligent reading focuses on two key allegories in the series: the song 'The Hanging Tree' that becomes the ballad of the revolution in *The Hunger Games*, and the existence of the 'Mockingjay' birds which become the emblems for nation-wide resistance. They read *The Hunger Games* as *political action* able to help young people think through the dilemmas posed by neo-Liberalism, to reinvent themselves in the process, and resist, when they can, those socio-economic conditions that we are raised to believe are inevitable.

In Chap. 3, Julia Coffey draws on data from a qualitative study to explore the ways in which moral imperatives of health and well-being shape young people's negotiations of health and body work practices. Julia suggests that body work practices such as diet and exercise, and those practices that modify the body's form or appearance, are a central way in which young people are encouraged to be increasingly responsible for their own health and well-being. Deploying a Deleuzo-Guattarian theorisation of health as an assemblage, Julia analyses the ways in which moral imperatives function through discourses and affects associated with neo-Liberal conditions—such as in the importance of 'looking' and 'feeling' healthy, and the 'worry' associated with becoming overweight. From this perspective, health as an assemblage 'works' through discourses of individualised self-responsibility and bodily perfection, as well as through affects that mediate a body's capacities.

In a provocative Chap. 4, Deirdre Duffy argues that happiness is a central theme in the current well-being agenda for young people: both implicitly, when it is couched in the language of therapy and ensuring contentment, and explicitly, through the adoption of 'happiness measures' and the emergence of Happiness Studies. Drawing on the particular context of the UK post-GFC, and after the implementation of a Conservative–Liberal Democrat government austerity programme from 2010, Deirdre suggests that the happiness agenda operates not as some sort of vague, well-intentioned support, but as a form of affective governance. In this sense, the happiness project represents the production and regulation of neo-Liberal subjects through the regulation of 'affect', 'emotion' and 'futurity'. This form of governing orients subjects towards ways of being by connecting them to desired emotional states (joyfulness, pride, happiness) that are felt viscerally before they are subjected to reflection. In this chapter, Deirdre suggests that contemporary populations of young people in the UK are readily 'governable' in these ways, as their ways of being in the present are already oriented towards ways of being in the future. As a consequence, the promotion of happiness in discourses of well-being is part of a strategy of both orienting young people towards particular ways of being and, in doing so, regulating young people in the present: a present that is marked by crisis and austerity.

Lucas Walsh in Chap. 5 suggests that in the moral economies of neo-Liberalism and austerity, young people, in transition from school to work, are entering both new and familiar territories. In his chapter, he highlights the ways in which business mantras about skills shortages, wider orthodoxies about the value and purpose of education, and entrenched forms of inequality and marginalisation collide with recent social, economic and geographic impacts of the GFC and various policy responses to them. At these intersections, young people are encouraged to develop what Lucas identifies as a form of 'adversity capital'—the skills and literacies that promise to produce young people who are more adaptive, flexible and resilient. His chapter critically explores the conceptual and practical possibilities—and potential limitations—of 'adversity capital', and how it might build on a notion of 'resilience' that is located in a wider social ecology beyond the individual capabilities of young people.

Part II: Young People, Austerity and the Moral Geographies of Disadvantage

Part II presents a series of chapters that explore diverse aspects of young people's marginalisation, their differing experiences of marginalisation and some of the health and well-being consequences of what we are calling moral geographies of disadvantage. In different spaces—cities, regions, nation states—neo-Liberalism and austerity give a particular shape, a certain character to the practices, the processes, the situations, the norms, the values, the choices made by the State and its agencies, by organisations, businesses, communities, families and individuals that give form to young people's experiences of disadvantage and injustice, and their health and well-being.

Portugal, and Portuguese young people, have been hit hard by the GFC and its downstream effects. For example, in Portugal in 2014 young people were registered as unemployed at double the rates of their older counterparts: 34 % of young people between 15 and 24, and 25 % of young people between 15 and 29, against 15 % for the general population. It is in this context that Magda Nico and Nuno de Almeida Alves present data from a number of studies they have undertaken, data that they interpret and analyse using two key concepts: the importance of cultural and historical location to the examination of young people's life course, to the 'historicality of the individual', and the so-called accumulation of inequalities in which moments of crisis encounter national and individual social, cultural, economic and political histories. From this perspective, Chap. 6 by Magda and Nuno powerfully demonstrates the long-term, corrosive effects on young people's well-being, their life chances, life choices and life courses, of a declining welfare state when it is combined with an economic crisis and the austerity measures introduced in its name.

Chapter 7 by Giuseppina Cersosimo and Maurizio Merico explores how, over the last decade, Italy has witnessed a significant increase in the prevalence of childhood and juvenile obesity. They suggest, as much as other research does, that the incidence of childhood and juvenile obesity can produce serious consequences for the physical health and well-being of young people, now and in their futures. Indeed, the GFC has exacerbated these health challenges for many regions in Italy by contributing to a decline in food quality, a deterioration in eating habits and a decrease in State funding of primary and preventative health care. Giuseppina and Maurizio's contribution to thinking about these challenges is to propose a social epidemiological framework that articulates with an analysis of the transformations in the process of socialisation of children and young people. They suggest that in an age of austerity this kind of approach compels us to take into consideration the need for new relationships between the different actors and agencies engaged at different levels, and with different roles, in addressing this complex issue.

Kerry Montero in Chap. 8 draws on research undertaken in a secondary school-based young driver health education programme to explore wider concerns about the health and well-being of young people growing up on the margins, at the 'interface' of the urban and rural. As she demonstrates, in the Australian context of growing populations on the expanding urban–rural interface areas of large cities, areas that are notoriously transport and infrastructure poor, 'healthy', 'responsible' alternatives and choices do not always exist for many young people. Here, 'safe transport options' for young people are fundamentally shaped by spatial geographies that are linked to economic and social disadvantage. In a time of neo-Liberal reform agendas, incremental government withdrawal from support services and programmes, and measures to shift the burden of economic crisis onto those who are already struggling, young people who depend on these services and supports are further disadvantaged. Kerry powerfully argues that many young people are growing up in a 'perfect storm' of historical neglect of basic infrastructure and community amenities, and public policies driven by market forces indifferent to their needs.

Jade is a 14-year-old white, working class girl from the north of England. In Chap. 9 by Louise Laverty, we are introduced to Jade through an account of Louise's ethnography of a youth club in a disadvantaged area of a northern English city. Louise's discussion focuses on aspects of Jade's experience of her sexuality, and the responses of other young people and youth workers to her apparent 'deviant' 'sluttishness'. Louise explores the social role of emotions in generating and regulating stigma and creating exclusion. As she argues, this is important to consider as stigma is increasingly utilised as an acceptable and necessary force to change behaviour in public policy. 'Slut-shaming' is a tactic that tries to reinforce certain sexual norms and punish deviance through evoking shame, disgust and guilt. In this sense, Jade is regarded as wholly responsible for her behaviours, a responsibilisation that leads to Jade's marginalisation, and which blames the individual for their 'deviance' or 'failure'. Louise suggests that beyond the experience of Jade, neo-Liberal austerity programmes in the UK mean that issues such as poverty are subject to similar moral discourses, via discourses of 'welfare-shaming'. In this context, we are likely to see similar experiences of exclusion and blame laid at the feet of individuals. Perhaps, asks Louise, we should be more concerned with questioning who is being shamed and stigmatised, by whom, and with what consequences.

In Chap. 10, John McKendrick builds on his previous work in Scotland and England on the ways in which the UK population understands, and wants the State and individuals to respond to, the problems of childhood poverty. In his discussion of an evolving policy framework, and of data from the British Social Attitudes (BSA) survey, John explores the unravelling of a consensus position that, under New Labour aspired to eradicate child poverty within a generation. He suggests that a post-GFC austerity agenda in the UK has provided the context in which, at first, a regressive neo-Liberalism dismantled this consensus, only to be itself challenged by thinking that appears even more progressive than that which previously prevailed. His analysis suggests that in the rise of the Scottish Nationalist Party, and in BSA data, there is evidence that the advent of austerity has not been accompanied by a strong reversal, but that the hardening of attitudes against the most vulnerable has been checked. For John, it is clear that social attitudes are malleable and that there is the basis for nurturing a moral economy of social justice that may open the policy space for more progressive interventions to tackle child poverty in the UK.

Chapter 11 by Kelley Moult and Alexandra Müller identifies that the provision of sexual and reproductive health services (SRH) for young people in South Africa is a complex landscape—balancing youth and human rights, numerous laws, legally and professionally mandated obligations, and a tenuous and resource-strained implementation context. These conflicts are compounded in neo-Liberal environments of limited infrastructure and resources, such as the South African public health system. Their chapter examines the decision-making processes of South African nurses providing SRH services to adolescents in health facilities in the public sector. Kelley and Alexandra explore the impact of extremely limited financial and human resources on nurses' decisions related to service provision, including the significant implementation gaps that exist in clinics. They analyse nurses' feelings about, and experiences of, policy changes, and describe a number of structural obstacles to involving nurses in policy processes, including a lack of communication about existing policies, new policy initiatives from 'top' to 'bottom' level and work load pressure due to understaffing. In the context of the provision of SRH services for young people in South Africa, Kelley and Alexandra powerfully argue that tightening the screws on service provision in a climate of austerity and resource scarcity increases the pressure on nurses, and constrains young people's lives, health and choices.

Part III: Young People, Welfare States and Their Futures

In Part III, contributors take up the challenges of examining aspects of young people's futures, their engagement with, and transitions out of, different education and training settings, and their movements into increasingly globalised and precarious labour markets and working environments. These engagements, these transitions, these movements take on different characteristics, different limits and possibilities in different settings. The role of the State and its agencies in regulating diverse and various aspects of the systems, practices and processes that shape education, training and work—and the relationships between them—is a central concern for our colleagues in this section. Welfare state futures and young people's futures are, they suggest, intimately connected, and continuously reassembled in the moral economies of neo-Liberal capitalism and austerity.

Annelies Kamp in Chap. 12 offers a post-critical reading of youth transitions in the Republic of Ireland. In her chapter, Annelies draws on the material semiotics of Actor Network Theory (ANT) to explore the 'pre-assemblage' of young people moving through, and beyond, second-level school in the post-austerity context of Ireland as it emerges from the management of its fiscal affairs by the *troika* of the International Monetary Fund, the European Central Bank and the European Commission. Her deployment of the material semiotics of ANT brings into focus actors, distant and local, human and non-human, who shape the movement of young people beyond a primary engagement with formal education, and the consequences of this for young people's health and well-being. The analysis here looks closely at one of the central techniques of transition in Ireland—colloquially referred to as 'the points race'—to consider how points have evolved to a 'black box' status, and to demonstrate their mediating role in enabling certain events to flow while others can only stutter. This work enables her to explore the potential for some form of reassemblage of what happens between school and work and the contribution such a rethinking might make to the health and well-being of the young people of Ireland.

Alan France in Chap. 13 draws on an extensive body of work in his examination of the ways in which, over the last three decades, welfare-to-work programmes in countries such as the UK, Australia and New Zealand have become a 'normal' part of how social welfare for the young unemployed is constructed. As Alan suggests, in these settings the 'workfare state' is at the heart of the neo-Liberal project and makes significant contributions to our understanding of citizenship for the young. In the aftermath of the GFC, and in the context of an austerity agenda that has developed in the Great Recession, welfare to work has further evolved as a way of not only getting people back to work, but as a means to reduce the social benefit budget. Its advocates suggest that welfare to work is the best way to tackle the 'problem' of dependency and worklessness among the young unemployed. Yet, as Alan makes clear, little evidence exists to suggest that such programmes are effective in getting young people into the labour market. Indeed, evidence suggests that most of these strategies are targeted at disciplining, regulating and controlling the poor, and operate to show that the state is doing something about the 'feckless', the 'work shy' and the undeserving. What we are seeing here is the embedding of a moral economy of unemployment that re-enforces individual responsibility and self-blame while also punishing those who are unable to access work (regardless of its quality and value).

In Chap. 14, Barbara (Barb) Chancellor and Marg Sellers illustrate the ways in which a particular 'Bush Kinder' (Bush Kindergarten) in suburban Melbourne (Westgarth, Australia) is a setting where young children's play is 'powerfully' arranged through particular moral geographies. They argue that these particular moral geographies promise to trouble or unsettle what can be called more 'traditional', more 'orthodox' power relations, and the spatial and moral dimensions of practices and responses of conventionally structured early childhood settings. Barb and Marg begin their engagement with these possibilities through what they describe as a Deleuzo-Guattarian 'and … and … and' conversational wondering/wandering about the space of Bush Kinder, the one in Westgarth in particular, but other (early) childhood spaces beyond the particular, and how these spaces relate to neo-Liberal programmes of early childhood provision in Australia: programmes that are increasingly privatised, commodified and shaped by commercial, rather than educational forces. Is the Bush Kinder a privileged space? If so, in what ways? What does the notion of privilege mean? In wondering/wandering that suggest that the moral project of the self in human and non-human relations becomes apparent in the Westgarth Bush Kinder, in ways that hold the promise for thinking differently about how we see and make the world of young children's well-being and learning in such spaces.

Chapter 15 by Jo Pike examines the shifting understanding of the State's role in the provision of school meals in the UK—and the roles that changing understandings of the concept of 'fairness' play at different times, with different consequences. Her chapter examines the policy shifts related to the provision of school meals of the Conservative–Liberal Democrat coalition government during the period of 2010–2015, a period when an austerity agenda in the UK saw significant cuts in government spending across a range of areas and programmes. Jo explores the ways in which policy decisions related to school meals, and more specifically the introduction in 2013 of a universal free school meals policy, were justified to the public, and how these debates are morally framed in public discourse. In doing this work, she pays close attention to the ways in which concepts of 'fairness' are deployed in response to questions regarding the obligations of the state and the family with respect to the well-being of children and young people. She argues that moral concepts such as fairness have become 'monetarised' in the context of neo-Liberalism and have replaced more welfarist perspectives premised on notions of 'public good'. In this sense, Jo questions whether school meals can be classified as a 'public good', and whether this 'rethinking' can shape debates about aspects of young people's health and well-being in the moral economies of neo-Liberalism and austerity in the UK.

At the start of the twenty-first century, the population demographics of many of the Middle East and North Africa (MENA) countries are, as Christoph Schwarz demonstrates, characterised by a 'youth bulge'. These young people have occupied a troubled/troubling presence in the West's imagination: prior to the uprisings of 2011, they tended to be discussed as a potential threat—associated with debates on terrorism—or as politically lethargic victims of failed policies of authoritarian regimes, and a premodern 'traditional Islamic culture'. Since 2011, explanations have been sought for their involvement in differing forms of protest across the MENA. In Chap. 16, Christoph uses this background to explore the usefulness, or otherwise, of the concept of 'waithood'—a form of social exclusion of the young through a particular 'political economy of marriage' that results in stalled transitions to adulthood—to examine the particular case of the Moroccan unemployed graduates movement. The movement provides an example of how young adults have addressed their economic situation, and have 'apolitically' protested in an authoritarian regime for over a decade before the 'Arab Spring'. Christoph's research and analysis suggests that, at least in the Moroccan case, the concept of waithood cannot be applied without discussing precarious work conditions in the private sector, and the changing character of State interventions and regulations. Indeed, the research presented here illustrates that the transition to adulthood, its intersection with the reproduction of social inequality and social exclusion, and the potential processes that the State develops to facilitate transitions always emerge from the particular intricacies and intimacies of the relationships between the State, the individual and the economy— and the choices, norms and values that shape and saturate these intricacies and intimacies.

References

Chakrabortty, A. 2016. We've been conned by the rich predators of Davos. *The Guardian*, January 19. Available from http://www.theguardian.com/commentisfree/2016/jan/19/davos-super-rich-wealth-inequality. Accessed 20 Jan 2016.

Dogan, M. 2010. When Neoliberalism Confronts the Moral Economy of Workers: The Final Spring of Turkish Labor Unions. *European Journal of Turkish Studies* [En ligne], 11 | 2010, mis en ligne le 05 octobre 2010, Consulté le 10 avril 2015. Available from http://ejts.revues.org/4321. Accessed 20 Jan 2016.

Elliott, L. 2012. Britain's richest 5% gained most from quantitative easing— Bank of England. *The Guardian*, August 23. Available from http://www.theguardian.com/business/2012/aug/23/britains-richest-gained-quantative-easing-bank. Accessed 20 Jan 2016.

Eurostat. 2015. Unemployment Statistics, December 2015. Available from http://ec.europa.eu/eurostat/statistics-explained/index.php/Unemployment_statistics. Accessed 20 Jan 2016.

———. 2016. Young people neither in employment nor in education and training by sex and age (NEET rates), January 2016. Available from http://ec.europa.eu/eurostat/en/web/products-datasets/-/EDAT_LFSE_20. Accessed 20 Jan 2016.

Fletcher, N. 2016. Sell everything ahead of stock market crash, say RBS economists. *The Guardian*, January 12. Available from http://www.theguardian.com/business/2016/jan/12/sell-everything-ahead-of-stock-market-crash-say-rbs-economists. Accessed 20 Jan 2016.

Foucault, M. 1983. The Subject and Power. In *Michel Foucault: Beyond Structuralism and Hermeneutics*, eds. H.L. Dreyfus and P. Rabinow, 208–226. Chicago: University of Chicago Press.

———. 1985. *The Use of Pleasure*. New York: Pantheon.

———. 1986. *The Care of the Self*. New York: Pantheon.

———. 1991. Governmentality. In *The Foucault Effect: Studies in Governmental Rationality*, eds. G. Burchell, C. Gordon, and P. Miller, 87–104. Hemel Hempstead: Harvester Wheatsheaf.

Frank, R. 2013. Druckenmiller: Fed robbing poor to pay rich. *CNBC*, September 19. Available from http://www.cnbc.com/2013/09/19/druckenmiller-fed-shifting-money-to-rich-from-poneo-Liberal ascendency or.html. Accessed 20 Jan 2016.

Gray, J. 2014. *The Silence of Animals: On Progress and Other Modern Myths*. London: Penguin.

Hall, S., D. Massey, and M. Rustin, eds. 2013a. *After neoliberalism? The Kilburn manifesto*, Soundings. London: Lawrence & Wishart.

———. 2013b. After neoliberalism: analysing the present. In *After neoliberalism? The Kilburn manifesto*, Soundings, eds. S. Hall, D. Massey, and M. Rustin. London: Lawrence & Wishart.

Harvey, D. 1996. *Justice, Nature and the Geography of Difference*. Oxford: Blackwell.

Kelly, P. 2013. *The Self as Enterprise: Foucault and the "Spirit" of 21st Century Capitalism*. Aldershot: Ashgate/Gower.

———. 2016. Growing up After the GFC: Responsibilisation and Mortgaged Futures. *Discourse*. doi:10.1080/01596306.2015.1104852.

Kelly, P., and A. Kamp. 2015. *A Critical Youth Studies for the 21st Century*. Amsterdam/Boston: Brill.

Lee, R. and Smith, D. (2011). Introduction: Geographies of Morality and Moralities of Geography, in R. Lee and D. M. (eds) *Geographies and Moralities: International Perspectives on Development, Justice and Peace*, Blackwell, Oxford, pp 1–12.

Max Planck Institute. 2016. The International Max Planck Research School for Moral Economies of Modern Societies. Available from https://www.mpib-berlin.mpg.de/en/research/research-schools/imprs-moral-economies. Accessed 20 Jan 2016.

Morrow, V. 2009. The global financial crisis and children's happiness: a time for re-visioning?, *Childhood* 16 (3) 293–298.

Nietzsche, F. 2003. *The Genealogy of Morals*. Mineola, NY: Dover Publications.

Oxfam. 2016. *62 people own same as half world—Oxfam*. Press release, January 18. Available from http://www.oxfam.org.uk/media-centre/press-releases/2016/01/62-people-own-same-as-half-world-says-oxfam-inequality-report-davos-world-economic-forum. Accessed 20 Jan 2016.

Pike, J., and P. Kelly. 2014. *The Moral Geographies of Children, Young People and Food: Beyond Jamie's School Dinners.* London: Palgrave.

Piketty, T. 2014. *Capital in the Twenty-First Century.* Cambridge, MA: Harvard University Press.

Proctor, J.D., and D.M. Smith, eds. 1999. *Geography and Ethics: Journeys in a Moral Terrain.* London: Routledge.

Rose, N., and P. Miller. 1992. Political Power Beyond the State: Problematics of Government. *British Journal of Sociology* 43(2): 173–205.

Sack, R.D. 1993. *Homo Geographicus: A Framework for Action, Awareness, and Moral Concern.* Baltimore: Johns Hopkins University Press.

———. 2003. *A Geographical Guide to the Real and the Good.* London: Routledge.

Saez, E. 2015. *Striking it Richer: The Evolution of Top Incomes in the United States.* Available from https://eml.berkeley.edu/~saez/saez-UStopincomes-2013.pdf. Accessed 20 Jan 2016.

Sayer, A. 2000. Moral economy and political economy. *Studies in Political Economy* 61(1): 79–103.

———. 2004a. Moral Economy. Available from http://www.comp.lancs.ac.uk/sociology/papers/sayer-moral-economy.pdf. Accessed 20 Jan 2016.

———. 2004b. Agendas for Moral Economy. *Moral Economy: Agendas for the Future.* Workshop held on July 6th 2004, at the Department of Sociology, Lancaster University, Lancaster LA1 4YD, UK.

Smith, D.M. 1997. Geography and ethics: a moral turn? *Progress in Human Geography* 21(4): 583–590.

———. 2000. *Moral Geographies: Ethics in a world of difference.* Edinburgh: Edinburgh University Press.

Stuckler, D., and S. Basu. 2013. *The Body Economic: Why Austerity Kills.* New Yok: Basic Books.

Thompson, E.P. 1971. The Moral Economy of the English Crowd in the Eighteenth Century. *Past & Present* 50(1): 76–136.

Thrift, N. 2005. *Knowing Capitalism.* London: Sage.

Weber, M. 2002. *The Protestant Ethic and the 'Spirit' of Capitalism: and Other Writings.* London: Penguin.

World Health Organization (WHO). 1946. Preamble to the Constitution of the World Health Organization as adopted by the International Health Conference, New York, 19–22 June, 1946; signed on 22 July 1946 by the representatives of 61 States (Official Records of the World Health Organization, no. 2, p. 100) and entered into force on 7 April 1948.

Part I

After Neo-Liberalism? Re-thinking Choices, Responsibilities and Young People's Futures

1

Young People's Marginalisation: Unsettling What Agency and Structure Mean After Neo-Liberalism

Peter Kelly

Introduction: Young People's Marginalisation and a Post-GFC World

In the days, months and years after many of the major institutions of globalised and financialised capitalism near froze, then went into melt-down in the later part of 2007 and the early part of 2008, and began to wreak havoc in spaces that, at first glance, had little direct relation to the worlds of US-based sub-prime mortgages, derivatives, Collateralised Debt Obligations, Credit Default Swaps, billion dollar profits and multi-million dollar bonuses, powerful, vested interests mobilised to reconfig-ure, to reimagine, the Global Financial Crisis (GFC) as being a crisis of sovereign debt, as signalling a need for massive reductions in state spend-ing, as creating an urgent need for austerity. As I have argued elsewhere

P. Kelly (✉)
RMIT University, Melbourne, VIC, Australia

© The Editor(s) (if applicable) and The Author(s) 2017
P. Kelly, J. Pike (eds.), *Neoliberalism, Austerity, and the Moral Economies of Young People's Health and Well-being*,
DOI 10.1057/978-1-137-58266-9_2

35

(Kelly 2013, 2016), the work done by conservative governments, the International Monetary Fund, *troikas*, think tanks, conservative commentators and media outlets has been largely successful in many of the Organisation for Economic Co-operation and Development/European Union (OECD/EU) economies in framing responses to the downstream effects of the GFC as being principally about State debt levels. In this discourse, those that depend most on State-provided services, payments and programmes have been the ones to carry the greatest burden as severe austerity measures are implemented to protect sovereign debt ratings, or to bail out banks and financial institutions.

On a Tumblr blog called *We are the ninety nine %*, thousands of young people, many of them from what might be called the American working class, have given voice to many of their frustrations with a post-GFC assemblage that loads them with large amounts of student debt for their college education, denies them access to universal health care, and then fails to provide them with access to jobs that could generate the income to service their debt and hold at bay the precariousness of a globalised, neo-Liberal, flexible capitalism (Kelly 2013). And, as we have witnessed from the streets of Ferguson (Missouri) to #BlackLivesMatter, this post-GFC assemblage is made more complex, precarious and possibly deadly, for many young people by the intersections of race, ethnicity, religion, sexuality and geography.

On the *We are the ninety nine %* blog, there is one post from a young woman, accompanied by a photo where she peers over the top of a sheet of ruled paper on which she has written about how she and her boyfriend struggle to survive on his '$8.50 an hour pay check', about how they 'barely have enough money to pay rent and bills', about carrying 'over $30,000 in college loans that I have to start paying back, but I cannot find a job' and about how all they are 'asking for' is a '**CHANCE** at the American Dream'.[1] Another young woman, aged 19, also peering over a handwritten note, tells us she that has 'no dad', but was raised by her 'single mom who tried her hardest'. Her mother always struggled, including having been 'arrested for not being able to pay my hospital bill' when

---

[1] http://wearethe99percent.tumblr.com/post/12030210178/my-boyfriend-and-i-are-currently-living-off-of-his

this young woman was 14. She tells us that she has 'had 7 jobs' and has 'worked for everything I have'. Yet, she is 'behind on [her] phone and car bills and can't afford car insurance', and is 'constantly worried about being pulled over'. She says that she suffers from 'severe anxiety and depression and can't afford my medicine'. Under these circumstances, she tells us that she is too 'scared to even attempt going to college because I will never be able to pay back my student loan'.[2]

In this space, the stories of marginalisation, of precarious lives, of physical and mental health and well-being challenges, of young people struggling to imagine a more secure, less parlous future in the aftermath of the GFC are legion. The tragic dimensions of these sorts of stories include that they are so many, and that in their multitude they have become 'mundane' in community, policy and academic spaces that take some interest in explaining or analysing or responding to them. My aim in this chapter, then, is to open up spaces in which young people's marginalisation of the kind made clear in these Tumblr posts can be rethought in ways that are productive for Youth Studies at the start of the twenty-first century. I want to suggest that concepts such as *structure* and *agency* do not well capture what it is that these two young women, and millions more like them, or in more dire circumstances, in the overdeveloped, developing and underdeveloped economies of a globalised capitalism are giving voice to, are experiencing.[3] In doing so, I want to locate Youth Studies' diverse interests in young people's marginalisation in cultural, social, economic and political contexts that are global, that are characterised by increasing wealth and poverty, and a widening gap between them, by the remaking of the markers of marginalisation in which some forms appear to wane while new forms seem to emerge; in the 'opportunistic political economy

---

[2] http://wearethe99percent.tumblr.com/post/12030253648/i-have-no-dad-a-single-mom-who-tried-her-hardest

[3] In an article in *The Guardian* from 2013, Andris Piebalgs, the then EU Commissioner for Development, in a discussion of the ways in which global concerns about youth unemployment are informing discussions on a post-2015 development agenda, suggested that 'To a degree, the problem of youth unemployment is understood in different ways depending on where you are. In Europe, youth unemployment is seen as a welfare problem, in that you still have a minimum welfare system to protect unemployed young people'. In the developing world, 'youth unemployment is seen more explicitly in relation to its direct political and security repercussions on the country ... in the latter, young people often have no access to social protection and basic services, such as health and education' (Young 2013).

of bio-genetic capitalism' where, as Rosi Braidotti (2013, p.61) argues 'Life/*zoe*—that is to say human and non-human intelligent matter' is turned 'into a commodity for trade and profit'. A point of departure here will be Stuart Hall, Doreen Massey and Michael Rustin's (2013a) *After Neo-Liberalism? The Kilburn Manifesto* in which they and their colleagues explore the challenges and opportunities for intellectual and political practice in the context of the renewed ascendency of neo-Liberalism in a post-GFC environment of sovereign debt crises, austerity and the Great Recession. Drawing on these ideas, and Hall's direct association with the legacy of the Centre for Contemporary Cultural Studies at Birmingham, Michel Foucault's work on apparatus (*dispositif*), together with Bruno Latour's work on *Reassembling the Social,* and the critical post-humanism of Rosi Braidotti and others, I will argue that 'after neo-Liberalism' is a space of possible futures. From where we currently stand some of these futures look—troublingly—more probable than others. In the context of these probable futures, Youth Studies need to develop tools capable of rei-magining young people's marginalisation, and the possible physical and mental health and well-being consequences of marginalisation, beyond an 'orthodoxy' shaped by ideas of *structure* and *agency*.

After Neo-Liberalism? The Kilburn Manifesto and Framing the Crisis

Neo-Liberalism is a much used, possibly little examined concept, even orthodoxy, in current sociological discourse. Elsewhere I have developed a detailed account of neo-Liberalism that draws on Foucault's (1991) work on governmentality, and the literature that has taken up and worked with some of these ideas (Kelly 2013). In brief, my own sense of how it is that we need to understand neo-Liberalism is that it is a mentality of rule, a moral project, an art of governing at a distance, that increasingly make individuals responsible for the practice of freedom, for the exercise of choice and for the consequences of choices made and not made. As an art of government, neo-Liberalism is a vast assemblage, even apparatus (Foucault 1980; Agamben 2009), that brings together an array of political rationalities and governmental technologies in order to render 'reality' knowable, in ways that promise to make 'reality' governable (Rose and Miller 1992). In this sense, neo-Liberalism is so much more than political rhetoric, a political party, a parliamentary system.

But this is just one way to know neo-Liberalism. In their Introduction to the *Kilburn Manifesto—After Neoliberalism: Analysing the Present—* Stuart Hall, Doreen Massey and Michael Rustin (2013b) try to capture and analyse a sense of the moment, of our present, of young people's present that is more sociological, less genealogical. A sociological present that is marked by recession, sovereign debt crises, austerity and the language of *strivers and skivers* and *lifters and leaners*, as seemingly unproblematic ways of describing self-evident realities in human experience, circumstances and orientations to the conduct of a life. For Hall and the others (Hall et al. 2013b, pp.8–9), the 'current neoliberal settlement has … entailed the re-working of the common-sense assumptions of the earlier, social democratic settlement'. Drawing on an extensive, long-running thread in Hall's work they suggest that every 'social settlement, in order to establish itself, is crucially founded on embedding as common sense a whole bundle of beliefs'. This making of 'common sense' requires the articulation, the joining together, of 'ideas beyond question, assumptions so deep that the very fact that they are assumptions is only rarely brought to light'. The bundle of beliefs we name as neo-Liberalism 'revolves around the supposed naturalness of "the market", the primacy of the competitive individual, the superiority of the private over the public'.

For Hall et al. (2013b, pp.14–15), neo-liberal economic theories have, during the past 30 years or so, in different ways, in different countries, with different purposes, different outcomes, taken on an air of 'naturalness', of self-evident 'rightness', of inevitability. For Hall (1986) in particular, this work is ideological, the space in which 'no necessary correspondence' becomes 'necessary correspondence'. In these spaces, neo-Liberal discourses 'can claim to be implemented with popular consent, though they are manifestly partial and limited'. The drive to open, for example, 'public areas for potential profit-making is accepted because it appears to be "just economic common sense"'. It is in this sense that the 'ethos of the "free market" is taken to licence an increasing disregard for moral standards, and even for the law itself' (Hall et al. 2013b, pp.14–15).

[handwritten annotation:] Collapse of wealth with commercialism ... (neolib)

The ideological work here is not just at the level of making the theoretical and the abstract work at the level of common sense. It is also,
for Hall et al. (2013b, pp.14–15), something that works to reshape the
ethical, even moral, dimensions of the economic. To configure what a
neo-Liberal moral economy looks like, what it feels like (Sayer 2004).
So, neo-Liberal discourses have, for example, played a prominent role in
cultivating 'an ethos of corruption and evasiveness'. In these spaces, institutions such as banks, 'once beacons of probity', now 'rig interest rates,
mis-sell products, launder drug money, flout international embargoes,
hide away fortunes in safe havens'. In a similar vein, 'when private firms
that have been publicly contracted fail to meet targets they are allowed
to continue'. And graduates who find themselves 'stacking supermarket shelves are told they don't need to be paid because they are "getting
work experience"'. When an ethic of competition, profit and enterprise
colonises all relations and practices, then 'Commercialisation permeates
everywhere, trumps everything'. As the 'imperatives of a "market culture"
become entrenched, anything goes. Such is the power of the hegemonic
common sense' (Hall et al. 2013b, pp.14–15).

As I suggested in *The Self as Enterprise: Foucault and the 'Spirit' of 21st
Century Capitalism* (Kelly 2013), neo-Liberal arts of government also
remake ideas of what it is to be a person. These ideas of what a person is,
or should be, are always ethical, always moral. From a different perspective,
the *Kilburn Manifesto* suggests that the 'ideology of competitive individualism has also been imposed via the stigmatisation of the so-called "undeserving" poor'. The ideological work here seeks to label 'Welfare scroungers' as
'morally deficient—"idlers who prefer a lie-in to work", "living on benefits
as a 'life-style' choice"' (Hall et al. 2013b, pp.15–16).

For all of these neo-Liberal 'successes' in remaking the world and our
sense of what it is to be a person, many of the overdeveloped OECD
economies currently find themselves in deep trouble, and young people
are carrying a particularly heavy burden for their trouble. As Hall et al.
(2013b, pp.16–17) suggest

> This phase of free-market capitalism has now entered a serious economic
> crisis from which it cannot easily engineer an exit. But the shape of the
> crisis remains 'economic'. There are so far no major political fractures, no

unsettlings of ideological hegemony, no ruptures in popular discourse. The disastrous effects of the crisis are clearly evident; but there is little understanding of how everyday troubles connect to wider structures. There is no serious crisis of ideas.

What we see in the work begun under the *Kilburn Manifesto* is a powerful framing of the urgent need for rethinking the ways in which we respond to the crisis, the ways we reassemble the social, or imagine the futures that might lie beyond neo-Liberalism. These ideas of the ways in which the realm of the economic has been expanded to frame, make sense of and remake the social, the cultural, the political and the natural—from the nano-level to that of the infinitely immense—have been taken up in a number of fields. In Youth Studies, there have been tentative though limited steps to do some of this thinking. James Côté's (2014) *Towards a New Political Economy of Youth* is, possibly, the most significant example from the *Journal of Youth Studies*. In the space available here, I do not want to argue against the substance of the elements of the political economy that Côté identifies. There is much in his analysis of age-related distributions of educational and labour market inequalities and incomes that I find generative. I would, however, question whether the political economy of the reproduction of inequalities in America by Bowles and Gintis, even an updated version of their work from the 1960s, is well equipped to do the work that Côté identifies needs to be done in Youth Studies.[4] It is difficult to imagine how the work of Bowles and Gintis can capture the political economy of a capitalism that, among other things, is remaking the human and introducing a whole array of novel and powerful non-human actants or agents into the exchange relations that shape contemporary and future life: from bots to robots, from AI to social networking algorithms, from autonomous, privatised weapons systems, to autonomous vehicles (Braidotti 2013). In the *Self as Enterprise* (Kelly 2013), for example, I referenced Nigel Thrift's (2005) *Knowing Capitalism* and his framing of a new political economy, a political economy that would try to come to grips with some of the transformations that have reshaped the character of capitalism in the last 30 years. Writing before the GFC,

---

[4] For a fuller critique of Côté's argument, see France and Threadgold (2015).

Thrift identified three key elements of this political economy, including the *discursive power of the cultural circuits of capitalism*, in which capitalism endlessly commodifies the deconstruction and reassembling of capitalism's own failings, successes and dysfunctions—and feeds it to itself; the changing *form of the commodity*, a change possibly best exemplified by the monetization of the electronic traces we leave as we 'freely' roam the web—in ways that make the Mark Zuckerbergs of the world multi-billionaires, and in which *labour* consists largely of billions of users telling others what they *like*, and the ways in which time and space are reconfigured as a *productive grid of resources*, so that, for example, we can work, shop and play 24/7—in/from the office, our bedroom, the bus stop—and we and others (such as our managers) resent it when we do not, or cannot.

The limits and possibilities of this approach, and others, indicate that there is much work to do in Youth Studies if we are to contribute to a 'serious crisis of ideas' after neo-Liberalism. As part of that work, what options might exist for thinking beyond agency and structure in the doing of Youth Studies?

Structure and Agency and an Orthodoxy in Youth Studies

In the remainder of this chapter, I want to revisit a discussion I started to develop in a recent chapter in a collection on Australian Youth Subcultures (Kelly 2014). There, I reviewed recent debates in the *Journal of Youth Studies* about the usefulness or otherwise of Ulrich Beck and/or Pierre Bourdieu's work for understanding the problem of structure and agency in Youth Studies. At various times in those debates, Dan Woodman (2009, 2010), Steven Roberts (2010, 2012) and Steven Threadgold (2011) made the coupling of marginalisation/structure/agency central to the points they were trying to make. For example, Steven Threadgold (2011, p.388), who wanted to map and occupy a 'middle ground' through the use of Bourdieu's work, suggested that 'individual reflexivity can be understood as cultural capital: like language, everyone is using it, but some have the skills and resources to use it better than others'. In this sense, young people 'can be as reflexive as possible, but if they cannot put their choices into action, reflexivity becomes an intrinsic part of the reflexive experience of inequality'. For Threadgold, agency, the sense and experience of a capacity 'to put one's choices into practice, or not, can produce a whole gamut of emotions and feelings from confidence, joy and satisfaction to frustration, alienation and withdrawal'.

In doing this work, I want to foreground a number of concerns that are well captured by Julia Coffey and David Farrugia's (2014) argument that there is an orthodoxy in the sociology of youth that is structured through this agency/structure dualism, and which seems unable to find a way beyond it except by occupying some 'middle ground', an occupation that remains trapped within this dualism. And while orthodox sociologies of youth occupy this middle ground, a whole variety of work in the humanities and social sciences has long moved on—trying to think about, understand and assemble human behaviour in much more generative, even challenging ways. As Ian Hunter (1993, p.129) argued over 20 years ago:

> If by agency we mean human capacities for thought and action then, given the irreducible positivity, variety and dispersion of the technologies of existence and conducts of life in which such capacities are formed, it is implausible to assume that agency has a general form; and it is even more implausible to identify this general form with that special Western conduct that we call the formation of the subject.

John Law (2004), and others, might argue that the assemblage we name as the sociology of youth makes some things present, some things manifestly absent, and still more things absent as Other. Any assemblage, argues Law (2004, p.144), 'makes something present by making absence'. The idea of assemblage, in playing with the relations between presence, manifest absence and absence as Otherness, tries to make explicit and imagine the consequences of the 'crafting, bundling, or gathering of relations' between these elements. Between what Law identifies as 'in-here or present (for instance a representation or an object)', between what is 'absent but also manifest (it can be seen, is described, is manifestly

So my interest at this moment is in what we might make present, manifestly absent or absent as Other in assembling the social in ways that try to accommodate those things we call structure and agency. This is an ongoing challenge. A challenge that itself must be an assemblage. An assemblage that, possibly, has a number of 'lines of flight' by which new assemblages might be made to cohere, made to unsettle orthodoxy (Kamp and Kelly 2015).

In the space left, I want to turn to a sketch one possible line of flight. I want to revisit Foucault's work on apparatus (dispositif) to flag how it can be made to trouble these relations between presence, manifest absence and absence as Other in accounting for the biodiversity and materiality of human being in the world, in troubling the structure–agency couplet. John Law (2000), in an article called On the Subject of the Object: Narrative, Technology, and Interpellation, asks, at one point, 'Which story will I tell about Michel Foucault?' The story he tells is one in which Foucault is concerned with the arrangements of materials of all kinds, including discourses, systems of thought, rationalities, technologies. Of particular interest to Foucault are the possible relations between materialities and human bodies:

> Yes, there is no doubt: Foucault is particularly interested in bodies, bodies and souls. He is interested in how to separate them, how to keep them together; how they are overseen, how they are marked; how they are broken down into little components and then reassembled, pressed into disciplinary forms. (Law 2000, pp.12–13)

Law (2000, pp.12–13) argues that it is the ways in which materials and bodies relate that is important to Foucault:

> Bodies and souls, and then the other materials: talk; buildings; texts … maps; plans. Techniques for constituting materials and relating them together. For Foucault's archaeology is an attempt to decode the logics of relations, the spaces made available by those logics, the spaces, or at any rate the hints of the spaces, denied and made Other by such logics.

Foucault (1980, p. 194) clarified his use of the term *dispositif* (apparatus) in a 1977 interview published in the 1980 collection *Power/Knowledge*. For Foucault, an apparatus is the particular 'system of relations that can be established' between such things as discourse, institutions, systems of thoughts: 'in short, the said as much as the unsaid. Such are the elements of the apparatus'. In turn, what is of interest here is 'precisely the nature of the connection that can exist between these heterogeneous elements'. The work to be done in this sense is in identifying the character and the consequences of these connections (what Hall [1986] would call 'articulations'). As Foucault (1980, p.195) argues there is, 'between these elements, whether discursive or non-discursive', a 'sort of interplay of shifts of position and modifications of function which can also vary very widely'. Finally, Foucault (1980, p.195) suggests that in using the concept of apparatus he wants to point to, and examine, a 'formation which has as its major function at a given historical moment that of responding to an urgent need'. An apparatus, then, always 'has a dominant strategic function'.

Probably the most significant recent engagement with Foucault's work on these matters is by the Italian philosopher Giorgio Agamben. In his short essay titled *What is an Apparatus?* Agamben (2009, p.1) argues that Foucault's definition and the use of the concept of apparatus are central to his work on the 'government of men'. In providing a genealogy of the use of the term in Foucault's work, something that does not directly interest me here, Agamben (2009, p.13) proposes his own reading, his own definition of what an apparatus is and how it can be put to work in a contemporary research and political agenda:

> I wish to propose to you nothing less than a general and massive partitioning of beings into two large groups or classes: on the one hand, living beings (or substances), and on the other, apparatuses in which living beings are incessantly captured. On one side, then to return to the terminology of the theologians, lies the ontology of creatures, and on the other side ... [an economy] ... of apparatuses that seek to govern and guide them toward the good.

In this sense, argues Agamben (2009, p.14), we can assemble the materiality of human existence, human relations, human behaviours, dispositions and practices in terms of the complex relations between organisms, and the elements, functions and strategic priorities of an apparatus:

> To recapitulate, we then have two great classes: living beings (or substances) and apparatuses. And, between these two, as a third class, subjects. I call a subject that which results from the relation and, so to speak, from the relentless fight between living beings and apparatuses.

In relation to discourses of youth at risk, for example, I have used Foucault's work on governmentality and practices of the self to think about such things as the identification and analysis of systems of relations between young people, knowledge, institutions, practices, in their particularity and in their generality; the nature of the interplay of these diverse elements, and the consequences of this interplay; and the strategic function of an apparatus of risk, of youth at risk, particularly in the context of neo-Liberal arts of government (Kelly 2001, 2006, 2011).

In my more recent discussions of Youth Studies and the problem of agency and structure, I have suggested that Foucault's work, the work of Bruno Latour (2007) on actor-networks and the post-humanism of Rosi Braidotti (2013), with their indebtedness to Foucault's legacy, offer different, though related, ways of unsettling what it is that we make present, manifestly absent and absent as Other in terms of this problem, in terms of what we call agency and who has it, in what we call structure and what it is and what it does. My interest in this space is with the ways in which these different trajectories can trouble the character of sociological worlds and sociological humans, and the orthodoxies that assemble these worlds, these humans.

I have suggested elsewhere (Montero and Kelly 2016) that when we go looking in young people for that thing we call agency, when we imagine that the world does not have to just be as we encounter it, as it shapes us, as it sets limits and possibilities. We look to young people to be acting in and on the world in ways that we imagine signify that thing that we call agency, that thing which suggests a special, purposeful way of being, thinking, doing, acting in and on a world that does not have to be just as we find it.

It is the special character of this purposeful way of being, thinking and doing that is most problematic for Youth Studies researchers who are on the lookout for such things. Because that thing that they, that we, call agency is so special it is not to be found in the everyday, the mundane, the myriad acts of daily life, of survival. To be special, to *be* agency, it has to be something else. And if the being and thinking and doing is everyday, mundane, not special it cannot be that thing that they, that we, are looking for. It cannot be agency. But it is in the everyday, mundane acts of a life that the experience, and meaning, and limits and possibilities of a life emerge, are encountered, are made.

The question here, then, is not one of young people's agency, but one of the making, the assembling of thinking, acting and doing into something we can *recognise* as agency. Particularly when the question of young people's social, cultural, economic and/or political marginalisation, exclusion or disadvantage is the object of the doing of Youth Studies, and the explanation is to be found in the coupling of structure and agency.

The world as imagined in sociologies in general, in sociologies of youth in particular, is one that is inhabited and populated by humans—children, young people, adults. These humans have something called agency, and do and make things. These made things are, overwhelmingly, the *only* Others in this sociological world. These Others include cultures and subcultures, education and health systems, labour markets, a vast array of administrative, even governmental programmes, and diverse technologies (old and new, media-based, war oriented, biogenetic). The list here can be made long and complex. So, it is a heavily populated world. But if we go into the world—the 'real' world (the 'scare marks' are deliberate, ironic and ambiguous)—then the world of sociologies of youth looks underpopulated, even barren. The non-sociological world is much more biodiverse, and richly populated with non-human Others: the subatomic and atomic, proteins and hormones, viruses and bacteria, animals, plants, geology, clouds; ocean depths and wilderness. Again, the list, and humans do like to catalogue, to classify these Others, can be made long, diverse and complex. And that is without leaving the planet and venturing into the vastly non-human scale of the cosmos.

Rosi Braidotti (2013, p.55) suggests that George Eliot, in her novel *Middlemarch*, 'has authored [her] favourite sentence in the English language':

> If we had a keen vision and feeling of all ordinary human life, it would be like hearing the grass grow and the squirrel's heart beat, and we should die of that roar which lies on the other side of silence. As it is, the quickest of us walk about well wadded with stupidity.

Humans—child, youth, adult—can, then, be made to look different to sociological humans, particularly if they are imagined as interacting and being shaped by these non-sociological Others (How does the warmth of the sun on your back make you feel, make you think, make you act?)

It is in this sense that I have argued that when young people encounter and are represented by sociologists, what often emerges, at least in the published accounts of these encounters in which questions of choice and agency are said to be important, is an overwhelming sense of the young person as a more or less rational being, devoid of emotions or ambivalence: pain, hurt, hunger, despair, anxiety, decisiveness, uncertainty, ambiguity, irony, humour, longing, desire, loneliness, companionship and love. If we want to, we can say that many of these things shape and enable choice or agency. Though these things might be of interest to Youth Studies, they are not matters, solely, of sociological concepts such as class or individualisation or habitus or reflexivity. Such things can be readily experienced or felt or considered without recourse to any of these concepts, or to the wider institutionalised systems of thought from which they emerge and to which they give shape (Kelly 2014).

In this unsettling, would structure and agency still be appropriate terms, appropriate concepts? What sorts of thinking, doing, being should sociologies of youth be concerned with? What relationships, practices, functions and consequences, what organisms, substances and apparatuses can be made present, manifestly absent, absent as Other in the doing of this work? Who or what might have that thing called agency in the twenty-first century, biogenetic, digital capitalism in which human exceptionalism looks increasingly problematic and provisional?

None of these approaches offer certainties in what is to be done in their name. But they are critical in their ethos. They are not *quietist*. Each, in different ways, argues that the world does not have to be as it is. A post-human ethics, for example, argues for the values of life forms and practices that might emerge beyond the tendency for globalised, technologised neo-Liberal capitalism to create and to destroy value only in the terms of endless, reflexive, autonomous, infinitely inventive and destructive cycles of profit. After neo-Liberalism is a space of possible futures. From where we currently stand, some of these futures look more probable than others. My provocation here is that the promise, the hope of remaking the world, cannot be invested in the autonomous, choice making, individualised human agent/subject. That is neo-Liberalism's game. It *owns* that subject. Structures and agency need to be reassembled in ways that are fit for our times, and for new ways of understanding what it is to be a truly networked organism (Braidotti 2013).

References

Agamben, G. 2009. *What is an Apparatus?* Stanford CA: Stanford University Press.

Braidotti, R. 2013. *The Posthuman*. Cambridge: Polity Press.

Coffey, J., and D. Farrugia. 2014. Unpacking the black box: The problem of agency in the sociology of youth. *Journal of Youth Studies* 17(4): 461–474.

Côté, J. 2014. Towards a new political economy of youth. *Journal of Youth Studies* 17(4): 527–543.

Foucault, M. 1980. The Confession of the Flesh. In *Power/Knowledge Selected Interviews and Other Writings*, ed. C. Gordon, 194–228. New York, NY: Pantheon Books.

———. 1991. Governmentality. In *The Foucault Effect: Studies in Governmental Rationality*, eds. G. Burchell, C. Gordon, and P. Miller, 87–104. Hemel Hempstead: Harvester Wheatsheaf.

France, A., and S. Threadgold. 2015. Youth and political economy: towards a Bourdieusian approach. *Journal of Youth Studies* 19(5): 612–628. doi:10.108 0/13676261.2015.1098779.

Hall, S. 1986. On Postmodernism and Articulation. *Journal of Communication Inquiry* 10(2): 45–60.

Hall, S., D. Massey, and M. Rustin, eds. 2013a. *After neoliberalism? The Kilburn manifesto*, Soundings. London: Lawrence & Wishart.

————. 2013b. After neoliberalism: analysing the present. In *After neoliberalism? The Kilburn manifesto*, Soundings, eds. S. Hall, D. Massey, and M. Rustin. London: Lawrence & Wishart.

Hunter, I. 1993. Subjectivity and Government. *Economy and Society* 22(1): 121–134.

Kamp, A., and P. Kelly. 2015. On Becoming. In *A Critical Youth Studies for the 21st Century*, eds. P. Kelly and A. Kamp, 16–24. Amsterdam/Boston: Brill.

Kelly, P. 2001. Youth at Risk: Processes of Responsibilization and Individualization in the Risk Society. *Discourse* 22(1): 23–34.

————. 2006. The Entrepreneurial Self and Youth at-Risk: Exploring the Horizons of Identity in the 21st Century. *Journal of Youth Studies* 9(1): 17–32.

————. 2011. Breath and the truths of youth at-risk: allegory and the social scientific imagination. *Journal of Youth Studies* 14(4): 431–447.

————. 2013. *The Self as Enterprise: Foucault and the "Spirit" of 21st Century Capitalism*. Aldershot: Ashgate/Gower.

————. 2014. Youth Studies and the Problem of Agency: Foucault vs Marx, Tait vs Sercombe; Beck vs Bourdieu, Woodman vs Threadgold vs Roberts. In *Youth Cultures and Subcultures*, eds. S. Baker, B. Buttigieg, and B. Robards, 21–30. Aldershot: Ashgate.

————. 2016. Growing up After the GFC: Responsibilisation and Mortgaged Futures. *Discourse*. pp. 1–13. doi:10.1080/01596306.2015.1104852.

Latour, B. 2007. *Reassembling the Social: An Introduction to Actor-Network-Theory*. Oxford: Oxford University Press.

Law, J. 2000. On the Subject of the Object: Narrative, Technology, and Interpellation. *Configurations* 8(1): 1–29.

————. 2004. *After Method*. London: Routledge.

Montero, K., and P. Kelly. 2016. *Young People and the Aesthetics of Health Promotion: Beyond Reason, Rationality and Risk*. London: Routledge.

Roberts, S. 2010. Misrepresenting choice biographies?: a reply to Woodman. *Journal of Youth Studies* 13(1): 137–149.

————. 2012. One step forward, one step Beck: a contribution to the ongoing conceptual debate in youth studies. *Journal of Youth Studies* 15(3): 389–401.

Rose, N., and P. Miller. 1992. Political Power beyond the State: Problematics of Government. *British Journal of Sociology* 43(2): 173–205.

Sayer, A. 2004. Moral Economy [online]. Available from http://www.comp.lancs.ac.uk/sociology/papers/sayer-moral-economy.pdf Accessed 25 Apr 2015.

Threadgold, S. 2011. Should I pitch my tent in the middle ground? On 'middling tendency', Beck and inequality in youth sociology. *Journal of Youth Studies* 14(4): 381–393.

Thrift, N. 2005. *Knowing Capitalism*. London: Sage.

Woodman, D. 2009. The mysterious case of the pervasive choice biography. *Journal of Youth Studies* 12(3): 243–256.

———. 2010. Class, individualisation and tracing processes of inequality in a changing world: A reply to Steven Roberts. *Journal of Youth Studies* 13(6): 737–746.

Young, H. 2013. Andris Piebalgs on a truly global crisis—youth unemployment. *The Guardian*, [online]. Available from. http://www.theguardian.com/global-development-professionals-network/2013/nov/14/youth-unemployment-global-development. Accessed 21 Sept 2015.

2

'Wear a Necklace of h(r)ope Side by Side with Me': Young People's Neo-Liberal Futures and Popular Culture as Political Action

Luke Howie and Perri Campbell

An Introduction: to the Risks of Neo-Liberalism

Occupy your heart. Another world is possible, make ready your dreams (banner at an Occupy rally. In Chomsky 2012, pp. 20–21).

The Occupy movements, according to Noam Chomsky (2012, p. 54), were the:

first major public response … to about thirty years of a really quite bitter class war that has led to social, economic and political arrangements in which the system of democracy has been shredded.

L. Howie (✉)
Monash University, Melbourne, VIC, Australia

P. Campbell
Lartrobe University, Melbourne, VIC, Australia

© The Editor(s) (if applicable) and The Author(s) 2017   **53**
P. Kelly, J. Pike (eds.), *Neoliberalism, Austerity, and the Moral Economies of Young People's Health and Well-being*,
DOI 10.1057/978-1-137-58266-9_3

For Wendy Brown (2015), these 'arrangements' are what we have come to call *neo-Liberalism*. Neo-Liberalism is the catchphrase, the ideological label, we give to conditions of economic, social and cultural marginalisation, disadvantage and uncertainty born of a fetishistic version of the so-called free-market capitalism. It is a condition where the money-making logic has no stopping point and has the capability to destroy anything in its path—the environment, democracy, people. 'The institutions and principles aimed at securing democracy', argues Brown (2015, p. 17), 'are challenged by neo-Liberalism's "economization" of political life and of other heretofore noneconomic spheres and activities'. Neo-Liberalism, in this view, is an extension of rational, utility maximising economics into the everydayness of social and cultural belonging. It can even be said that neo-Liberalism produces its own type of 'common-sense' which encourages us to understand ourselves, our lives and each other as consumers and market competitors, dragging us further and further away from 'collectivist attitudes that underpinned the welfare state era' (Hall and O'Shea 2013, p. 11). This type of common-sense encourages fierce individualisation, competitiveness, entrepreneurialism and servitude to the so-called *realities* of the market.

Pop culture in a time of neo-Liberalism, especially since the 2007–2008 Global Financial Crisis (GFC), has played a significant role in representing and questioning these arrangements, this neo-Liberal common-sense (Hall and O'Shea 2013). These moments in pop culture often feature young characters and are made, mostly, for young audiences.[1] In this chapter, we want to examine *The Hunger Games* novels and films and the story of a teenager named Katniss Everdeen as an artefact of a neo-Liberal, post-GFC world. *The Hunger Games* refers to a popular three-part book series: *The Hunger Games* (2008), *Catching Fire* (2009) and *Mockingjay* (2010); and four-part film series: *The Hunger Games* (2012), *Catching Fire* (2013), and *Mockingjay* Part 1 (2014) and Part 2 (2015). The movies and books gained significant global attention. Mockingjay Part 1 had the biggest opening weekend at the box office of 2014. More than 36.5 million copies of the book series went to print in the USA alone. *The Hunger Games* series asks its audiences to consider what the world would

---

[1] Although there have been some surprising viewership outcomes. See Daily Mail Australia, 2012.

look like if we imagined it in other terms. What if we replaced the status quo with a world of our own making? What *sacrifices* would this require?

The Hunger Games novels and films can be read as *moments that imagine the future in other terms* and are, therefore, possible catalysts for change. This reading requires diligent viewing and a little imagination. We have organised this chapter around two sections. In the first, we describe key allegories from *The Hunger Games Mockingjay Part 1* that we believe have the capacity to inform and influence how young people imagine their futures. We focus on the song 'The Hanging Tree' that becomes the ballad of the revolution in *The Hunger Games*, and the existence of the 'Mockingjay' birds which become the emblems for nation-wide resistance. In the second section, we analyse these allegories in relation to contemporary social theory and youth studies that has explored the roles of young people in times of socio-economic uncertainty, especially as they relate to themes of neo-Liberalism and the GFC. In this section, we also provide examples of the impact of *The Hunger Games* in post-GFC societies. We want to read *The Hunger Games* as *political action* able to help young people think through the dilemmas posed by neo-Liberalism, to reinvent themselves in the process, and resist, when they can, those socio-economic conditions that we are raised to believe are inevitable. In this way, we do not wish to shy away from the possibility that rethinking neo-Liberalism may require a *revolution*—perhaps a revolution of imagination.

Katniss Everdeen's Panem

Are you, are you, coming to the tree?—Katniss Everdeen.

The Hunger Games is set in the not-too-distant future in a nation called *Panem*. It is a nation built out of the ashes of present-day North America. It tells a well-worn dystopic tale. The history of Panem is a story about division, war and its fallout, and the ushering in of a functioning totalitarianism where the affluent flourish at the expense of the huddled, 'silent' majority (Baudrillard 1983). For more than 70 years, this order is maintained in the realm with vicious peacekeeping troops and the annual 'Hunger Games' where each segregated 'district' must offer two children—one girl and one boy—to participate in a fight-to-the-death, gladiatorial event which is beamed into households across Panem as a spectacularised sporting event (Collins 2008, p. 21). *The Hunger Games* tells the story of Katniss Everdeen and her life in 'District 12', an impoverished region of *Panem*. In this hyper-mediated, hyper-surveilled dystopia, the whole nation witnesses Katniss time and again show courage beyond her age and social status and it inspires insurrection in the most desperately marginalised sections of the population.

The Hanging Tree

The song 'The Hanging Tree' tells the story of an alleged criminal, captured and sentenced to hanging, who cries out to his missing lover and co-accused. Katniss' father sung it to her as a child. In *Mockingjay Part 1*, Katniss, sitting beside a lake, sings it for the media team charged with following her around to capture moments that could be used as propaganda to inspire the resistance movements. The video becomes the 'spark' that leads to violent rebellion during the uprising. In *Mockingjay Part 1*, revolutionaries are depicted singing this song as they launch an attack against a water catchment that serves the population in the affluent 'Capitol'. This attack costs many of the revolutionaries their lives. One particular verse of this song stands out as the call to revolution and becomes an allegory for the ambivalence inherent in any attempt to create significant socio-economic change. This is how the lyrics appear in the novel:

> Are you, are you, coming to the tree?
> Wear a necklace of rope, side by side with me.
> Strange things did happen here, no stranger would it be,
> If we met at midnight at the hanging tree (Collins 2010, p. 139).

Katniss—as the narrator of the novels—speaks at length about the ambivalence inherent in the song, the uneasy feelings it sparked within her and her mother's intense reaction when her father sung it. It is Katniss' musings on the song's shifting meaning as she transitioned from childhood to adulthood that illuminates some of the revolutionary character of *The Hunger Games* series:

> At the beginning, it sounds like a guy is trying to get his girlfriend to secretly meet up with him at midnight … but it's not until the third verse that "The Hanging Tree" begins to get unnerving. You realize the singer of the song is the dead murderer. He's still in the hanging tree. And even though he told his lover to flee, he keeps asking if she's coming to meet him … at first you think he's talking about when he told her to flee presumably to safety. But then you wonder if he meant for her to run to him. To death … it's clear what he's waiting for. His lover, with her rope necklace, hanging dead next to him in the tree. (Collins 2010, pp. 140–141)

Plutarch Heavensbee—a double agent and architect of both the 'Hunger Games' and the revolution—sees enormous potential in this song as a propaganda weapon, but with one small change. One should change the 'necklace of rope' to a 'necklace of hope'. The change is dramatic. In one, the uprising requires that civil unrest ends in almost certain death for the revolutionary, but perhaps we should pay such a price for meaningful change. In the other, all that is required is *hope*. Perhaps all one needs to rebel is to simply *want* change? We believe that all we need is hope despite knowing that hope will never be enough, the sacrifice will be far greater. Thoughts do not secure change, but action might. In a further twist, the official song that hit the global charts and features on the motion picture soundtrack to *Mockingjay* is the version with 'hope'. We, as consumers of *The Hunger Games* franchise, consume the propaganda version of the song.

Katniss wonders whether it may be better to die rather than live under the Capitol's rule. Indeed, in *The Hunger Games* films, suicidal resistance is a central theme. The song becomes a tool of the rebellion—come and join Katniss in certain death and face the possibility of freedom. In the water reservoir scene, the rebels can be seen charging with rudimentary weapons at peacekeepers with machine guns. Their sheer numbers see them win the day. A key feature of their attack is the use of rebels to shield a large bomb and those carrying it. Suicidal violence is inscribed into the revolutionary message again when Katniss ends a furious and uplifting speech with the phrase 'If we burn you burn with us' (Collins 2010, p. 119).

The Mockingjay

The second story we want to focus on is the birth of what came to be called the 'Mockingjay'. *Mockingjay* is the title of the third book, the third and fourth films (the *Mockingjay* book in two parts), and a type of bird that can be found in many parts of Panem. It was the symbolism around which the icon of Katniss Everdeen was built and which served as a recognisable symbol of the uprisings that spread throughout the nation. The imagery of the Mockingjay appears again and again as an antagonism to those in power and as a symbol of non-compliance and resistance. Symbols of the Mockingjay are subsequently banned throughout Panem.

In the films, the symbol of the Mockingjay is rendered abstract. Little is explained of their existence and much is made of their trait of imitating sounds. Katniss' three-toned whistle used to communicate with allies during the Hunger Games is imitated by the birds and spread throughout the forest. But in the books, the birds have a history bound to oppressive governmental policies, unfair working conditions, marginalisation, surveillance, violence, genetic engineering and nature's accommodating and adapting tendencies. Mockingjays began their species as 'Jabberjays'—creatures that were genetically engineered by the government ('mutts', as they are known in *The Hunger Games* universe) to spy on rebels during the first uprising 74 years before the events in the books take place. Jabberjays repeat whatever they hear. As such, jabberjays would fly in to listen to secret meetings and report back to the government and military. The irony of these creatures is that their failure leads ultimately to the destruction of the authoritarian rulers who created them (although this destruction takes three-quarters of a century to transpire). In short, the jabberjays mate with the native Mockingbirds and create a new species dubbed 'Mockingjays' that, instead of repeating words, repeat sounds and tunes in melodic tones (Collins 2010, p. 137). These tones become a resource for the impoverished District 8 and a tool for the nature-savvy competitors in the Hunger Games arena. In the arena of the Hunger Games, Katniss and her District 9 ally Rue use the Mockingjays to communicate and signal the next stage of their plan. The existence of Mockingjays literally mocks the supposedly powerful Panem rulers and becomes an emblem of the government's weakness and vulnerability. A powerful weapon of the government is transformed into a weapon of the resistance. And as a material force, an inspiration, a revolutionary symbol that inspires the events leading up to the building of an army, the storming of the Capitol and the removal of the totalitarian government bunkered there. The tragic irony, from the perspective of the denizens of the Capitol, is that their special weapons, science and tricks are what made them vulnerable. Their attempts to defeat the rebels made the rebels stronger, delivering them the tool and symbol that would help them realise victory.

These stories are rich in allegory, but they should not be read in abstraction. At its heart, *The Hunger Games* is a story of *revolution*. It is about rising up, shedding the shackles of unfreedom, much of which is emotional and psychological. As the story continues to unfold, we begin to learn that the dystopia that Collins is describing shares many socio-economic similarities to the world in which we live. One might even argue that we find ourselves, in the second decade of the twenty-first century, in a situation that is *proto*-Hunger Games. The economic inequality, the social and biological engineering, the cultural domination, the competitivism—it is all there. All we need now, perhaps, is some sort of military catastrophe or misplaced aggression. Or, so the story goes.

Precariousness: Imagined and Unimaginable Futures

Recent youth studies scholarship has been heavily influenced by Guy Standing's (2014) work on *the Precariat*. It comes on the back of two decades of youth studies scholarship that has explored the meanings of risk particularly in the contexts of participation in the labour market and how young people manage 'transitions' from childhood to adolescence to the so-called adulthood (see Furlong and Cartmel 2007; Kelly 2006; Wyn and White 1997).

In the aftermath of the 2007–2008 GFC, understanding how young people find their way into various versions of adulthood has taken on dangerous dimensions. There was a 'deadly time bomb' that loomed over the world, 'more destructive and dangerous' than anything an international terrorist could muster:

Ticking time bombs, social dynamite, boiling-over frustrations, pent-up anger, violent conflicts, political insurrection and instability, disease and death. These are some of the representations of youth that are now being widely circulated, as youth returns to centre stage in poverty and development discourse in global centres of power and across the developing world. (*The Hindu* in Sukarieh and Tannock 2008: 301)

There is a second portrayal of young people at work in these dangerous times, and that is young people as 'agents of change', as 'citizens and leaders' and as a nation's 'most important assets'. We view young people in their positivity when they 'stand inside this system as willing and enthusiastic participants'. But when young people stand 'outside this system' and question and doubt 'its basic precepts and promises' (Sukarieh and Tannock 2008: 302), they become subject to discourses of being dangerous, 'at-risk' (Kelly 2006; Harris 2004), not fully developed in their brains and bodies (Bessant 2008). Here, we find intervention strategies designed to correct the supposedly bad choices they have made, such as in the case of counter-radicalisation programmes that have been *en vogue* since the rise of the Islamic State (Schmitt 2015).

These framings of young people as a problematic and dangerous population have a long history (see for instance: Bessant 2008: 348 and Harris 2004: 13). Kelly (2006) has argued that 'young people'—as a discursive category—have been institutionally produced as a dangerous and at-risk population that should be made subject to a range of narratives and social engineering interventions that sit among neo-Liberal imperatives of transitioning from education to the labour force, from idleness to productivity, and from family- and school-based dependency to individualism. But these narratives were based on assumptions about the reliability and continuity of the institutions that structure everyday neo-Liberal realities. That hard work and education will result in stable employment. That avoiding risky habits surrounding sex and drugs will ensure mature adult relationships. That a positive attitude would ward off collapsing mental health and well-being.

In the aftermath of the GFC, Walsh (2015, p. 57) argues that young people face 'an increasingly fluid workforce that is … insecure and precarious'. We might say that for young people, there is increasingly a 'grey area between employment and unemployment' (Furlong 2007, p. 102). 'The Precariat' is Guy Standing's (2014) name for a generation and a class that is characterised by under- and unemployment, perpetual and structural disadvantage, perpetual uncertainty and marginalisation:

> Youth are entering labour markets in some disarray, many experiencing status frustration, feeling economically insecure and unable to see how to build a career. Their predicament in many countries is compounded by unemployment. The financial meltdown hit young people hard. Millions lost jobs, millions more could not enter the labour market, and those who did found they had lower wages than their predecessors. (Standing 2014, p. 132)

While Standing's argument runs the risk of essentialising the experiences of a diverse and complex population, it is evident that the 2007–2008 GFC has exacerbated the already existing conditions of disadvantage and youth marginalisation. A situation that is coupled with the phenomenon of older people re-entering the labour market, working longer and doing so in lower-skilled jobs that may have otherwise been occupied by under-skilled young people (Standing 2014, pp. 135–137). 'Dismal prospects' is how Standing (2014, pp. 133–134) describes these multitude of challenges facing young people as they enter the 'precarity trap'. A life shaped by the incentives of neo-Liberalism—the encouragement to be employable 'to be made *presentable and flexible* in any number of ways'—and the need for a sense of social belonging. These conditions, along with 'exposure to a commodifying education system', give rise to a 'status frustration' (Standing 2014, pp. 133–134, our emphasis).

Against the neo-Liberal common-sense, this 'status frustration' could be viewed as a positive development, since dissatisfaction with the status quo may prove to be the seed of meaningful change. Career/life/identity/self-status frustration may come to represent the base from which the future can be imagined in other terms (see Howie and Campbell 2015). This might be the seeds of the Mockingjay—a predicament created by the powerful that may lead to uprising and change among those who do not benefit under neo-Liberalism. This, one might say, was the essence of the activities pursued by the Occupy movement in protests against austerity and globalisation around the world.

For Wendy Brown (2015, p. 30), 'Intensified inequality, crass commodification and commerce' and 'ever-growing corporate influence in government' are among the consequences of neo-Liberalism and among the chief grievances of post-GFC protest movements. What these movements understand better than most people is that 'Citizenship in its thinnest mode is mere membership' (Brown 2015, p. 218). What many young activists also seem to understand is that *patriotism* is not the only form that activism might take (although, for a whole range of reasons, right-wing movements are particularly prominent in Western countries at the time of writing). But what form can and should their *action* take?

> Today, as economic metrics have saturated the state and the national purpose, the neoliberal citizen *need not stoically risk death on the battlefield*, only bear up uncomplainingly in the face of unemployment, underemployment, or employment unto death. The properly interpellated neoliberal citizen makes no claims for protection against capitalism's suddenly burst bubbles, job-shedding recessions, credit crunches, and housing market collapses, its appetites for outsourcing or the discovery or pleasure and profit in betting against itself or betting on catastrophe. (emphasis added, Brown 2015, p. 218)

Defined in this way, the task in developing a disposition suited to neo-Liberal times becomes to be 'dispossessed' of one's neo-Liberal citizenship (see Butler and Athanasiou 2013, pp. ix–xi). Part of simply *being* a neo-Liberal citizen, in this view, is doing nothing, accepting the world as it is, living happily (or not) among the status quo. It may be that doing *something*, resisting in any meaningful or perhaps non-meaningful way, are the building blocks for resisting the injustices of neo-Liberalism. It may be the basis of imagining a future in other terms. This might be the moment that young people decide if their necklace is one of rope, or one of hope.

How 'Generation K' Imagines the Future

The Hunger Games have been, in recent times, the most read and most watched novels and films in the youth culture literary and film genre. As a 'franchise' it has, in undoubtedly diverse and complex ways, inspired young people in a post-GFC world to think and act in other terms. Evidence of this can be found in many places. Hughes (2015) argues that the 'generation who came to Katniss as young teens and have grown up ploughing through the books and queuing for the movies respond to her story in a particularly personal way'. The generation of young people born between 1995 and 2002, according to Noreena Hertz (2015), can be referred to as 'Generation K'—a generation of young people raised with social networking technologies and some of the worst disasters since the Second World War. 9/11, the GFC, Wikileaks and Snowden and looming environmental catastrophe have characterised the first 16 years of the twenty-first century, with few signs that a belief in imminent disaster is fading: 'They are a group for whom there are disturbing echoes of the dystopian landscape that Katniss encounters in *The Hunger Games*'s District 12. Unequal, violent, hard' (Hertz 2015). The consequence of this is a generation living under a siege mentality, a generation that labours under a belief that anxiety, uncertainty and doubt are inevitable consequences of imagining a future. The character of Katniss Everdeen shows us that maybe there is reason for hope if we are willing to do what it takes. We may, perhaps, have to wear a necklace of rope (or hope) before change is secured, but fire, rage and desire have the potential to overthrow an unjust and immoral system.[2]

Recent protests and civil disruptions in Hong Kong in 2014 provide some merit to the idea of a revolution born of Generation K. They were protests partially inspired by *The Hunger Games* books and movies. The 'pro-democracy protesters' even adopted the 'three-fingered salute' championed by Katniss. In the Hunger Games' universe, this salute is about defiance and represents a 'screw you' attitude towards people with impossible power (Sim 2014a). The salute was used by protesters in Thailand prompting the Thai government to declare that if people continued to make the salute while part of a large group, then military police 'will have to make an arrest' (Sim 2014b). In late 2014, the Thai police and military made good on this threat by arresting several student protesters, and a

---

[2] This is the essence of what Khader (2014) has described as the effects of 'Mockingjay delusions': romantic or tangential storylines are read as an example of Hollywood surplus enjoyment that provides the audience with a way to disengage from the traumatic true message of a film.

cinema chain pulled *The Hunger Games: Mockingjay Part 1* movie from their screens (Mydans 2014). Katniss' salute had evolved into a symbol of real, violent uprising.

Katniss Everdeen, we argue, helped provide a narrative for these protesters to imagine their futures on other terms. The three-finger salute is not simply a pop-cultural tribute or a playful representation of civic rights. Revolution was on Katniss' mind and she asked her followers to wear not only a necklace of hope but also one of ropes. Violence, the Thai police and government likely feared, may soon follow the salute. This, for Žižek (2012), is the effect of a superhero. It is the 'outcasts, freaks' who take action when injustice reigns and where 'superheroes have to enter precisely when normal society cannot do it'. But change does not happen overnight. The seeds of change are often laid well before change is realised. As Žižek (2014, p. 20) argues: 'People do not rebel when 'things are really bad' but when their expectations are disappointed'. This is perhaps one of the key messages of The Hunger Games novels and films and the message that has contributed to the mobilisation of 'Generation K'. The first step towards change is knowing, and believing, that changed is needed.

Conclusion: Do - Something

The point we make here is that action, activism and resistance take many forms. And doing *something* in a neo-Liberal system that hopes we do *nothing* is potentially the most rebellious act of all. Danger and risk in their *negativity* can be reimagined as opportunities for actions in their *positivity* (see Kelly 2006, p. 18). It is a space where neo-Liberal power can be redirected to benefit those without power. We witness this in protesters in Thailand who deploy a revolutionary symbol they found in a billion-dollar Hollywood franchise. This was their *Mockingjay*. It is in this moment that neo-Liberalism might merge with the movements that resist it.

We want to conclude by highlighting the tragic plight of some of the highest achieving young people in the USA. Silicon Valley, in the

bohemian 'Bay Area' of Northern California, is the corporeal and geographical home of the social media revolution. It is also home to what is
known as a 'suicide cluster'—a concentration of suicides in a particular
geographic region, often linked by particular socio-cultural conditions
(Rosin 2015). Indeed, it is also home to an 'echo cluster'—an extraor-
dinarily rare occurrence where the same geographical location is subject
to a second suicide cluster within a decade. These clusters were found
in local high schools where the demands imposed by Silicon Valley
parents—many of whom moved to the area to give their children elite
education and employment opportunities—were, simply put, push-
ing their children over the edge through a 'competitive insanity' that
'breeds competition, hatred, and discourages teamwork and genuine
learning. ... We are sick. ... Why is that not getting through to this
community?' (Walworth in Rosin 2015). The favourite method for
suicide among young people in this region was to throw themselves
in front of the *Caltrain*. One student compared the train's 'warning
whistle' to the 'cannon that goes off in *The Hunger Games* every time a
kid dies' (in Rosin 2015).

Perhaps, the money making, the stress and anxieties it induces, and
the neo-Liberal systems that hold it all together conspire to make many
of us desperately depressed, making our world competitive, hellish and
hopeless. Perhaps, we live in a world where the only choice many can see
is death, but at least a death of their choosing. Perhaps, it is, as Schrecker
and Bambra (2015) have argued that neo-Liberalism makes us sick.
Obesity, mental illness, austerity and inequality are all perhaps as much a
part of thriving in neo-Liberalism as profits, market share and entrepreneurialism and innovation. When framed in these ways, neo-Liberalism
is almost certainly not something we hope for young people who face a
future of uncertainty (Bauman 1998), precariousness (Standing 2014;
Turner 2006) and anxiety (Stossel 2014). But what could be done about
this? How do young people survive such hostile conditions? The Occupy
movement asks questions like these, as do the activists of the Arab Spring.
So too did protesters in Thailand and China in 2014. The existence of
these social movements suggests that something is being done in neo-
Liberal times, within/against neo-Liberal common-sense.

References

Baudrillard, J. 1983. *In the shadow of the silent majorities—or the end of the social and other essays*. New York: Semiotext(e).

Bauman, Z. 1998. What prospects of morality in times of uncertainty? *Theory, Culture and Society* 15(1): 11–22.

Bessant, J. 2008. Hard wired for risk: Neurological science, 'the adolescent brain' and developmental theory. *Journal of Youth Studies* 11(3): 347–360.

Brown, W. 2015. *Undoing the demos: Neoliberalism's stealth revolution*. Brooklyn: Zone Books.

Butler, J., and A. Athanasiou. 2013. *Dispossession: The performative in the political*. Cambridge: Polity.

Chomsky, N. 2012. *Occupy*. London: Penguin Books.

Collins, S. 2008. *The hunger games*. London: Scholastic.

———. 2009. *The hunger games: Catching fire*. London: Scholastic.

———. 2010. *The hunger games: Mockingjay*. London: Scholastic.

Daily Mail Australia. 2012. 'Girls' very unlikely demographic: How more men over 50 are watching hit HBO series than actual twenty-something girls. *Daily Mail Australia*, 19 June. Available from http://www.dailymail.co.uk/femail/article-2161274/Girls-unlikely-demographic-How-men-50-watching-hit-HBO-series-actual-girls.html. Accessed 4 Jan 2016.

Furlong, A. 2007. The zone of precarity and discourses of vulnerability: NEET in the UK. *The Journal of Social Sciences and Humanities* 381: 101–121.

Furlong, A., and F. Cartmel. 2007. *Young people and social change: New perspectives*, 2nd edn. Maidenhead: Open University Press.

Hall, S., and A. O'shea. 2013. Common sense neoliberalism. *Soundings: A Journal of Politics and Culture* 55: 8–24.

Harris, A. 2004. *Future girl: Young women in the twenty-first century*. New York: Routledge.

Hertz, N. 2015. Generation K: What it means to be a teen [online]. Available from http://www.noreena.com/wp-content/uploads/2015/04/Generation-K.jpg. Accessed 14 Dec 2015.

Howie, L., and P. Campbell. 2015. Guerrilla selfhood: Imagining young people's entrepreneurial futures. *Journal of Youth Studies* [online first] 19(7): 906–920. doi:10.1080/13676261.2015.1123236.

Hughes, S. 2015. In debt, out of luck: Why Generation K fell in love with The Hunger Games [online]. *The Guardian*, November 1. Available from http://www.theguardian.com/film/2015/oct/31/hunger-games-mockingjay-teenage-anxiety. Accessed 4 Dec 2015.

Kelly, P. 2006. The entrepreneurial self and 'youth at-risk': Exploring the horizons of identity in the twenty-first century. *Journal of Youth Studies* 9(1): 17–32.

Khader, J. 2014. Mockingjay delusions: *The Hunger Games* and the postcolonial revolution to come [online]. *The Postcolonialist*, January 27. Available from http://postcolonialist.com/civil-discourse/mockingjay-delusions-the-hunger-games-and-the-postcolonial-revolution-to-come/.

Mydans, S. 2014. Thai protesters are detained after using 'Hunger Games' salute [online]. *The New York Times*, November 20. Available from http://www.nytimes.com/2014/11/21/world/asia/thailand-protesters-hunger-games-salute.html?_r=0. Accessed 21 Apr 2015.

Rosin, H. 2015. The Silicon Valley suicides [online]. *The Atlantic*, December. Available from http://www.theatlantic.com/magazine/archive/2015/12/the-silicon-valley-suicides/413140/. Accessed 17 Nov 2015.

Schmitt, E. 2015. ISIS followers in U.S. are diverse and young [online]. *The New York Times*, December 1. Available from http://www.nytimes.com/2015/12/02/us/politics/56-arrests-in-us-this-year-related-to-isis-study-says.html?_r=0. Accessed 1 Dec 2015.

Schrecker, T., and C. Bamber. 2015. *How politics makes us sick: Neoliberal epidemics*. Houndmills: Palgrave Macmillan.

Sim, D. 2014a. Hong Kong: Defiant protesters give Hunger Games' three-fingered salute as police clear camp [online]. *International Business Times*, December 11. Available from http://www.ibtimes.co.uk/hong-kong-defiant-protesters-give-hunger-games-three-fingered-salute-police-clear-camp-1479120. Accessed 21 Apr 2015.

———. 2014b. Thailand: Anti-coup protesters adopt Hunger Games' three-fingered salute. *International Business Times*, June 3. Available from http://www.ibtimes.co.uk/thailand-anti-coup-protesters-adopt-hunger-games-three-fingered-salute-1451036. Accessed 21 Apr 2015.

Standing, G. 2014. *The precariat: The new dangerous class*. London: Bloomsbury.

Stossel, S. 2014. *My age of anxiety: Fear, hope, dread and the search for peace of mind*. London: William Heinemann.

Sukarieh, M., and S. Tannock. 2008. In the best interest of youth or neoliberalism? the World Bank and the new Global Youth Empowerment Project. *Journal of Youth Studies* 11(3): 301–312.

Turner, B. 2006. *Vulnerability and human rights*. University Park, PA: The Pennsylvania State University Press.

Walsh, L. 2015. *Educating generation next: Young people, teachers and schooling in transition*. Basingstoke: Palgrave Macmillan.

Wyn, J., and R. White. 1997. *Rethinking youth*. St Leonards: Allen & Unwin.
Žižek, S. 2012. Slavoj Žižek on The Avengers (2012) [online]. Available from https://www.youtube.com/watch?v=tP4pcDLI57c. Accessed 11 May 2015.
———. 2014. *Trouble in paradise: From the end of history to the end of capitalism.* London: Allen Lane.

3

Youth, Health and Morality: Body Work and Health Assemblages

Julia Coffey

Introduction

In the current neo-Liberal context, individuals are both required and expected to be responsible for managing the health and well-being of their bodies (Moore 2010). A range of sociological work has argued the current emphasis on individual responsibility for managing health and the body is indicative of the ways in which neo-Liberal rationality permeates contemporary social life (Rose 1996; Lupton 1999). This chapter draws on data from a qualitative study to explore the ways in which moral imperatives of health and well-being shape young people's negotiations of health and body work practices. Body work practices, which include diet, exercise and all practices aimed at modifying the body's form or appearance, are a central way in which young people are encouraged

J. Coffey (✉)
University of Newcastle, Newcastle, NSW, Australia

© The Editor(s) (if applicable) and The Author(s) 2017   **69**
P. Kelly, J. Pike (eds.), *Neoliberalism, Austerity, and the Moral Economies of Young People's Health and Well-being*,
DOI 10.1057/978-1-137-58266-9_4

to be increasingly responsible for their own health and well-being. The moral and individualistic dimensions of 'health' were apparent in many instances in interviews with young people. Many spoke of how they felt 'lazy' or 'slack' if they had not been exercising regardless of the broader contexts of their lives such as long working hours in casualised industries. Where 'fit, healthy' bodies were broadly described as 'deserving of respect', people with 'overweight' were described as moral failures, lacking in self-esteem and self-restraint. The chapter combines a Deleuzo-Guattarian theorisation of health as an assemblage to analyse the ways in which moral imperatives function through discourses and affects associated with neo-Liberal conditions. From this perspective, health as an assemblage is comprised (among numerous other things) by discourses, such as those which emphasise individualised self-responsibility and bodily perfection in Western, neo-Liberal contexts, as well as through affects which mediate a body's capacities (what a body can do) (Coffey 2014). The examples and analysis aim to show the ways in which moral imperatives of health function through discourses of neo-Liberal self-responsibility, and through affect and embodied sensations, such as in the importance of 'looking healthy' and 'feeling healthy' and 'worry' associated with becoming overweight.

Health and Well-being as Moral Imperatives

Neo-Liberalism is commonly understood as 'a political and economic approach which favours the expansion and intensification of markets, while at the same time minimizing government intervention' and is 'inherently social and moral in its philosophy' (Ayo 2012, p. 101). The social and moral implications of neo-Liberal rationality can be seen in approaches to public health, health promotion and health education which 'serve to individualise, responsibilise and moralise health[y] conduct' (Leahy 2014, p. 172). Further, the pursuit of 'health' and the desire to 'be healthy' is a key quality defining the self, central to modern identity (Crawford 2006, p. 402). Crawford uses the term 'healthism', defined as the primary preoccupation with personal health as the achievement and definition of well-being, to describe the ways that solutions to health 'rest within the individual's determination' (Crawford 1980, p. 368). Health and working on the body are promoted as consumer choices, 'choices' essential to general well-being and success and the 'quest to fulfil themselves' (Rose 1996, p. 162). Rose argues that health is ensured through consumption, as 'individuals will want to be healthy, experts will instruct them on how to be so, and entrepreneurs will exploit and enhance this market for health' (Rose 1996, p. 162). This can be seen in the growth and profitability of the health, beauty and fitness industries in Australia (Australian Centre for Retail Studies 2005; Australian Bureau of Statistics 2009).

At the same time as promoting particular individualised responses to managing health, the neo-Liberal project has informed the reshaping of working conditions in Australia towards short-term or casual individual employment contracts known as 'flexible regulation' (Quinlan and Johnstone 2009). These new regimes:

> may offer productivity benefits to employers and to some employees, but generate a stratum of workers who are poorly paid, lack job security, lack predictable work times and have limited or few social benefits. (Dixon et al. 2014, p. 462)

Young Australians are predominantly employed under these 'flexible' arrangements, characterised by conditions of casualisation and precarity. Though young people aged 18–24 make up 21 % of the workforce, 40 % are casual employees (Australian Bureau of Statistics 2008). The sectors in which the largest numbers of young people are employed (retail trade and accommodation [47 %], cafes and restaurants [40 %]) are also those which employ the highest proportion of casual workers (45 % and 59 %, respectively). The implications of working under these 'flexible' or precarious working conditions, in which employees lack job security and control over their hours, are considered a modern structural determinant of health. The demands of these structural conditions dovetail with the individualisation of health and broader individual management of social risks. Young people are required to take increased responsibility for managing risks while 'inequalities are rendered invisible' (Wyn 2009, p. 6).

Sociological analyses have also focused on the politics of health promotion in relation to the self-management of health (Petersen 1996) in which 'duty and deservedness' are core moralities understood as necessary to experiencing 'good health' (Broom et al. 2012, p. 13). The body's corporeality is perhaps most visible as an object of scrutiny and concern in discussions of the 'obesity epidemic' (Lupton 2013). Critical writers on fatness and the body (Gimlin 2002; Grimshaw 1999; Crossley 2006b; Lupton 1996; Lupton 2013) situate the current pathologisation of fatness within the socially and culturally constructed context of current biomedical and public health knowledge systems.

The strength of health as a moral imperative takes a specific form in discussions of youth. Young people's bodies are typically understood and managed through a 'risk' framework in policy and developmental approaches (Coffey and Watson 2015). The 'youth at risk' discourse frames public discussions of youth in a range of interconnected ways, from concerns that young people are not 'transitioning' successfully through traditional pathways from education to employment (Wyn and Woodman 2006). This is linked to health issues such as poor mental health outcomes, substance use, crime and delinquency, and even teenage pregnancy (Harris 2004; te Riele 2006; Kelly 2001). For example, as Pike (2015, p. 89) has shown, encouraging young people to engage in self-formation practices through eating behaviours are 'part of a broader moral enterprise'. The emphasis placed on health and meeting normative goals also reveals anxiety about particular dangers young bodies pose to society in the present and in future adulthood. In countries such as Australia, the UK and the USA, this has centred around so-called lifestyle (and by implication preventable), health issues such obesity, mental illness, eating disorders and alcohol (particularly binge drinking) and other drug use.

Alongside this, body image is a key concern for youth that centres on idealised constructions of the body. Body image is a term that has links with psychology and medicalised definitions of health, since a person's body image is thought to be 'strongly influenced by the psyche and may or may not reflect a realistic interpretation of our actual bodies' (Centre for Health Promotion 2010, p. 6). Whether or not a person's 'body image' is deemed 'realistic', and if a person is 'satisfied' with their body, determines if their body image is 'healthy'. Unhealthy 'body image' is popularly understood as a problem primarily affecting young women and girls. This is due to the greater prevalence of eating disorders in young women and girls. However, surveys show that body image is a major concern to a large proportion of both young women and men, as it has consistently ranked in the top three issues of most concern for young women and men (Mission Australia 2014). Young people's concern about the body's appearance can be understood in the context of increased individualisation of health and marketing of health as an 'image' that can be made visible through the body's shape, size or appearance (Featherstone 2010).

The practices aimed at crafting the 'healthy' body and self-responsible citizen are also strongly delineated by gender (Moore 2010). Though men are now argued to be suffering the 'dubious equality' as consumers of health, fitness and cosmetic products (Featherstone 1982), the idealised physical dimensions of the body are gendered in ways which link with traditional gendered hierarchies and inequalities (Moore 2010). The idealised 'healthy' woman's body in this context remains slender (Bordo 2003), while the idealised man's body is toned and muscular (Crossley 2006a). Moore (2010) argues that traditional ideas about gender underpin the particular attitude to the body found in contemporary health promotion. The body consciousness and self-awareness demanded in new paradigms of health are attributes that have historically been associated with femininity (Moore 2010, p. 112).

Health Assemblages and Affect

Exploring how young people live their bodies and explain their practices of body work is crucial for understanding how health is lived and produced. A Deleuzo-Guattarian (1987) perspective approaches the body as an 'assemblage' that is in active engagement with the social world, rather than as a discrete entity that is passively produced by social or cultural norms. This is a particular ontological perspective which understands bodies as processes of relations, rather than pre-formed entities (Goodchild 1997). Bodies are understood as produced by engagements with other bodies and forces, including discourses, affects, ideals, norms, practices and institutions. Health assemblages are one such aspect which bodies engage with, and which compose bodies. Health assemblages are 'a function of encounters between bodies, between forces and between practices' (Duff 2014, p. 186). From this perspective, health as an assemblage is comprised by discourses, such as those which emphasise individualised self-responsibility and bodily perfection in Western, neo-Liberal contexts, as well as through affective relations which may register as embodied sensations and mediate a body's capacities (what a body can do) (Coffey 2014). Affects are 'felt bodily intensities' and are particularly relevant to understanding the dynamics by which consumer culture images affect or impact upon people and identities:

> Other bodies and the images of other bodies in the media and consumer culture may literally move us, make us feel moved, by affecting our bodies in inchoate ways that cannot easily be articulated or assimilated to conceptual thought. Here we think of the shiver down the spine or the gut feeling. Affect points to the experience of intensities, to the way in which media images are felt through bodies. (Featherstone 2010, p. 195)

Affect is also important in understanding the particular gendered images of health in the landscape of consumer culture (Coffey 2016).

This approach can assist in making sense of the dynamic ways in which bodies are actively produced against and alongside the current socio-cultural conditions, such as the heightened focus on image-based notions of health, which arise from the intersections between neo-Liberal and consumer culture imperatives. It broadens an understanding of health as multiple, including its force as a 'culturally sanctioned way of being' in contemporary, neo-Liberal Western economies such as Australia (Crawford 1987; Featherstone 1982; Featherstone 2010). Empirically, this perspective also enables a focus on the practices understood to denote health (such as diet and exercise), and its embodied and affective dimensions of the 'experience' of health. As such, health may be better conceptualised as an active process rather than as a static image or state of being that can be attained (Coffey 2014; Featherstone 2010). The affective and embodied aspects of 'health' are as important as discursive framings of health in understanding the significance of health and well-being as moral imperatives of contemporary life.

The following analysis draws from a qualitative study of young people's body work practices related to gender, health, identity and the body. These themes were explored through 22 in-depth semi-structured interviews with young men and women aged 18–33 in Melbourne, Australia, in 2010. A broader age range was included aligned with other research on body image and identity, which holds that that those aged roughly 18–35 in Western cultures have grown up in the context of consumer and neo-Liberal imperatives vital to understanding the types of body work that are pervasive in contemporary Western contexts (Gill et al. 2005; McRobbie 2009). I recruited the sample through asking personal contacts to forward electronic advertisements to their friends (not known to me) through Facebook and email, which enabled participants to self-select. Participants were mainly white, middle class and heterosexual; but they came from a range of professions and education levels. Participants discussed a range of body work practices related to their identities such as exercising through jogging, attending classes at a gym or weights training, as well as diet, wearing make-up, tattooing and cosmetic surgery (Coffey 2013a; Coffey 2013b; Coffey 2014). The aim was to explore how body work is done and how understandings of bodies are produced through these practices.

Health as an Individual, Moralised Responsibility

The following examples explore the ways in which moral imperatives of health assemble: first, through discourses of individual responsibility and participants' judgments of their and others' bodies, and in a later section, through affective relations.

The moral and individualistic dimensions of 'health' discourses were repeated throughout the interviews. Many spoke of how they felt 'lazy' or 'slack' if they have not been exercising. Health or practices that were considered to lead to 'health', such as exercise, were discussed as though they were a common requirement, which, if not being met, warranted explanation and justification. For example, Steph discusses how her work hours have increased, and she is no longer at college where she used to play organised team sports:

> Julia: *Before you were saying that you would want to exercise more if you weren't working so much?*
> Steph: *Yeah, it's probably a pretty shit excuse to be honest! [laughs]*
> Julia: *What do you mean?*
> Steph: *Oh, like everybody works and heaps of people find time to work out.*
> (Steph, 21, server)

Steph says that working long hours is a poor 'excuse' for not exercising, illustrating the moralised dynamics of individual responsibility for health (Lupton 1995; Crawford 1980). That the physical and emotional toll associated with working long hours in the service industry is not seen as an understandable hindrance to the time and energy required for 'working out' shows the primacy of individual responsibility for health and appearance. The structural impediments, such as the 'flexible', casualised employment conditions which characterise the service industry in Australia, are not discussed by Steph, and her lack of time for exercise due to work is framed as her own individual failing.

Others' bodies were discussed as a way of defining or demarcating 'health' based on what activities or health practices they did or did not undertake, such as exercising:

> Victoria: *I'm not the sort of person who would just sit there. I don't know, like my sister for example. Sometimes she's a bit lazy and wouldn't do anything.*
> Julia: *Wouldn't exercise?*
> Victoria: *Yeah wouldn't exercise and that sort of thing. Sometimes I don't have sympathy for people who don't, who complain about where they're at [laughing] Like, what are you there for, why don't you do something about it, sort of thing! People complain, and I just want to say, why don't you get off your ass and do something, you know! [laughing]. (Victoria, 25, marketing)*

The expectation that someone should be self-motivated to 'do something about it' is undoubtedly a moral judgement drawn from the broader neo-Liberal ethos of self-responsibility for health and the body's appearance. Many other participants speak with similar disapproval of those who do not 'take care of themselves' in supposedly appropriate ways. In Adam's example, he equates a person's 'body type' with the amount of respect he affords them and type of person he deems them to be:

Yeah, I think you can read straight into someone with their body type. I think when I look at [athletes] I automatically have respect, because I think, ok, obviously what you do, you take kind of seriously, and therefore you take a lot of things seriously in your life, you respect your body. For me, I like people who respect their health and their body. (Adam, 23, footballer and university student)

'Health' was also frequently described as in opposition to 'fat'. Simon, for example, describes athletic bodies as ideal for men and women because 'it all comes down to health':

If you're free to move and stuff, if you're fit you can run and stuff and you have stamina and all those kind of skills, and stuff. Um yeah, I guess that's healthy. And just not lazy I guess, I don't know, I associate fat with laziness. (Simon, 18, University student)

Being 'active' was broadly understood as being important and essential to health, while 'laziness' was criticised and associated with a range of other negative traits such as a lack of self-esteem or self-respect. These descriptions were often attributed to others they deemed to be overweight or fat. Participants deemed those who were 'fat' or 'overweight' as 'definitely not healthy', and as seriously contravening health as an idealised 'state' of being and image. Participants described those who are 'fat', 'overweight' or 'obese' as lazy, lacking self-esteem and self-restraint, and deserving of the increased surveillance and criticism they receive.

I think that if you're incredibly overweight and obese you need to do something about it. There was a girl at my school as an example, she has dropped out now, but she was huge and she was always saying 'I'm so fat, I need to lose weight, I need to do exercise', and we said 'we'll support you, we'll help you' and then the next second she'd be buying cheese jaffles, a Big M and a massive Freddo Frog for breakfast every morning at school. And it's kind of the point where, it's ridiculous, you're not being healthy, you're not doing anything to help yourself. (Clare, 18, school student)

Clare is most critical of the girl's individual failure of responsibility to 'do anything to help herself'. Tom makes similar generalisations about his housemate's lack of self-discipline and assumes that she would like to lose weight, even though in a later section of the interview Tom says he has never actually discussed this with her:

My housemate, she's overweight; she knows that she's overweight, but she's lazy. Despite the effort, you know, or she wants to do something about it but at the same time, does nothing. So, she'd be quite happy to eat what she eats in the quantity that she does, but there's no effort or commitment to a plan. And no drive I suppose. Whereas, I think if you look at confident people, most of them are probably pretty fit kind of people, fairly driven sorts of people. And this is just generalisations as well, I'm sure there are exceptions to the rule, but overweight people are generally, I find, more shy. Or withheld. I think it would be true to say, to generalise again, that a lot of people that are overweight have some self-esteem issues. (Tom, 25, firefighter)

The moral implications of health are most evident in statements such as these, which attach a negative moral judgement of 'lazy', or positive judgements of 'healthy', to specific body shapes. As many others have argued (Gimlin 2002; Grimshaw 1999; Crossley 2006b; Lupton 1996; Lupton 2013), being 'fat' is culturally stigmatised and comes to symbolise a range of other negatively inscribed aspects of self, such as laziness, poor 'self-esteem' and a 'lack of effort or commitment'— the opposite of successful and 'driven' and other characteristics most valued in a neo-Liberal context. Those deemed 'fat' are also subjected to greater surveillance, such as when Clare lists the different sorts of food eaten by the 'huge' girl at her school, or when Tom emphasises the quantity of food his housemate consumes. Where looking or being 'fat' was considered 'unhealthy' and linked to a range of other moralised statements such as lack of effort or motivation, and condemned by participants as a result, individualised self-discipline through body work regimes was celebrated. Adam and Victoria both equated body work, through physical exercise and maintenance of body weight, with earning or being worthy of 'respect'. As Dworkin and Wachs (2009, p.138) describe, 'while the fat body remains stigmatised as lazy, undisciplined, or as a poor member of the social body, the fit body becomes a metaphor for success, morality and good citizenship'.

These examples illustrate some of the regulatory discursive framings associated with 'healthism' (Crawford 1980) in a neo-Liberal context. The moral and symbolic order underpinning the notion of respect for others who 'respect their own bodies' through undertaking 'healthy' activities is gendered, classed and racialised (Dworkin and Wachs 2009), in the process, marginalising corporeal forms that are not white, middle class or slim. The expectation that 'everyone should make time to be healthy' obscures the classed and structural aspects of health and body work, such as socio-economic, living and working conditions. The primary consumers of health and fitness products such as magazines are 'white and middle class'. The constitution of emphasised masculinity and femininity (Connell 1987) through body work practices of this dominant group intersect with class and race privilege (Dworkin and Wachs 2009, pp. 162-163). In this neo-Liberal context in which individual responsibility for health and the body is intensified, health is increasingly tied to appearance in 'looking like' a good citizen (Gill et al. 2005). Moralised dimensions of this neo-Liberal health discourse positions bodily discipline as imperative without regard or sympathy for the broader structural conditions such as increased hours or precarious working conditions that shape their lives. As the following section discusses, the responsibilities associated with feeling and looking healthy operate through both discourses and affect.

Health, Affect and Image

The affective and embodied aspects of 'health' are also crucial in understanding the significance of health and well-being as moral imperatives of contemporary life. Paul, for example, discusses that 'taking care of himself' through going to the gym enables him to 'feel better' in his body:

I try and ... maintain a level of fitness when I'm taking care of myself. I've always gone to the gym a little bit. Mostly just to, you know, stay active and feel better ... about ... I mean partly physically, but ... partly the way I look, but also partly the way I feel ... about inhabiting my flesh. (Paul, 32, film and TV editor)

Kate also refers to health as a 'feeling' or an idealised state of 'being' that she 'should' aspire to:

Kate: I wouldn't do it [exercise] to improve my body to get a six-pack or to get toned. I'd do it more just to feel good. ... I think I focus more on looking healthy, but as far as feeling it, I don't think I feel it as much as I should. I definitely should get out and do more exercise. I feel so much better when I do. (Kate, 24, administration assistant)

The appearance of health is not enough. Kate explains that she wants to focus more on *feeling* healthy: 'I don't think I feel it as much as I should'. The feeling of health in this example is described as another aspect with moral dimensions that 'should' be attained as an ideal state.

Health is assumed to be not only a practice or appearance, but also valued as an embodied sensation that can be 'felt'. Most participants broadly agreed that their 'exercise' practices linked to the way their body feels. Anna discusses how she used to play in team sports at college but no longer does because her circumstances have changed: she has finished her undergraduate University degree and is working full-time hours as a server to save money to travel overseas. She says:

I normally feel, like, a lot better if I have been exercising, but just, like, little things if I do them now I'm like, 'Phew! That was a bit of a struggle! That's a bit embarrassing!' But um, yeah I generally do like it when I am exercising a little bit more. Although a lot of the times I can't really be bothered but I know, you do, you do feel a little bit better if you know that you're doing something, but I have been very slack the last couple of months. (Anna, 21, server)

Again, Anna does not see working long hours as an adequate 'excuse' for not finding the time to exercise. Despite the significant physical demands of service work, Anna describes herself as having been 'slack' in her exercise routine lately. Many participants agreed that doing exercise equated with 'feeling good' or 'feeling better' in some way. As Anna explains, 'I think you just generally feel better for it [exercise] because you don't feel like you're lazing around and being a bit of a couch potato'. Exercise here has a moral dimension in ways similar to those described in the previous section and enables her to feel moral satisfaction related to physical activity, though there are numerous times she 'can't really by bothered'. 'Knowing you're doing something', related to exercise specifically, is also an important aspect of body work. Because 'looking healthy' was also equated with looking good or attractive, this also motivated participants towards body work practices such as exercising.

> *The best way you can look is if you're healthy I think ... Just someone who looks like they take care of themselves I guess. Ummm ... how to describe it without sounding like an asshole? ... I just don't want to be overweight. And that, much as I hate to say it, is a concern for me. Like it's something that I am consciously worried about. Like, I'm by no means skinny, I don't wanna be any more overweight than I am right now. It's something that, like, I worry about. I don't know if it's even really worth worrying about ... but it's something that is on my mind a lot.* (Steph, 21, server)

Steph's worrying about becoming overweight can be understood in the broader context of consumer culture images that privilege 'skinny' body shapes. These images are affective and carry particular intensities related to 'worry' about becoming overweight and the imagined shame of inhabiting a fat body. This can help to explain and contextualise the examples in which Steph, Anna, Kate and Paul described activities related to health as associated with 'feeling better'.

These examples suggest the ways moral imperatives of health function through affect and embodied sensations such as in the dynamics of 'looking healthy' and 'feeling healthy', and the fear of becoming overweight ('it's something I worry about'). In the health assemblage (Duff 2014), health can be understood to be produced by health discourses and also by felt bodily intensities or affects (and myriad other aspects, including objects, images, others' bodies and spaces). These intensities form what a body can do. In other words, they can assist our understanding of *why* the young people in these examples say they want to exercise, and 'feel better' when they do. Combined with the discourse of health and its prioritisation of neo-Liberal values of self-responsibility and 'no excuses', young people such as Anna and Steph are left with few options other than to understand themselves as 'slack' if they do not exercise (and feel 'worried' about becoming overweight), regardless of the broader conditions which shape their lives. Since these conditions include structural labour market forces which shape service work as an industry characterised by low pay, lack of job security and lack of predictable work hours, individualised notions of health can be seen as particularly punishing and problematic.

The consumer culture image of health presents work on appearance as an 'imperative or duty, and casts those who become fat, or let their appearance go, or look old before their time, as not only slothful but as having a flawed self' (Featherstone 2010, p. 195). The young body is also laden with additional cultural dimensions and affective intensities as it is seen to epitomise health (Atkinson and Monaghan 2014). In these examples, the 'image' of health works alongside the 'feeling' of health as being an important motivator for body work practices. Both carry affective charges which assist in understanding the ways in which health currently assembles for young people, and the problematic ways by which health imperatives function. The analysis assists understanding the ways that neo-Liberal health demands register and operate both discursively and affectively.

Conclusion

This chapter has aimed to show the ways in which health assemblages are produced through engagement with health discourses that are edged with associations with morality and good citizenship, and through affect. Participants described those who are 'fat', 'overweight' or 'obese' as lazy, lacking self-esteem and self-restraint, and deserving of the increased surveillance and criticism they receive. Participants were often pitiless in their criticism of their own and others' bodies for their perceived 'laziness' or 'slackness'. This has implications for 'non-conforming bodies' in particular, as those who fail to live up to the imperative of perceived self-care in the form of body and weight management are seen as having a 'flawed self' (Featherstone 2010, p. 195). These examples illustrate regulatory discursive framings associated with 'healthism', youth and the body. Neo-Liberal rationality is also present in the moral and symbolic order which underpinned participants' descriptions of which bodies were worthy of 'respect' because they 'respect their own bodies' through undertaking 'healthy' activities. Such notions of 'respect' have significant gendered, classed and racialised dimensions (Dworkin and Wachs 2009), and marginalise corporeal forms that are not white, middle class or slim in particular.

This has particular implications in the context of efforts to address 'unhealthy' body image as a key concern for youth. It suggests that a key cause for body image distress or 'worrying' about the body's appearance is linked to the broader pathologisation of overweight bodies, and moralising messages that certain bodies are more deserving of respect and recognition as 'selves' than others.

Aligned with this, many participants saw doing exercise as a way of warding off negative associations of the self as 'lazy', and they equated body work practices such as going to the gym with 'feeling good' or 'feeling better' in some way. Health as a moral imperative operates through discourses as well as at the level of affect through bodily intensities and sensations. Health was described as 'felt' as an embodied sensation. From a conceptual perspective, a focus on embodied sensations assists in explaining the ways in which health assemblages are engaged with and produced through the body. Indeed, the discursive and regulatory aspects of health assemblages are so potent *because* of their affective, intensive properties and the ways in which they register in the body as embodied sensations. These twin dimensions are important because they assist in understanding the strength or power of 'health' to motivate different actions and activities. Importantly, affect operates beyond (or beneath) the register of 'consciousness' or 'choice'. In the examples of many of the participants in this chapter, affects served to encourage them towards greater surveillance and regulation of their bodies towards a narrow image of health.

Importantly, this perspective highlights that there is nothing essential or pre-given in how health assemblages are comprised or affect particular bodies. From a Deleuzo-Guattarian perspective, health is profoundly embodied and affective, which means that the ways that health assembles in relation to social context may be different for each person. This perspective enables the complex and specific ways in which engagements between bodies and the world are productive rather than purely regulatory or repressive. It is about examining how particular contexts are assembled and actively lived: in this case, the ways in which neo-Liberal regimes are implicated in the production of moral imperatives of health, and the ways in which these regimes assemble in young people's understandings of health and the body. A focus on the discursive and affective dimensions by which moral imperatives of health function can contribute to understanding the ways in which neo-Liberal contexts are engaged with and lived by young people. The examples in this chapter show both the strength of those discourses of health, and the specific ways in which health assembles in relation to neo-Liberal notions of morality in a context such as Australia.

References

Atkinson, M., and L.F. Monaghan. 2014. *Challenging Myths Of Masculinity: Understanding Physical Cultures*. Dorchester: Ashgate Publishing, Ltd.

Australian Bureau of Statistics. 2008. Measures Of Casual Employment. *Australian Labour Market Statistics Cat. No. 6105.0.*

Australian Bureau of Statistics. 2009. Feature Article 2: Health and Fitness Centers and Gymnasia, 4156.0.55.001. *Perspective on Sport May 2009*, Canberra. www.abs.gov.au/AUSSTATS/abs@.nsf/Lookup/4156.0.55.001Feature+Article2 May%202009.

Australian Centre for Retail Studies. 2005. Australian Health and Beauty Report (B.a.E. Department, Trans.) *ACRS Secondary Research Report*, Monash University, Australia.

Ayo, N. 2012. Understanding Health Promotion In A Neo-Liberal Climate And The Making Of Health Conscious Citizens. *Critical Public Health* 22(1): 99–105.

Bordo, S. 2003. *Unbearable Weight: Feminism, Western Culture And The Body*, 10th Anniversary edn. California: University Of California Press.

Broom, A., C. Muerk, J. Adams, and D. Sibbritt. 2012. My Health, My Responsibility? Complementary Medicine And Self (Health) Care. *Journal of Sociology* 504: 515–530.

Centre For Health Promotion. 2010. *Absolutely Every Body: Achieving A Body-Image Friendly School*. Government of South: Australia.

Coffey, J. 2013a. Bodies, Body Work And Gender: Exploring A Deleuzian Approach. *Journal Of Gender Studies* 22(1): 3–16.

———. 2013b. Body Pressure: Negotiating Gender Through Body Work Practices. *Youth Studies Australia* 32(2): 39–48.

———. 2014. As Long As I'm Fit And A Healthy Weight, I Don't Feel Bad': Exploring Body Work And Health Through The Concept Of 'Affect. *Journal of Sociology* 51(3): 613–627.

———. 2016. 'She Was Becoming Too Healthy And It Was Just Becoming Dangerous': Body Work And Assemblages Of Health. In *Learning Bodies: The Body In Youth And Childhood Studies*, eds. J. Coffey, S. Budgeon, and H. Cahill. New York: Springer.

Coffey, J., and J. Watson. 2015. Bodies: Corporeality And Embodiment In Childhood And Youth Studies. In *Handbook of Children And Youth Studies*, eds. J. Wyn and H. Cahill. New York: Springer.

Connell, R. 1987. *Gender And Power: Society, The Person And Personal Politics*. Cambridge: Polity Press.

Crawford, R. 1980. Healthism And The Medicalisation Of Everyday Life. *International Journal Of Health Services* 10(3): 365–388.

———. 1987. Cultural Influences On Prevention And The Emergence of A New Health Consciousness. In *Taking Care: Understanding And Encouraging Self-Protective Behavior*, ed. N. Weinstein, 95–114. Cambridge And New York: Cambridge University Press.

Crawford, R. 2006. Health as a meaningful social practice. *Health* 10(4): 401–420.

Crossley, N. 2006a. In The Gym: Motives, Meaning And Moral Careers. *Body and Society* 12(3): 23–50.

———. 2006b. *Reflexive Embodiment In Contemporary Society*. Berkshire: Open University Press.

Deleuze, G., and F. Guttari. 1987. *A Thousand Plateaus: Capitalism And Schizophrenia*. Edinburgh: Edinburgh University Press.

Dixon, J., D. Woodman, L. Strazdins, C. Banwell, D. Broom, and J. Burgess. 2014. Flexible Employment, Flexible Eating And Health Risks. *Critical Public Health* 24(4): 461–475.

Duff, C. 2014. *Assemblages of Health*. New York: Springer.

Dworkin, S., and F. Wachs. 2009. *Body Panic: Gender, Health And The Selling Of Fitness*. New York & London: University of New York Press.

Featherstone, M. 1982. The Body In Consumer Culture. *Theory, Culture And Society* 1: 18–33.

———. 2010. Body, Image And Affect In Consumer Culture. *Body And Society* 16(1): 193–221.

Gill, R., K. Henwood, and C. Mclean. 2005. Body Projects And The Regulation Of Normative Masculinity. *Body And Society* 11(1): 37–62.

Gimlin, D. 2002. *Body Work: Beauty And Self Image In American Culture*. Los Angeles: University Of California Press.

Goodchild, P. 1997. Deleuzean Ethics. *Theory, Culture & Society* 14(2): 39–50.

Grimshaw, J. 1999. Working Out With Merleau Ponty. In *Women's Bodies: Discipline And Transgression*, eds. J. Arthurs and J. Grimshaw. London And New York: Cassell.

Harris, A. 2004. *Future Girl: Young Women In The Twenty-First Century*. New York: Routledge.

Kelly, P. 2001. Youth At Risk: Processes Of Individualisation And Responsibilisation In The Risk Society. *Discourse* 22(1): 23–33.

Leahy, D. 2014. Assembling A Health [Y] Subject: Risky And Shameful Pedagogies In Health Education. *Critical Public Health* 24(2): 171–181.

Lupton, D. 1995. *The Imperative Of Health: Public Health And The Regulated Body*. London: Sage.

———. 1996. *Food, The Body And The Self*. Thousand Oaks: Sage.

———. 1999. *Risk*. London: Routledge.

———. 2013. *Fat*. London: Routledge.

Mcrobbie, A. 2009. *The Aftermath Of Feminism: Gender, Culture And Social Change*. London: Sage.

Mission Australia. 2014. *Youth Survey*. Australia: Mission Australia.

Moore, S. 2010. Is The Healthy Body Gendered? Toward A Feminist Critique Of The New Paradigm Of Health. *Body And Society* 16(2): 95–118.

Petersen, A. 1996. Risk and the regulated self: the discourse of health promotion as politics of uncertainty. *Journal of Sociology* 32(1): 44–57.

Pike, J. 2015. Young People And Food: The Moral Project Of The Healthy Self. In *A Critical Youth Studies For The 21st Century*, eds. P. Kelly and A. Kamp. Leiden And Boston: Brill.

Quinlan, M., and R. Johnstone. 2009. The Implications Of De-Collectivist Industrial Relations Laws And Associated Developments For Worker Health And Safety In Australia, 1996–2007. *Industrial Relations Journal* 40(5): 426–443.

Rose, N. 1996. *Inventing Our Selves: Psychology, Power And Personhood*. Cambridge: Cambridge University Press.

Te Riele, K. 2006. Youth 'At Risk': Further Marginalizing The Marginalized? *Journal Of Education Policy* 21(2): 129–145.

Wyn, J., and D. Woodman. 2006. Generation, Youth And Social Change In Australia. *Journal Of Youth Studies* 9(5): 495–514.

Wyn, J. 2009. *Youth Health and Welfare: The Cultural Politics of Education and Well-being*. Melbourne: Oxford University Press.

4

Get on Your Feet, Get Happy: Happiness and the Affective Governing of Young People in the Age of Austerity

Deirdre Duffy

Introduction

Happiness is a central theme in the current well-being agenda both implicitly—when couched in the language of therapy and ensuring contentment (Ecclestone and Hayes 2009; Brunila 2012)—and explicitly—through the adoption of 'happiness measures' and the emergence of Happiness Studies (Ahmed 2007/08). However, this chapter suggests that the happiness agenda, which dominates neo-Liberal well-being discourses, operates not as vague well-intentioned support but as a form of affective governance. The happiness project represents the production and regulation of neo-Liberal subjects through the manipulation of emotion and futurity. The term affective refers to the 'pre-reflexive and preconscious [...] embodied encounters that influence the capacity

D. Duffy (✉)
Manchester Metropolitan University, Manchester, UK

© The Editor(s) (if applicable) and The Author(s) 2017   **87**
P. Kelly, J. Pike (eds.), *Neoliberalism, Austerity, and the Moral Economies of Young People's Health and Well-being*,
DOI 10.1057/978-1-137-58266-9_5

of the mind and body to act' (Pimlott-Wilson 2015, p. 3). This form of governing orients subjects towards objects or ways of being by connecting them to desired emotional states (e.g., joyfulness, pride, happiness) that are felt viscerally before they are subjected to reflection. The actions of subjects are thus pre-consciously governed by the potential possessions or ways of being of the future (Berlant 2011; Staunæs 2011; Sellar 2014; Bjerg 2013). Under neo-Liberal austerity these 'happy objects' are principally financial stability, employment and economic success (Ahmed 2007/08)—artefacts of the moral economy. Young people, the chapter proposes, are particularly susceptible to this phenomenon, as their ways of being in the present are already oriented towards ways of being in the future. As a result, the chapter concludes, the promotion of happiness under the discourse of well-being is part of a strategy of both orienting young people towards particular ways of being and, in doing so, regulating young people in the present.

Happiness and Governing

While the concepts applied in this chapter are not common in discussions of youth well-being, the notion that emotion can be used to govern subjects is. Siivonen and Brunila (2013) and Ecclestone and Hayes (2009), for example, consider how the neo-Liberal subject's actions are restricted not just through their construction as self-propelling and enterprising (Kelly 2013), but also through their construction as self-responsible and emotionally reserved. Kulz (2013), in a study of the governance of subjects through academies in the UK, notes how young people police their own speech, particularly speech that vocalises complaints through internalising notions that successful students are emotionally controlled and contained.

Moreover, the notion that discourses of 'acceptable' emotional expression are used to govern (predominantly) female subjects and People of Colour has been a central proposition of feminist theorists such as Lorde (1984), Campbell (1994) and Boler (1999). In *Sister, Outsider* (1984), Lorde documents how liberal and cultural feminist understandings of progressive, 'feminist' emotional expression sought to rob her of her ability to vocalise her experience of race-based oppression. According to Lorde, angry speech was constructed as characteristic of the unresolved and regressive subject through the command that angry speakers should 'move on'. This left her silenced, and made her history of race-based discrimination invisible. Campbell (1994) expands on this, describing how phrases such as 'don't be bitter', and notions of progressive emotional expression are part of a strategy of silencing victims of oppression. In addition, Boler (1999) positions discourses of emotional literacy and intelligence as an extension of gendered regulation. *C(llcur)*

Commentaries on how political resistance is policed have also highlighted how emotion is used to construct the resisting subject as unreasoned and interruptive. Lyman (1981, 2004) and Bauman (2012), for example, explore how the construction of 'good' and 'bad' emotion and the 'domestication' of emotion (Lyman 2004: 133) serve to limit radical political action. In a similar way to the feminist theorists listed above, Lyman and Bauman focus upon anger, which they position as the 'essential political emotion' (Lyman 1981, p. 61). For Lyman, the construction of anger as a 'bad' emotion by philosophers from Aristotle to Sartre (1962) to Nietzsche (1967) has undermined the ability of angry subjects to express their complaints. These thinkers have proposed that anger is antithetical to reasoned and productive debate, and facilitated the performative construction of angry subjects as political inhibitors. Discourses of emotion have, as a result, undermined radical political action. Furthermore, Bauman (2012, pp.35–36) argues that the delineation of 'good' and 'bad' anger is directed by class-based prejudices of 'good' and 'bad' expression: *Goo is bad angr.*

> the angry rich [...] have the right to be angry; they are allowed to pump their anger through loudspeakers installed on public squares in front of the offices of supreme powers—without any fear of being charged with selfishness, breaking solidarity, anarchy, anti-Americanism, or the mentality of a Luo tribesman.

Combined, these commentaries illustrate how constructions of emotion as good or bad, controlled or uncontrollable, are employed in order to silence and control subjects. However, in terms of developing an understanding of how happiness governs subjects, their usefulness is somewhat undermined by their shared assumption that the 'emotional governance' of particular discourses, of progressive politics for example or of self-propulsion constitutes the process of limiting subjects from feeling or expressing particular emotions (usually anger). All of these theorists implicitly and explicitly suggest that anger is discursively regulated through the construction of the angry subject as inhibitive, interruptive and violent. As a result, the reasons why subjects feel anger (their complaints or experiences of oppression) are rendered invisible and silenced. This follows a governmentality perspective of the impact of performativity and the formation of the subject on the actions of the subject.

What I want to argue here is that the process of emotional governing facilitated by happiness, and how happiness regulates, is much more complex. Centrally, what I contend is not that discourses of neo-Liberal performativity prevent subjects from expressing unhappiness, it is that these discourses orient subjects towards particular states of being that under neo-Liberalism are projected as happy-making. The dynamic of governance in relation to happiness is thus quite different to the dynamic relating to anger. Anger, through its construction as interruptive, uncontrolled and resisting, is positioned as separate from neo-Liberal performativity by both its opponents and proponents. It is a way of being which falls outside neo-Liberal selfhood. Happiness, on the other hand, orients subjects in a particular direction through manipulating their formation at a visceral level. It makes them desire particular objects and in doing so facilitates their movement towards neo-Liberal performativity. In other words, happiness is neither *regulated* nor *used* to *regulate* the subject, it is *regulating*. The key difference here is that, unlike anger, happiness is not policed or used to police subjects. Happiness involves the *production* of policed subjects whose performativity is always oriented towards subjectivities and performativities considered desirable under neo-Liberalism.

Adopting an *affective* governance framework involves positioning happiness not as a performativity that aligns to neo-Liberal performativity (i.e., a happy subject is a neo-Liberal subject), but as a performative technology of neo-Liberalism (i.e., subjectification is oriented towards neo-Liberal sub-jectivities through a discourse which constructs these as happy futurities). This technology operates at the level of bodily intensities and felt tem-poralities. This provocative interpretation of happiness was first proposed by Sara Ahmed in *The Cultural Politics of Emotion* (2004). In this work, Ahmed positions happiness not as a feeling external to the subject which is expressed or not expressed by the subject, but as a process which orientates subjectification towards a particular way of being through the manipu-lation of desire. This requires the acceptance of the idea that emotions are not '*vented* by already existing subjects' but that emotions 'help bring subjects into being, or help *make subjects*' (Sparks 2014, p. 34, emphasis in original). Happiness, according to Ahmed, involves the 'orientation [of the subject] towards the future' (Ahmed 2007/08, p. 12) or directing the formation of the subject towards a particular subjectivity through the pre-sentation of this futurity as a desirable.

There are two arguments at play here: first, that happiness governs through positioning a particular state or object as a 'hap' (Ahmed 2004), which, when occupied or possessed, is a manifestation of 'being happy'. Second, that as we do not yet possess the 'hap', happiness governs through directing us towards a future self who possesses the 'hap' and is happy. As Ahmed (2007/08, p.12, emphasis added) suggests, 'happiness operates as a *futurity*, as something that is hoped for; creating a political and personal horizon that gives us an image of the good life'.

The invocation of these imagined futurities, according to Ahmed, and the creation of a horizon between the present and the future, opens up possibilities for regulating the subject in the present through directing subjectification. Importantly for neo-Liberal governmentality, as Berlant (2011) argues, the impact of this imagined future happiness does not depend on the 'good life'. The fact that we do not know what happi-ness will be like or whether we will indeed be happy does not lessen the good life's influence on the subject. A practical application of these arguments on the process of regulation through imagined futurity and happiness is provided by Staunæs (2011). Exploring the contemporary approaches of managers in educational settings, Staunæs (2011, p.244) argues that education management is increasingly 'based on the potential, on that-which-is-not-there'. In other words, through centring on students' potential for possessing 'the good life' in the *future*, managers are able to direct students towards particular ways of acting in the *present*. As Staunæs (2011, p.245) explains:

> The future thereby becomes an instrument of modulating the present and an opportunity to change and create policies about what is already here; an opportunity not only to make the future governable but also to govern the present.

Moreover, as Sellar (2014) suggests, again in the context of education, the connection to 'the good life' (and risks to it) is felt emotionally and viscerally before it is interpreted cognitively. 'The good life' evokes bodily reactions before conscious responses and as such its precise meaning matters little (see also: Pimlott-Wilson 2015). To explore this argument, Sellar analyses the impact of performance indicators such as test scores on student's behaviour, proposing that the potency of performance indicators, as the quantitative commensuration of learnedness, lies not in what they actually mean but in how they are felt. As performance indicators are, fundamentally, over-simplified abstractions that cannot and do not represent the student's skills and abilities *in totalis*, Sellar suggests that their constituent power rests not in their 'digital' substance (what they say about the student) but in their 'analogue' impact (how the student feels or is felt). As Sellar (2014, p.133) suggests:

> Test results are always met with a complex of feelings by students—pride, disappointment, relief. These feelings are likely to be the primary effect of the data and may feed into increased or decreased motivation in the future. Students may undertake a conscious inquiry into their score and how it was produced, but their first reaction is likely to be a visceral one.

In terms of understanding how happiness can assist in the formation of neo-Liberal subjectivities, the interjections of the above commentators are crucial. Combined, they indicate that by associating particular ways of being with 'the good life', to use Ahmed's phrasing, presenting them as a 'hap' or a maker of happiness, the *promise* of happiness is able—and used—to direct the actions of subjects in the present. Importantly, this does not depend on the 'what' of happiness as this is interpreted viscer; before it is considered actively.

In adopting this conceptual framework, as Ahmed (2007/08, p.10) notes, we can understand better 'how claims to happiness make certain forms and personhood valuable', and the process through which these personhoods are constructed as the norm. Within the current socio-political context, the substance of 'the good life'—and what constitutes happiness—is characterised by forms of personhood valued under neo-Liberalism (i.e., economically self-sufficient, educated and part of a 'stable' family). This is reflected in the inclusion of financial stability and employment opportunities in global happiness indicators such as the Global Youth Well-being Index (GYWI), and in the positioning of citizens in economically dominant countries as happier. The resonance between happiness and neo-Liberal personhood is made explicit in the following description cited in Ahmed's (2007/08, p.9) critique of the 'happiness turn':

> happy persons are more likely to be found in the economically prosperous countries, where freedom and democracy are held in respect and the political scene is stable. The happy are more likely to be found in majority groups than among minorities and more often at the top of the ladder than the bottom. They are typically married and get on well with families and friends.

Furthermore, affective governmentality has already, some commentators suggest, been adopted by neo-Liberalism. As Staunæs (2011, p.229) argues:

> It is possible to identify the impact of the affective trend in buzzwords like 'emotional leadership' [...] and 'management of relations'. Indeed, these new terms are now often found in policy documents and handbooks. [...] [T]he affectivisation of educational leadership is spoken into existence as a promising path toward the future—a way of learning, transforming human capital and employing this in generating economic growth. Leadership and management—often using (what is recognised as) good and positive feelings (for instance joy and happiness)—seem to be key objectives of current edifying approaches to educational leadership and development.

Youth Well-being and the Affective Governmentality of Happiness

Thus far, this chapter has positioned the discourse of happiness as the governing of the present through the manipulation of emotion and temporality, labelling this as affective governmentality. It has suggested that the promise of happiness, and of 'getting happy', is deployed as a means of directing subjectification and subject-action through creating an emotional connection between the subject and an imagined futurity. It has also proposed that because this connection is emotional, the *substance* of this futurity and whether the subject in futurity will actually be happy is irrelevant. As such, the content of happiness is open to manipulation and, at present, has principally been projected as characterised by forms of personhood valued by neo-Liberalism. As Ahmed writes, 'the face of happiness is also the face of privilege' (2007/08, p.9).

What I now want to do is apply this broad argument to an exploration into the presence of this neo-Liberal affective governmentality in the current discourses of youth well-being. Specifically, I want to demonstrate how the discourse of youth well-being in its policy-based and institutional manifestations, interlaces with the neo-Liberal affective governmentality of happiness outlined in the previous section. To do this, I will highlight (i) the 'promise'-oriented nature of the youth well-being narrative and (ii) how the 'good life' presented to young people is characterised by neo-Liberal ideals of selfhood, particularly employment and economic independence. Having shown this, I will suggest that this affective governmentality is gaining increasing traction due to the effects of post-Global Financial Crisis (GFC) austerity.

The 'Promise' of Well-being

Commenting on the overall health of young people, Eckersley (2011) observes that, while globally young people's physical health is improving, their mental and emotional health is rapidly declining. Furthermore, reviewing the findings of the Australia21 report on young people's well-being, Eckersley et al. (2006, p.11) state that:

> a fifth to a third of young people are experiencing significant psychological
> stress and distress at any one time. [...] Young people are experiencing
> higher rates of mental health problems than other age groups.

At present, state-centric and global estimates suggest that the most significant health challenge facing young people relates to their mental and emotional well-being (Eckersley 2011).

Although the decline of young people's mental health and well-being has been directly linked to the economic, social, educational and political pressures they face (Furlong 2013), the well-being agendas proposed in countries such as the UK and Australia do not focus on unsettling the structural forces at the root of the noticeable decline in young people's health and well-being. Despite the actuality of young people's emotional precarity and the pressures they experience, the responses to these pressures are not focussed on addressing this actuality. This is reflected in the emphasis on supporting young people to 'become somebody well' (Wyn 2007: 35) and on their aspirations. As Pimlott-Wilson (2015, p. 2) highlights:

> Despite ubiquitous disparities [...] a powerful rhetoric of 'aiming higher'
> and personal responsibility for well-being and social cohesion persists.
> Political leaders place the onus on the individual to 'aspire' to dominant
> visions of adulthood rather than on the Government to address broader
> inequalities and barriers that young people face.

Applying the conceptual lens of affect, this points to the prioritisation of an imagined futurity above a lived actuality. Like Ahmed's reading of happiness, well-being serves to create a topology of subjectification and subject-action where the potential to achieve a present state, for example, the promise of well-being, is used to divert attention towards 'anticipated future emotions' (Pimlott-Wilson 2015, p.3).

The focus on futurities is made overt in national and international policies relating to young people's well-being and improving young people's well-being. For example, in its Youth Strategy, the European Union's (EU) indicators for assessing the health and well-being of young people within the EU are oriented not at the *present* situation for young people but whether and how effectively young people's *future* well-being will be achieved. While recognising the current difficulties facing young people, the EU's health and well-being agenda is framed in terms of bringing a particular futurity into being.

According to Pimlott-Wilson, Staunæs and others, this is indicative of the governing of young people's present using the promise of a particular futurity. Through orienting their strategies towards the 'promise of well-being', policy-makers limit opportunities for discussing the present actuality of precarity at an institutional level. Their interest is in young people's future circumstances not their current problems.

The Neo-Liberal 'Good Life'

The second element of the current discourse of well-being that reflects an affective neo-Liberal governmentality is the characteristics of the 'good life' that young people are oriented towards. Despite using the terminology of mental and emotional wellness, the 'hap' or future selfhood promoted by policy discourses of well-being is typified by 'ideals of neo-Liberal citizenship', including self-reliance, flexibility, mobility and 'fulfilment through material consumption' (Pimlott-Wilson 2015, p. 2). As UK Prime Minister David Cameron (2012) stated in 2012, the 'good life' for the ideal young person consisted of 'their first pay cheque, their first car, their first home'.

The promotion of a neo-Liberal 'good life' is reflected in the indicators for well-being and the rationale for the lack of emotional well-being presented in both policy and academic writing. For example, in the 40 indicators used by the GYWI (Youth Index 2015), there is a particular emphasis on young people's economic development and growth. This resonates with Cameron's promotion of employment and financial stability as central to well-being. Furthermore, not only is access to economic opportunities in itself an indicator of the 'good life', it also protects against other problematic futurities. As the GYWI's summary of 'economic opportunities' illustrates:

> Access to viable economic opportunities is critical to youth well-being and national growth. When youth are employed, earning and have access to financial institutions, they are less likely to rely on government support, more likely to be healthy, and less likely to be involved in criminal activity. With a stable economic foundation, youth tend to be optimistic and proactive in other areas of their lives. (Youth Index 2015)

The conflation of future emotional well-being and future employment is also manifested in the health and well-being indicators adopted by the EU's 2009 Youth Strategy. As the European Commission's Youth Dashboard implies, the successful attainment of a 'healthy' outcome for young people in the EU can be assessed by 'transition from education and training and the labour market' (EC 2011, p. 4) and 'integration into the labour market, either as employees or entrepreneurs' (EC 2011, p. 5) as much as by their physical health or 'political solidarity' (EC 2011, p. 8).

The dominance of neo-Liberal visions of the 'good life' in discussions of both the current and future state of young people's emotional well-being is also highlighted by critics of the 'therapisation' of education. By problematising the rise of the therapeutic ethos of producing self-reliant and resilient young people through education (Ecclestone and Hayes 2009; Furedi 2004; Brunila 2012), this body of literature argues that the ends of contemporary emotional work (Hochschild 1983) in education are protecting vulnerable young people against a 'bad life' of unemployment and economic exclusion (Brunila 2012). The valorisation of a socially included futurity—with inclusion understood as employment and financial stability versus the socially excluded situation of unemployment (Brunila 2012; Amsler 2011)—is, according to therapisation critics, fundamental to the 'pedagogy of comfort' (Amsler 2011, p. 47), which dominates understandings of the goals of education systems and projects.

In each of these examples, the imagined 'good life' which desirable emotions are connected with is decidedly neo-Liberal. The happy futurity that young people are oriented towards is one predominantly characterised by economic stability and employment.

Conclusion: 'Get Happy' and the Affective Production of Neo-Liberal Youth Subjectivity Under Austerity

Given the fluidity and becoming-ness of youth subjectivity (Jeffrey 2010; Kelly and Kamp 2015), it is perhaps unsurprising that affective, future-oriented governance has such traction. The construction of the young person as an immanent subjectivity is well established within policy and academic writing, the most obvious example of this being the 'youth as transition' model. However, applying the critiques of Ahmed and others, such presentations afford opportunities for invisibilising and regulating young people's actions in the present through orienting their subjectification towards a neo-Liberal futurity. Well-being operates as a 'promise', limits the possibilities for dealing with young people's current challenges and, exemplified within current policy discourses, is resolutely neo-Liberal in its characteristics. Employment and economic independence are emblematic of the 'good life'.

The arguments of affective governmentality have applications beyond the present socio-political moment. However, the neo-Liberal futurity imposed has arguably gained more ground since the GFC and emergence of the politics of austerity that represent the beginnings of the Age of Austerity. There are a number of reasons behind the synchronicity of affective governmentality and austerity. First, there is the future-oriented character of governmentality under neo-Liberalism. This point is raised by Newman (in Ayres 2014) who argues that the central difference between the pre- and post-austerity era (the start of which in the UK is marked by the election of the Conservative–Liberal Democrat Coalition in 2010) is the emphasis on design and planning about outcomes and evidence. According to Newman, the pre-GFC promotion of producing outcomes and evidence-based practice has been replaced by the prioritisation of programme design and pre-implementation targets. In the UK context, this is reflected in the emphasis on the future economy by George Osborne. In his 2015 Budget Statement, Osborne justified austerity on the basis that it protected the UK's future, asserting that, rather than returning to 'the mistakes of the past', he was making a 'critical choice' of 'the future' (Telegraph, March 2015).

Second, the proximity between austerity politics and the presentation of the discourse of happiness as neo-Liberal affective governmentality is reflected in the construction of full employment and individual economic stability as synonymous with the 'good life' or the 'hap'. By promoting economic self-reliance and entrepreneurialism as indivisible from contentment (Brunila 2012), and by portraying employed people as more contented through publicity documents such as those produced by the Department for Work and Pensions (2015), austerity politics in the UK is able to reinforce a particular characterisation of the 'good life', and of occupying this 'good life', as happiness.

Combined, the affective governmentality model presented by Ahmed (2004, 2010a) and others, and the current discourse of austerity demonstrates that the regulation of young people through contemporary discourses of well-being is more complex than the established arguments on emotional governance suggest. This is not simply a discursive separation or blockading of particular emotional registers (Boler 1999; Lyman 2004), it is an express manipulation of young people's subjectification through a publicly negotiated discourse of emotion (Sparks 2014). By constructing a neo-Liberal futurity as a manifestation of a desirable emotional state, the subject's thought is oriented towards the performativities of that futurity and its achievement rather than the realities of the present. The promise of future happiness regulates and renders invisible the present. Moreover, this operates at a visceral level, meaning that the substance of that futurity matters little, and can itself be manipulated by political discourses and elites. Young people, due to their becoming-ness, are already vulnerable to this kind of affective governmentality, something that the neo-Liberal politics of austerity is undoubtedly aware of and has used to its advantage.

References

Ahmed, S. 2004. *The cultural politics of emotion*. New York: Routledge.

———. 2007/08. The happiness turn. *New Formations* 63(1): 7—14.

———. 2010a. *The promise of happiness*. Durham: Duke University Press.

———. 2010b. Killing Joy: Feminism and the History of Happiness. *Signs: Journal of Women in Culture and Society Signs* 35(3): 571–594.

Amsler, S.S. 2011. From 'therapeutic' to political education: The centrality of affective sensibility in critical pedagogy. *Critical Studies in Education* 52(1): 47–63.

Ayres, S., ed. 2014. *Rethinking policy and politics: Reflections on contemporary debates in policy studies*. Bristol: Policy Press.

Bauman, Z. 2012. *This is not a diary*. Cambridge, UK: Polity Press.

Berlant, L.G. 2011. *Cruel optimism*. Durham: Duke University Press.

Bjerg, H. 2013. Staging the future—potentializing the self. *International Journal of Qualitative Studies in Education* 26(9): 1169–1191.

Boler, M. 1999. *Feeling power: Emotions and education*. New York: Routledge.
Brunila, K. 2012. From risk to resilience–The therapeutic ethos in youth education. *Education Inquiry* 3(3): 451–464.
Cameron, D. 2012. *Speech to Conservative Party Conference*. Birmingham: Conservative Party Conference.
Campbell, S. 1994. Being Dismissed: The Politics of Emotional Expression. *Hypatia* 9(3): 46–65.
Ecclestone, K., and D. Hayes. 2009. *The dangerous rise of therapeutic education*. London: Routledge.
Eckersley, R., W. Ani, and W. Johanna. 2006. Success and Well-being: A Preview of the Australia 21 Report on Young People's Well-being. *Youth Studies Australia* 25(1): 10.
Eckersley, R. 2011. A new narrative of young people's health and well-being. *Journal of Youth Studies* 14(5): 627–638.
European Commission, 2011. On EU indicators in the field of youth—Commission Staff Working Document [SEC(2011)401]. Available from: http://ec.europa.eu/youth/library/publications/indicator-dashboard_en.pdf Accessed 12 Nov 2015.
Furedi, F. 2004. *Therapy culture: Cultivating vulnerability in an uncertain age*. London: Routledge.
Furlong, A. 2013. *Youth studies: An introduction*. New York: Routledge.
Hochschild, A.R. 1983. *The managed heart: Commercialization of human feeling*. Berkeley: University of California Press.
Jeffrey, C. 2010. Geographies of children and youth I: eroding maps of life. *Progress in human geography* 34(4): 496–505.
Kelly, P. 2013. *The self as enterprise: Foucault and the spirit of 21st century capitalism*. Gower: Farnham.
Kelly, P., and A. Kamp. 2015. *A Critical Youth Studies for the 21st Century*. Brill: Leiden.
Kulz, C. 2013. 'Structure liberates?': Mixing for mobility and the cultural transformation of 'urban children' in a London academy. *Ethnic and Racial Studies* 37(4): 685–701.
Lorde, A. 1984. *Sister outsider: Essays and speeches*. Trumansburg: NY. Crossing Press.
Lyman, P. 1981. The Politics of Anger: On silence, ressentiment and political speech. *Socialist Review* 57: 55–74.
———. 2004. The Domestication of Anger: The Use and Abuse of Anger in Politics. *European Journal of Social Theory* 7(2): 133–147.

Nietzsche, F.W., W.A. Kaufmann, and R.J. Hollingdale. 1967. *The will to power.* New York: Random House.

Pimlott-Wilson, H. 2015. Individualising the future: The emotional geographies of neo-Liberal governance in young people's aspirations. *Area.* doi:10.1111/area.12222.

Sartre, J.-P. 1962. *Sketch for a theory of the emotions.* London: Methuen.

Sellar, S. 2014. A feel for numbers: Affect, data and education policy. *Critical Studies in Education* 56(1): 131–146.

Siivonen, P., and K. Brunila. 2013. The making of entrepreneurial subjectivity in adult education. *Studies in Continuing Education* 36(2): 160–172.

Sparks, H. 2014. Mama Grizzlies and Guardians of the Republic: The Democratic and Intersectional Politics of Anger in the Tea Party Movement. *New Political Science* 37(1): 25–47.

Staunæs, D. 2011. Governing the potentials of life itself? Interrogating the promises in affective educational leadership. *Journal of Educational Administration and History* 43(3): 227–247.

Telegraph.Co.UK. 2015. *Budget 2015: Full text of George Osborne's speech.* [online]. Available from: http://www.telegraph.co.uk/finance/budget/11480319/Budget-2015-Full-text-of-George-Osbornes-speech.html. Accessed 12 Nov 2015.

Wyn, J. 2007. Learning to 'become somebody well': Challenges for educational policy. *The Australian Educational Researcher* 34(3): 35–52.

Youthindex. 2015. *The Global Youth Well-being Index.* [online]. Available from: http://www.youthindex.org/. Accessed 12 Nov 2015.

5

Treading Water? The Roles and Possibilities of 'Adversity Capital' in Preparing Young People for Precarity

Lucas Walsh

Introduction

The impact of the Global Financial Crisis (GFC) of 2007–8 on young people, both seeking and in work was immediate and typically disproportionate to older age groups (OECD 2010). The impact of precarious work, and particularly unemployment, on young people's mental health and well-being is widely documented—including depression, loss of hope, isolation and financial insecurity, among others (Hillman and McMillan 2005). These impacts were sometimes ironically compounded and intensified by neo-Liberal economic and political responses to the GFC (Walsh 2016). For David Harvey (2005, p.2):

> Neoliberalism is in the first instance a theory of political economic practices that proposes that human well-being can best be advanced by

L. Walsh (✉)
Monash University, Melbourne, VIC, Australia

© The Editor(s) (if applicable) and The Author(s) 2017
P. Kelly, J. Pike (eds.), *Neoliberalism, Austerity, and the
Moral Economies of Young People's Health and Well-being*,
DOI 10.1057/978-1-137-58266-9_6

liberating individual entrepreneurial freedoms and skills within an institutional framework characterized by strong private property rights, free markets, and free trade.

In the moral economies of neo-Liberalism and austerity, young people in transition from school to work are entering both new and familiar territories. Well-trodden business mantras about skills shortages, wider orthodoxies around the value and purpose of education, and entrenched forms of inequality and marginalisation intersect and collide with recent social, economic and geographic impacts of the GFC and various policy responses to them. In a very profound way, these conditions are challenging a key assumption and promise that education and training will lead to a better life. One outcome of this is a need to develop critical responses to these conditions—both to critically analyse them and come up with practical responses.

Accompanying the challenges of workforce marginalisation are proposals in many OECD economies to reinforce and extend the development of the competencies, skills and dispositions to navigate changing worlds of work. As the challenges, concerns and lifestyles of young people have become enmeshed in the global so too, it is argued, there is a need to foster the literacies necessary for them to understand and participate in the contemporary fluid workforce. Serving as a kind of 'adversity capital', these skills and literacies enable young people to be more adaptive, flexible and resilient.

This discussion locates proposals to develop these literacies within a wider context of neo-Liberal policy responses to youth unemployment and precarity. It began with my efforts as an educator to grapple with conceptualising ways of enabling young people to navigate the material realities of contemporary working life, while theorising possibilities for resilience and critical responses to the pervasive effects and ideological dominance of what Harvey (2005) identifies as neo-Liberalism. Continuing this line of inquiry, this chapter explores the theoretical concept of 'adversity capital' as a basis for critically understanding the recent move from 'risk to resilience' (Rose 2014).

This form of capital also offers scope for resistance to responsibilisation, to challenge certain moral norms underpinning neo-Liberalism. As Sayer (2007, p. 261) suggests: 'Moral norms are not merely conventions, but embody assumptions about what well-being consists in, and these can be evaluated'. Adversity capital consequently builds on a notion of resilience that is located within a wider social ecology beyond young individuals, but which also sees them as agents of possible change. Using Sayer's approach to moral economy as critique, this chapter critically explores the conceptual and practical possibilities—and potential limitations—of adversity capital.

Old and New Features of Precarity

The impact of the GFC was both familiar and new. It was familiar in so far as economic recessions typically have an often immediate and lasting effect on young people seeking work, or in work. In Indonesia, Australia and Japan, for example, recessions of the 1990s were acutely felt by many young people (Vickers 2013). Accordingly, following the GFC, the Organisation for Economic Co-operation and Development (OECD) reported that negative effects of the GFC were disproportionately experienced by the young (OECD 2010). These effects manifest in a variety of forms including financial deprivation, insecurity, alienation and depression. At the extreme end are those young people who are not in employment, education or training (NEET). This number is growing throughout the world—in 2014, it was estimated to be over 35 million people aged 16–29 in OECD economies alone (OECD 2015).

But there is arguably something new about the broader effects of the GFC on young people that need to be understood in a wider context. Structural changes to both local and global economies over the last 30 years have meant that recent generations of young people enter worlds of work that are more fluid and often insecure. 'Precarity' has entered the wider lexicon describing the working and unemployed lives of young people. Though not a new term (see Chomsky 2011), it has greater salience within a global context in which young people in developed economies must make do with more casualised, contract-based and temporary work along with a diminished social safety net. In less developed economies, the nature of work is characterised by poor quality, informal and subsistence jobs (ILO 2013).

Career pathways for young people have also changed. Most notably, the notion of a lifelong career has been replaced by more fluid life trajectories featuring multiple employment pathways. Alongside the roll-back of welfare states and associated social safety nets, it is argued that in economies such as the USA there is less investment by employers in staff than there was 40 years ago. Staff deemed to be 'redundant' are replaced rather than 'up-skilled' or retrained (Cappelli 2012).

Many young people are forced to make do with less work (Walsh 2016). As persistent underemployment trends indicate, young people express a desire to work more but cannot because of labour force volatility and increasingly pervasive fluidity. Opportunities for full-time work among teenagers, for example, have steadily declined (Lamb and Mason 2008). Some of these young people are instead staying in school or taking up other forms of study or training. The level of school completion in Australia has recently reached an historic high (Robinson and Lamb 2012). But again, this promise of education for a better life is challenged by conditions to which we will return below.

A related disconnect is emerging in what commentators have referred to as 'credential inflation' (Ortleib 2015) where some employers are seeking increasingly higher qualifications from employees. A perverse outcome of this development is the emergence of the 'Dutch' or reverse auction, in which employers in Germany, for example, are advertising jobs in which candidates must demonstrate that they have higher levels of experience and qualifications and are willing to take less pay in highly competitive labour markets (Brown et al. 2011). The conventional promise that education will lead to the good life is increasingly challenged by the precarity experienced by young people in their working lives throughout the world.

A final disconnect arises from claims that young people do not have the appropriate work-ready skills that businesses claim they need. Surveys of business consistently identify a lack of suitable 'work-ready' skills in young people (Stanwick et al. 2013; Mourshed et al. 2012). Ironically, some businesses struggle to describe what their workforce will be like in the future (Walsh 2016). The changing nature of economies, such as the decline of manufacturing in Australia and technological disruption to certain professions, partly explain why this is the case.

Policy Responses: Aspirations and Hard Realities

Governments throughout the world turn to education and training as a means of preparing young people for work and to address entrenched problems of youth precarity. Returning to the Australian example, government targets to increase school completion have arguably peaked (Keating and Walsh 2009). Other strategies are consequently sought to address educational participation, such as focusing on changing levels of resources to disadvantaged students and redeveloping initial teacher education (see Gonski et al. 2011; DET 2015).

The importance to policy makers of responding to problems of precarity relates to the futurity associated with young people (Black and Walsh 2015). They embody hope, possibility and the future—and yet their treatment is not without tension. The wider policy discourse has been somewhat confused in the way it treats young people—particularly those who are seen to be 'at risk'. In Australia, these populations include those who leave school early, come from Indigenous backgrounds, live in regional and remote communities, and those with a disability (Lamb and Mason 2008).

But the calculation of those 'at risk' extends more widely beyond youth transition. Young people as the subjects of policy are often regarded as suspect *because they are young*. Contradictory messages are sent to young people about their role and place in society. In Europe, this has been referred to as the 'yo-yo-isation' of young people in which young people are compelled to live adult and young lives simultaneously (Walther et al. 2001).

Young people notice a related bind: for example, teenagers who must work and pay taxes as adults are paid less and denied the opportunity to vote for the representatives who legislate the conditions in which they must work and pay taxes (Warnock, cited in Walsh 2012). The value of their participation (in political and economic ways) is fraught with contradiction.

Compounding these contradictions inherent in the moral economies of youth participation is the demonisation of young people by governments. In 2010, the Conservative–Liberal Democrat coalition government in the

UK explicitly sought to promote 'strivers', not 'skivers' and 'scroungers' as part of its austerity drive (Jowit 2013). Even in Australia, where the effects of the GFC were far less pronounced, the conservative Liberal–National Party coalition government followed a similar pathway, announcing that Australia needed 'lifters, not leaners' (Hockey 2014). In both countries, these responses targeted the young through punitive measures such as work for the dole schemes, reductions to the social safety net, and a pervasive, suspicious and deficit view of young people (Walsh 2016).

Moral Economies of Youth Transitions

The concept of 'moral economies' provides a useful way of thinking about young people's well-being in the context of young people's transitions from school to work and/or further study and training after the GFC, and in consequent policy measures seeking austerity. Following Sayer (2005a, p. 1), the concept of 'moral economy' assists in analysing and understanding how young people's transitions 'are influenced and structured by moral dispositions, values and norms, and how in turn these are reinforced, shaped, compromised or overridden by economic pressures'. These norms, values, dispositions and commitments comprise 'what is just and what constitutes good behaviour in relation to others, and implies certain broader conceptions of the good or well-being' (Sayer 2005a, p. 1). Notions of transitions as economic practices and relationships, such as between young people and older members of economy and society, employers, policy makers and each other, are shaped by and embody internal and external moral values, ethical considerations, external obligations, rights and entitlements (Sayer 2005b; Sanghera and Satybaldieva 2009).

The moral economies of young people are shaped by tensions between their relationship to futurity on the one hand, and their location as individuals as part of 'the problem' that austerity measures seek to address, on the other. As Wyn (2015 p. 56) suggests, this focus 'tends to be one-sided because it focuses on individual youth at the expense of recognising societal and economic change'. This individualisation of youth policy transitions is a pathological by-product of neo-Liberalism, and one that has become normalised. Sayer (2007, p. 263) argues that once:

economic institutions and practices have become established, these normative questions tend to be forgotten, and a shift takes place from the normative to the normalised or naturalised. Indeed, legitimations of the arrangements may scarcely be needed.

Following on from above, young people find themselves caught between being viewed by policy makers as part of the problems of society writ large, and their own responsibilisation to get themselves out of precarity. Recent research into young people has found that they have largely come to accept that it is up to them as individuals to figure out how to negotiate insecure labour markets (Wyn and Cuervo 2014). Young people also find themselves at the interstices of youth and changing markers of adulthood. Returning to 'the metaphor of "yo-yo" transitions they face the "either-ors" and "neither-nors" of ... living adult and young lives simultaneously' (Stein et al. 2003, p. 6).

There are other tensions and ambivalences evident in the perspectives of young people themselves. The moral economies of young people also feature varying degrees of 'post-materialism', in which some people aspire to gain both interesting well-paid work that does not become the centre of life at the expense of other lifestyle choices. Comparisons of youth surveys in recent years suggest swings in attitudes between concern for the environment on the one hand (Robinson et al. 2010), and increasing the economy and financial matters on the other (Mission Australia 2012). As unemployment 'results in a lack of hope' (UNRIC 2012) at one extreme, increasing numbers of young people overall believe that their future prospects will be worse rather than better (Ipsos MORI 2014)—even in countries that are faring relatively well economically such as Sweden and Germany.

From Risk to Resilience

Sociologists such as Rose (2014) have noted a shift in how young people are both treated as objects of contemporary governance and understood more generally. Where young people have been previously (and continue to be) treated as both sources of risk and at-risk, there has been greater emphasis on developing resilience in young people. Resilience relates to young people's capacity to 'bounce back' in the face of adversity. This capacity ranges from coping with the financial deprivation associated with underemployment and unemployment ('underutilisation'), to developing work-ready skills and further education and training, as well as becoming more entrepreneurial in how they attempt to 'lift' themselves out of precarity. Given the disconnects between business expectations of what skills are required by young people to work, this third point is significant. Within the pervasive neo-Liberal frame of Australian and UK policy, young people are responsibilised to navigate their way out of adversity by becoming more resilient. The individualised nature of this responsibilisation is well documented and theorised (Kelly 2013).

Recently, however, sociologists such as Rose (2014) and Ungar (2013) have challenged this individualised notion of resilience. Recent research into resilience has found that its development occurs, and must therefore be understood, within a wider social ecology. Social support networks and peers play an important role in developing resilience. The development of resilience is grounded in other relations, such as family, through schooling and through socially responsible activity. To these last two relations, Rose (2014) highlights that 'compensating experiences outside of home' are important for a range of reasons, such as building self-esteem. The work of Ungar (2013, p.1) and others draws on research that

> has shown that the resilience of individuals growing up in challenging contexts or facing significant personal adversity is dependent on the quality of the social and physical ecologies that surround them, as much, and likely far more, than personality traits, cognitions or talents.

Rose (2014) raises another important point: neo-Liberalism is not totalising as the framing prism through which policy responses are viewed and young subjectivities are located. There are other spaces, moments and factors in building resilience. It is argued that because resilience has no single form of logic, the 'polyvalence of resilient strategies' resists the simple reduction of resilience to the individuated notion underpinning neo-Liberalism (Rose 2014). Ungar (2013, p.1) suggests that the problem with this individualistic view of resilience is partially the result of a dominant view of resilience as something individuals have, rather than as a process that families, schools, communities and governments facilitate. Because resilience is related to the presence of social risk factors (we can only speak of resilience in the presence of at least one stressor), there is a need for an ecological interpretation of the construct that acknowledges the importance of people's interaction with their environments.

Building Adversity Capital

It is in this context that it becomes possible to articulate the concept of adversity capital as a basis for conceptualising a response to precarity. The fluidity of contemporary working life requires young people to 'become skilled at navigating a sea of uncertainty' (Wyn 2009, p. iii) and harness the necessary skills and competencies to interact with and potentially shape their environments. In a fluid and uncertain global economy, the need for soft skills has renewed significance.

Setting aside the problematic nature of the 'mismatch between skills and jobs', there is a renewed interest in developing foundation and soft skills in young people. The term 'soft skills' is confusing as it is used interchangeably with labels such as 'non-cognitive skills' and 'competencies' (Kahn et al. 2012, p. 8), 'generic and basic skills' (Roberts and Wignall 2010, p. 1), as well as '21st-century skills' and competencies to reflect

> the needs of the emerging models of economic and social development [rather] than with those of the past century, which were suited to an industrial mode of production. (Ananiadou and Claro 2008, p. 5)

These skills include social intelligence, emotional resilience (Roberts 2009), problem solving, oracy, self-discipline (IYF 2013), critical thinking, communication, creativity, information literacy, global awareness, and financial, cross-cultural and environmental (or ecological) literacies (Partnership for 21st Century Skills 2009; Hannon et al. 2011; Zhao 2009). More than just educational buzzwords, these skills and literacies have tangible properties through which young people can fluently comprehend and express themselves (Hannon et al. 2011). Soft skills feature in education and training systems throughout the world either implicitly or explicitly, but the argument here is to widen and conceptualise them in a more sophisticated way as key components of adversity capital.

Pavlidis (2009) proposes the idea of adversity capital in other domains of young people's lives, and this concept, reconstructed, may be applied to the context of labour force precarity. In her use of the term, Pavlidis (2009, p.9) writes that

> an individual's ability to negotiate risk depends on their ability to distance risk from themselves and their body—to overcome or negotiate the structures of society—and depends on their reflexive capacity.

The development of soft skills proposed here explicitly seeks to build this reflexive capacity. In addition to this, and following on from my discussion of resilience, adversity capital as a basis for responding to precarity requires consideration of the wider social ecologies in which young people live and develop. It consists of the collection of social and reflexive capacities to negotiate contemporary worlds of work.

As I have previously proposed, 'adversity capital' is a deliberately loaded concept (Walsh 2016). It firstly suggests that in an increasingly fluid and uncertain workforce, young people need to develop capabilities and dispositions to be economically mobile. The concept, secondly, includes the ability for young people to critically navigate different cultural, mediated and non-mediated contexts. Not only

> will these skills help young people get a job; it describes them as subjects potentially confronting a life of vulnerability and precarity. It is a form of capital that can be productive of other forms of capital upon which young people can critically confront and navigate precarity and potentially build a better life. (Walsh 2016, p. 90)

Adversity capital includes the capacity to navigate a changing workforce and critically engage the related contexts, practices and values of work, to challenge wider norms related to working life and life in general. This includes the knowledge and ability to question dominant discourses such as neo-Liberalism. But this concept of adversity capital is, arguably, problematic in at least three ways.

Firstly, the concept of adversity capital presented in this chapter relies in part on an instrumental view based on the metaphor of capital adopted by Bourdieu (see Bourdieu 1986). Sayer (2005b) is rightly critical of Bourdieu's use of the economic metaphor of capital and the orientation of his analyses towards structural explanations (although there are structural characteristics to the challenges faced by young people in transition, such as their location and socio-economic status). And, following Sayer, where the need for adversity capital is driven by a desire to accumulate capital, it needs to be understood in a wider context. But, as we shall see below, international surveys suggest that young people as social actors seek more from life than just work, and hold post-material values within their moral outlooks. This is why adversity capital contains both instrumental (Bourdieu) and critical dimensions drawing on young people's reflexivity as agents. Beyond Bourdieu, and consistent with Sayer, class-based dimensions of inequality remain important. Given the relationship of socio-economic status to transitions outcomes, class is salient in reconfigured ways. Standing (2012, p.590) evokes the notion of the precariat to refer to the emergence in Britain of groups of people characterised by

> casual, short-term, or temporary jobs, [with] none of the forms of labor security that the working class and the salariat acquired in the welfare-state era, and have relatively low and insecure earnings.

Secondly, discussions around soft skills need to be understood within a wider reorientation of the relationship between education and the workforce towards 'the knowledge society', which has been met with caution on the basis that they risk reducing education to a narrow vocationalism in lieu of other forms of lifelong learning (Andres and Wyn 2010). These soft skills include the ability to critique forces of domination and precarity, to understand the historical and contingent nature of these as a relatively recent development, and to realise that they are not as totalising as the neo-Liberal outlook seems to be. The concept of adversity capital presented here only seeks to address part of the concerns and challenges faced by young people after the GFC, and relies on other support mechanisms within the social ecology (e.g. an adequate social safety net).

A third danger here is that developing these skills reinforces the individualised, responsibilised subjectivities fostered by neo-Liberalism. The development of these skills as a form of adversity capital may be seen to reflect a shift in focus in education towards developing the 'entrepreneurial self', in which subjectivity is characterised by responsibility, reflexivity and individual self-management (Kelly 2013). Routinely included under the umbrella of soft skills are enterprise and self-discipline. A problematic aspect of adversity capital is that preparing young people to navigate seas of uncertainty reinforces responsibilised and individualised notions of young people's transitions from education and training to work. Indeed, much of the discourse around soft skills valorises self-discipline and entrepreneurialism that are normatively linked to neo-Liberalism. Consequently, developing these soft skills needs to be located within a wider social ecology in which resilience is developed and harnessed, and which connects these individualised dimensions to wider social frames of reference.

The concept of adversity capital proposed in this chapter is perhaps best understood within a political economy of youth that challenges the assumptions, values and impacts of neo-Liberalism. Sayer (2007, p.268) proposes a critical moral or political economy that

> turns questions of economic behaviour back into questions of validity, by asking not only what happens but on the basis of what kinds of legitimation, and it assesses those legitimations.

Developing adversity capital includes developing a '"critical emancipatory" position that helps those who might be accepting their exploitation as "normal" to see how they can overcome their false consciousness', and to enable them to critique 'free-market logics as the root of many social problems and seeking radical alternatives to correct capitalism's dehumanising tendencies' (Côté 2013, p. 3).

Conclusion

Many governments around the world base their youth transition policies on the assumption that sufficient levels of education and training will lead to a better, secure life, and consequently have targeted school completion as a major policy objective. It has increased the mobility of young people, such as those who move to urban areas and cities, to undertake study and training. But as Wyn (2015) suggests, policy has also intensified inequalities between those who have access to the economic and social resources to move to where the study opportunities exist, and those who do not. Wyn (2015, p. 54) also highlights how transitions regimes shape the life courses of young people through

> the institutional process, practices and discourses of education systems, labour markets and welfare systems that shape the meaning and experience of youth through the implementation of standard institutional transition points and statuses, such as the completion of secondary education or the entry into full-time employment.

Other conventional markers are changing, such as if and when young people purchase their home or start a family (Woodman 2012). In the context of ageing populations throughout the developed world, a question emerges as to the social, political and economic inheritance of young people today, and whether this inheritance includes a better world. In the context of the UK, Howker and Malik (2010) suggest the emergence of an 'age apartheid' or demographic discrimination favouring older groups of people at the expense of the young. This discrimination arises from a decline in the benefits enjoyed by the post-world war generation, such as affordable housing, secure employment, free tertiary education and a welfare safety net. Broader politics has shifted towards attempting to meet the satisfaction of short-term goals and the false empowerment of individuals (Howker and Malik 2010). In part, they argue that a focus on individual rights and self-expression has drawn the focus away from 'social inheritance', which 'has led us to assume that doing the best for ourselves will always be best for others, [which] is demonstrably untrue' (Howker and Malik 2010, p.202).

The distortion and possible rupturing of these transitions regimes has immediate and significant implications for the moral economies of young people. On the one hand, there is the intensification and 'credential inflation' of qualifications as labour markets become more competitive and precarious. On the other, there are sociological changes to the nature and markers of youth and meanings of adulthood that lie beyond 'youth'.

The tensions arising from this shifting terrain suggest a possibility and necessity to rethink the moral economies of young people and how policy makers, organisations and people such as educators can respond.

Perhaps, above all else, in the starkest of instrumental terms, education, training and soft skills do not matter much if *desirable* jobs, or at the very least, paid work, are not available. Andreas and Wyn (2010) have found that the types of qualifications held by young people are only tangentially related to the jobs they attain post-education and training. And for those that are out of work, or seeking more work, or finding themselves somewhere between unemployment and employment (Furlong 2007), adversity capital may only provide a basis for treading water on the wider seas of uncertainty described by Wyn (2009) and Bauman (2000).

Adversity capital only provides a starting point for responding to the challenges facing young people in the labour market. It aims to be both a conceptual and practical 'tool box' of resources from which young people can draw to navigate the fluidity of modern life. But it also includes the capacity to actively critique forces of domination and precarity under the ideological veil of 'flexibility' and 'enterprise'. Returning to Harvey's (2005) definition at the start of this chapter, the concept of adversity capital seeks to respond to the effects of neo-Liberal policies and practices by providing a basis for young people to navigate fluid labour markets while promoting a deeper, critical emancipatory approach that resists the belief

> that human well-being can best be advanced by liberating individual entrepreneurial freedoms and skills within an institutional framework characterized by strong private property rights, free markets, and free trade. (Harvey 2005, p. 2)

But, again, it is only a starting point. A wider set of conditions and support mechanisms to nourish the social ecologies around young people must be fostered in concert with these skills and competencies to have meaningful effect. This includes a continuing role for the state, rights and community-based responses deeply rooted in notions of social justice that seek to promote the common good beyond economistic, individualised ways of knowing and being.

References

Ananiadou, K., and M. Claro. 2008. 21st Century Skills and Competences for New Millennium Learners in OECD Countries. *OECD Education Working Papers No. 41.* Paris: OECD Publishing. [online]. Available from: http://www.oecd.org/officialdocuments/publicdisplaydocumentpdf/?cote=EDU/WKP(2009)20&doclanguage=en. Accessed 24 May 2015.

Andres, L., and J. Wyn. 2010. *The Making Of A Generation: The Children of The 1970s In Adulthood.* Toronto: University of Toronto Press.

Bauman, Z. 2000. *Globalization: The Human Consequences.* New York: Columbia University Press.

Black, R., and L. Walsh. 2015. Educating the Risky Citizen: Young People, Vulnerability and Schooling. In *Interrogating conceptions of 'vulnerable youth' in theory, policy and practice,* eds. K. Te Riele and G. Radka. Netherlands: Sense.

Bourdieu, P. 1986. The forms of capital. In *Handbook of Theory and Research for the Sociology of Education,* ed. J. Richardson, 241–258. New York: Greenwood.

Brown, P., H. Lauder, and D. Ashton. 2011. *The Global Auction: The Broken Promises of Education, Jobs, and Incomes.* USA: Oxford University Press.

Cappelli, P. 2012. *Why Good People Can't Get Jobs: The Skills Gap and What Companies Can Do About It.* Philadelphia: Wharton Digital Press.

Chomsky, N. 2011. The 'Great Moderation' and the International Assault on Labor. *In These Times,* May 2. [online]. Available from: http://inthesetimes.com/article/7264/the_great_moderation_and_the_international_assault_on_labor. Accessed 24 Aug 2015.

Côté, J.E. 2013. Towards a new political economy of youth. *Journal of Youth Studies* 17(4): 527–543.

DET (Australian Government Department of Education and Training). 2015. *Teacher Education Ministerial Advisory Group: Action Now: Classroom Ready Teachers. February 2015. Australian Government Response.* Canberra: Australian Government.

Furlong, A. 2007. The zone of precarity and discourses of vulnerability: NEET in the UK. *The Journal of Social Sciences and Humanities* 381: 101–121.

Gonski, D., K. Boston, K. Greiner, C. Lawrence, B. Scales, and P. Tannock. 2011. *Review of Funding for Schooling. Final Report. December 2011.* Canberra: Department of Education, Employment and Workplace Relations.

Hannon, V., A. Patton, and J. Temperley. 2011. Developing an Innovation Ecosystem for Education. Cisco White Paper December 2011. [online].

Available from: http://www.cisco.com/web/strategy/docs/education/ecosystem_for_edu.pdf. Accessed 2 June 2014.

Harvey, D. 2005. *A Brief History of Neoliberalism*. Oxford: Oxford University Press.

Hillman, K., and J. Mcmillan. 2005. *Life Satisfaction of Young Australians: Relationships between further education, training and employment and general and career satisfaction*. Victoria: Australian Council for Educational Research.

Hockey, J. 2014. Joe Hockey: We are a nation of lifters, not leaners. *The Australian Financial Review*, May 14. [online]. Available from: http://www.afr.com/news/policy/tax/joe-hockey-we-are-a-nation-of-lifters-not-leaners-20140513-ituma. Accessed 14 Sept 2014.

Howker, E., and S. Malik. 2010. *Jilted Generation: How Britain Has Bankrupted Its Youth*. London: Icon Books.

ILO (International Labour Organisation). 2013. *Global Employment Trends for Youth 2013: A Generation at Risk*. Geneva: International Labour Office.

IPSOS MORI. 2014. Ipsos MORI Global Trends Survey. 14 April 2014. [online]. Available from: https://www.ipsos-mori.com/researchpublications/researcharchive/3369/People-in-western-countries-pessimistic-about-future-for-young-people.aspx#gallery[m]/0/. Accessed 30 Jan 2014.

IYF (International Youth Foundation). 2013. Getting Youth in the Door: Defining Soft Skills Requirements for Entry-level Service Sector Jobs. [online]. Available from: http://library.iyfnet.org/library/getting-youth-door-defining-soft-skills-requirements-entry-level-service-sector-jobs. Accessed 1 May 2015.

Jowit, J. 2013. Strivers v shirkers: the language of the welfare debate. *The Guardian*, January 9. [online]. Available from: http://www.theguardian.com/politics/2013/jan/08/strivers-shirkers-language-welfare. Accessed 14 Sept 2015.

Kahn, L., B. Mcneil, R. Patrick, V. Sellick, K. Thompson, and L. Walsh. 2012. *Developing skills for life and work: Accelerating social and emotional learning across South Australia*. London: Young Foundation.

Keating, J, and L. Walsh 2009. *Submission by The Foundation for Young Australians to the House of Representatives Standing Committee on Education and Training Combining School and Work: Supporting Successful Youth Transitions*, Submission 26, 16 January 2009.

Kelly, P. 2013. *The Self As Enterprise: Foucault and the Spirit of 21st Century Capitalism*. Surrey: Gower Publishing.

Lamb, S., and K. Mason. 2008. *How Young People Are Faring 2008*. Melbourne: The Foundation for Young Australians.

Mission Australia. 2012. *Mission Australia Youth Survey—2012*. Sydney: Mission Australia.

Mourshed, M., D. Farrell, and D. Barton. 2012. *Education to Employment: Designing a System that Works*. US: McKinsey Center for Government.

OECD (Organisation for Economic Co-operation and Development). 2010. *Off to a Good Start? Jobs for Youth*. Paris: OECD [online]. Available from: http://www.oecd.org/els/emp/46717876.pdf. Accessed 1 May 2015.

———. 2015. *OECD Skills Outlook 2015: Youth, Skills and Employability*. Paris: OECD Publishing. doi:10.1787/9789264234178-en.

Ortlieb, E. 2015. Just graduating from university is no longer enough to get a job. *The Conversation*, Feburary 12. [online]. Available from: http://theconversation.com/just-graduating-from-university-is-no-longer-enough-to-get-a-job-36906. Accessed 16 Feb 2015.

Partnership for 21st Century Skills. 2009. *P21 Framework Definitions*. Washington, DC: P21. [online]. Available from: http://www.p21.org/storage/documents/P21_Framework_Definitions.pdf. Accessed 25 May 2015.

Pavlidis, A. 2009. The diverse logics of risk: young people's negotiations of the risk society. *The Future of Sociology*. The Australian National University, 1–4 December 2009 Canberra.

Roberts, Y. 2009. *Grit: The Skills for Success and How They are Grown*. London: The Young Foundation.

Roberts, A., and L. Wignall 2010. *Briefing on Foundation Skills for the National VET Equity Advisory Council* (NVEAC). [online]. Available from: http://www.nveac.natese.gov.au/__data/assets/pdf_file/0008/56348/Briefing_on_Foundation_Skills_-_Roberts_and_Wignall.pdf. Accessed 18 Aug 2014.

Robinson, L., and S. Lamb. 2012. *How Young People Are Faring 2012*. Melbourne: The Foundation for Young Australians.

Robinson, L., S. Lamb, and A. Walstab. 2010. *How Young People are Faring 2010*. Melbourne: The Foundation for Young Australians.

Rose, N. 2014. *From Risk to Resilience: Responsible citizens for uncertain times*. Public Lecture, 28 August 2014, Ian Potter Auditorium, Kenneth Myer Building, Royal Parade, Parkville, Australia.

Sanghera, B., and E. Satybaldieva. 2009. Moral sentiments and economic practices in Kyrgyzstan: The internal embeddedness of a moral economy. *Cambridge Journal of Economics* 33: 921–935.

Sayer, A. 2005a. Agendas for Moral Economy, paper presented at Perspectives on Moral Economy: An International Conference, 25–27 August, Lancaster, UK, [online]. Available from: http://www.lancaster.ac.uk/fass/doc_library/

sociology/moraleconomyabstracts/Perspectives_on_Moral_Economy.doc. Accessed 28 Sept 2015.

———. 2005b. *The Moral Significance of Class*. Cambridge: Cambridge University Press.

———. 2007. Moral Economy as Critique. *New Political Economy* 12(2): 261–270. doi:10.1080/13563460701303008.

Standing, G. 2012. The Precariat: From Denizens to Citizens? *Polity* 44(4): 588–608.

Stanwick, J., T. Lu, T. Karmel, and B. Wibrow. 2013. *How Young People are Faring 2013*. Melbourne: The Foundation for Young Australians.

Stein, T.G., B. Stauber, and A. Walther. 2003. Misleading Trajectories? An Evaluation of the Unintended Effects of Labour Market Integration Policies for Young Adults in Europe. Institut fuer regionale Innovation und Sozialforschung. [online]. Available from: http://cordis.europa.eu/documents/documentlibrary/70601461EN6.pdf. Accessed 18 Aug 2014.

Ungar, M. 2013. Introduction to the Volume. In *The Social Ecology of Resilience: A Handbook of Theory and Practice*, ed. M. Ungar, 1–12. New York, London: Springer.

UNRIC (United Nations Regional Information Centre for Western Europe). 2012. Youth: the hardest hit by the global financial crisis. [online]. Available from: http://www.unric.org/en/youth-unemployment/27414-youth-the-hardest-hit-by-the-global-financial-crisis. Accessed 29 Jan 2015.

Vickers, M. 2013. Youth Transitions. In *Education Change and Society*, ed. R. Connell, 32–54. Melbourne: Oxford University Press.

Walsh, L. 2012. More mixed messages about youth participation. *Youth Studies Australia* 31(2): 3–4.

———. 2016. *Educating Generation Next: Young People, Teachers and Schooling in Transition*. Basingstoke: Palgrave Macmillan.

Walther, A., B. Stauber, A. Biggart, M.D. Bois-Reymond, A. Furlong, A. López Blasco, A. Mørch, and J.M. Pias. 2001. *Misleading Trajectories—Integration Policies for Young Adults in Europe?* Hechingen/Tübingen: Institute for Regional Innovation and Social Research.

Woodman, D. 2012. Life out of Synch: How New Patterns of Further Education and the Rise of Precarious Employment Are Reshaping Young People's Relationships. *Sociology* 46(6): 1074–1090.

Wyn, J. 2009. *Touching the Future: Building skills for life and work*. Melbourne: Australian Council for Educational Research.

———. 2015. Youth Policy and the Problematic Nexus Between Education and Employment. In *Interrogating conceptions of 'vulnerable youth' in theory, policy and practice*, eds. K. Te Riele and G. Radka. Netherlands: Sense.

Wyn, J., and H. Cuervo 2014. Pain Now, Rewards Later? Young Lives Cannot be Relived. *The Conversation*, June 16. [online]. Available from: https://the-conversation.com/pain-now-rewards-later-young-lives-cannot-be-relived-27376. Accessed 18 Aug 2014.

Zhao, Y. 2009. *Catching Up or Leading the Way: American Education in the Age of Globalization*. Alexandria, VA: Association for Supervision & Curriculum Development.

Part II

Young People, Austerity and the Moral Geographies of Disadvantage

6

Young People of the 'Austere Period': Mechanisms and Effects of Inequality over Time in Portugal

Magda Nico and Nuno de Almeida Alves

Introduction

At least since the *Children of the Great Recession* (Elder 1974), the long-term negative effects of deprivation, poverty, insecurity, and an abrupt and sharp decline in well-being in childhood or early adulthood have been documented and acknowledged. But it is also important to remember that the context of the times, along with geographical and political variations, is highly relevant to any understanding of these effects. This notion provides one of the theoretical premises of our chapter. The life course research principle of the importance of cultural and historical location to the examination of young people's lives is particularly important to the Portuguese context. Due to its peripheral positioning—both geographical and social—and the current post-Global Financial Crisis (GFC) context of what could be considered the blunt force of austerity,

M. Nico (✉) • N. de Almeida Alves
University Institute of Lisbon, Lisbon, Portugal

© The Editor(s) (if applicable) and The Author(s) 2017
P. Kelly, J. Pike (eds.), *Neoliberalism, Austerity, and the Moral Economies of Young People's Health and Well-being*,
DOI 10.1057/978-1-137-58266-9_7

Portugal constitutes a rich observatory for an understanding of how transitions to adulthood, especially school-to-work transitions, operate amid socially stratified dynamics. It is to be noted, in particular, that life courses are both incorporated into and formed by the historical times and places in which they are lived and experienced (Elder et al. 2002, pp. 11–14). This is even more so in the case of children and young people, whose options are limited, both objectively and subjectively, from an early 'start'. A period of crisis such as that precipitated by the 2008–2009 GFC illustrates, in this sense, the inescapable 'historicality of the individual' (Abbott 2005).

A second important premise in this chapter relates to what can be termed the 'accumulation of inequalities' (O'Rand 2009; Dannefer 2002). This is evident at two levels. The first lies within the national 'cultural and historical location', not necessarily having in mind exceptional or transitory historical moments. Although Portugal has had its post-1974 democratic transition well recognised in academic and public arenas, as well as the massification of higher education and the increase of middle classes, the relative positioning of Portugal in Europe is not as confident. For instance, even before the crisis, Portugal was clustered by youth researchers in a 'sub-protective regime', characterised by a non-selective school system, training systems with low average standards and coverage, and a closed, segmented and informal employment regime (Walther 2006). Portugal stood out in European Statistics with the highest ages of young people still living with their parents, atypical and precarious links to the labour market, increasing age at first child and decreasing number of children. The second level is the social location of each individual, in the sense that socio-demographic and educational variables accumulate, overlap and/or interact with each other over time in such a way that they determine the timing, the sequence and most importantly the 'success' of life courses and projects. We can illustrate these two layers of inequalities in relation to Portugal in the European context in Fig. 6.1.

In this chapter, we want to demonstrate the different mechanisms operated by these layers. The historical and cultural location has a direct and causal relationship with inequalities where the welfare, structural and economic Portuguese conditions determine to a high degree the amplitude and 'success of young people's life expectations and trajectories'. At

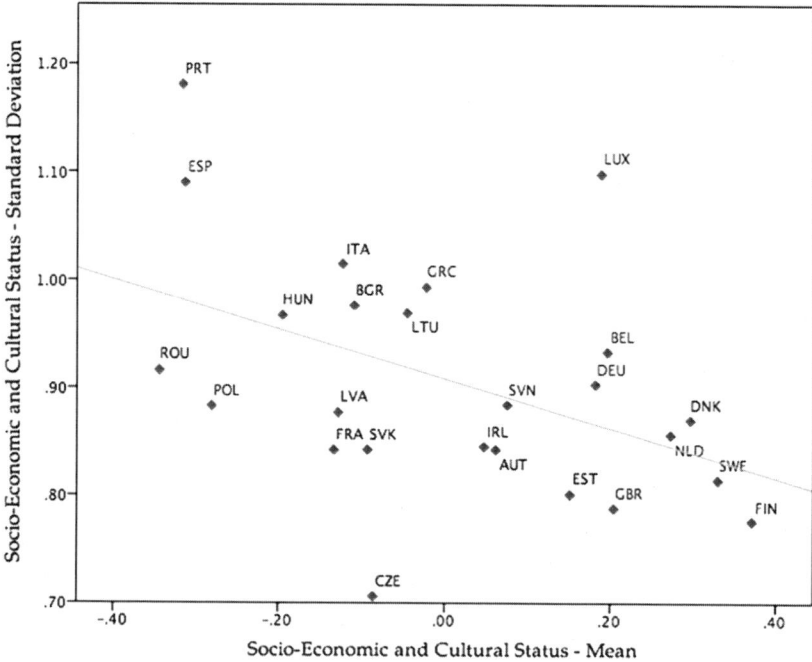

Fig. 6.1 Average and Standard Deviation of Social–Economic and Cultural Status in Europe (2009)

the same time socio-economic variables should be tackled in an interdependent and holistic approach. While statistics provide an overall understanding of the country in question, they do not provide a comprehensive picture of the extent and multiple effects of precarious labour in the current market, nor their influence on contemporary young people's lives. This is, in a way, our third premise: that the array of research chosen to 'put flesh on the bones' of our argument would have had to be necessarily qualitative. To describe and understand the effects and mechanisms of living with and through a difficult economic period and historic landmark such as the current dyad of crisis/austerity, it is crucial to draw on qualitative data that is capable of giving real, messy, complicated and intricate lives the analytical dignity they deserve.

The projects whose results we draw on here were carried out separately, with their 'distinctive strengths and potential', but our intent in this discussion is to mix the results and conclusions in a 'multidimensional logic' (Mason 2006: 9). One set of material to be discussed here is based on research into transitions to adulthood in Portugal and in Europe as a whole, from a life course perspective (Nico 2011, 2014a, b, 2015). The qualitative component of this research was vulnerable to the vagaries of the historical moment of the data collection, and thus 'blessed' with serendipity. Biographical and life calendar material was collected using a holistic and interdependent approach and included educational, sentimental, work and housing trajectories, among other turning points. As such, 52 life-grid interviews were carried out in a diversified group of 26- to 32-year-olds. The interviews were subjected to holistic form and content analysis. Another set of qualitative data included 80 semi-directive interviews with young people with precarious jobs in Portugal and covered the different modalities of precarious employment in Portugal (Alves et al. 2011; Carmo et al. 2014). This research covered several implications of this condition for the life courses of young people in Portugal, such as current and previous jobs, wages and life circumstances, housing arrangements, family prospects and conceptions of the future.

Recession and Austerity: Portugal and Its Historical Antecedents

During the twentieth century, Portugal has managed to add a political element to the geographical periphery in Europe. Throughout three quarters of the last century, Portugal was able to maintain its five centuries-long empire and escape almost untouched the devastating consequences of two European abased world wars. However, this century was not a politically and economically easy one for Portugal: the monarchic regime was overthrown in 1910 by a republican revolution which was later deposed by a military coup (1926) that produced a 48-year-long dictatorship, led by António de Oliveira Salazar. On 25 April 1974, the regime was overthrown by a military coup commanded by junior officers of the Portuguese Army, tired of a 13-year-long colonial war fought simultaneously in Angola, Mozambique and Guinea-Bissau. 'Empire' has always had a significant influence in the political and economic management of the country. The colonies were the most significant economic partners of the Metropolis and allowed the maintenance of a close interdependence between the dictatorship's most prominent dignitaries, the army's structure and the most notable/successful Portuguese entrepreneurs whose economic success was based on economic protectionism, absence of foreign competition and a tamed labour force with few political or social rights. The dictatorship envisaged Portugal as a rural country, with an economy based on agriculture and limited industrial development. For this limited economic market, the primary education of the (male) population was considered more than enough. This negligence in respect to education has left profound structural effects that last until today: 56 % of the working-age (15–64) population has less than 9 years of schooling (79 % in 2000) (Eurostat, Labour Force Survey (LFS), 2000; 2014).

After the revolution and following a short period of political unrest, the country was finally able to build a constitutional democracy based on the rule of law. However, from an economic and social perspective, Portugal was decades behind many European counterparts: the foundations of a welfare state needed to be built alongside the restructuring of economic production and the progressive raising of the standards of living of the mass of the population. The budgetary consequences of this process soon became apparent: the debt raised by this economic and social restructuration process caused two interventions of the International Monetary Fund (IMF [1977 and 1983]) followed by the austerity plans attached to it. In 1986, Portugal joined the European Economic Community. This was a crucial step for its further development on the infrastructural, economic and social fronts. This path of multidimensional development lasted until the country's inclusion in the European currency (Euro) in 2002. This adoption of the Euro led to a long economic stagnation due to the lack of competitiveness and low productivity of the Portuguese economy within a single currency market (Fig. 6.2).

The articulation of these factors with a long period of easy access to credit by public and private partners (including families) contributed to an economy highly levered on credit, compensated by annual public budgetary deficits. Such economic and financial conditions almost brought the country to a financial collapse in 2011, enforcing a third intervention of the IMF accompanied by fierce austerity measures in the form of

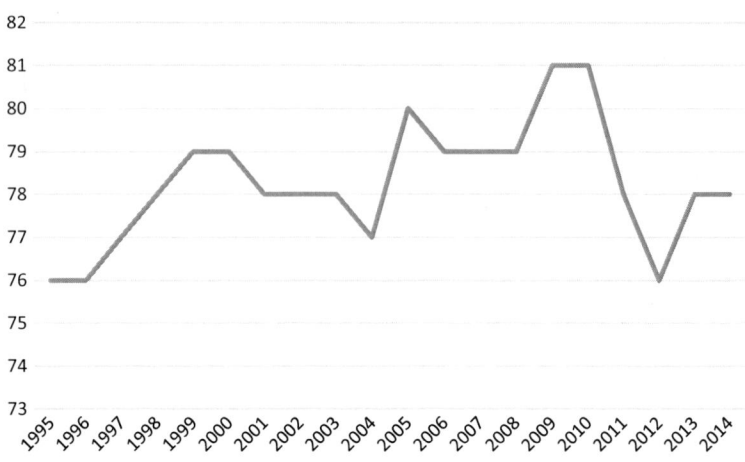

Fig. 6.2 GDP per capita in Portugal 1995–2014 (EU28 = 100)

budget cuts in welfare state provisions, reduction of wages and pensions, and rises in income and consumption taxes. Such fiscal conditions drove the country to a very significant rise in unemployment and a general degradation of employment. Young people were more seriously affected by this problem than older workers.

Young people are registered as unemployed at double the rates of their older counterparts—34 % of young people between 15 and 24, and 25 % of young people between 15 and 29 against 15 % for the general population in 2014 (Eurostat, LFS). Temporary employment affects more than twice as many young people as older workers—39 % of young people between 15 and 24, and 35 % of young people between 15 and 29, against 15 % for the general population in 2014 (Eurostat, LFS).

Is 'Precarious Well-being' a Contradiction in Terms?

We want to suggest in this section that there are three main messages to take home from the lives lived and stories told in the projects we discussed in the Introduction. These messages come from a starting point that precariousness, combined with a heavily informal labour market to begin with, and now affected by a financial crisis and the austerity measures taken on its behalf, is the predominant factor for determining low well-being during youth and early adulthood. One is that precariousness is a process, it is not a temporary event in one's life but it has longitudinal and long-term effects. Two, precariousness affects all social strata but is in itself a socially stratified phenomenon. Three, these effects are multiple not only across time but also across spheres of life.

Although not an entirely new phenomenon in Western societies, the precarious employment of the present day contrasts sharply with the standard employment structure of twentieth-century liberal democracies, capitalist economies and welfare societies. It signals the slow but steady dissolution of the balances achieved with the structuring of these three pillars in the decades following the Second World War. In broad strokes, precarious work refers to any atypical form of employment; this interpretation covers and extends to issues related to work, wages or entitlements. One of the most complete definitions of the situation is that formulated by Vosko (2010, p.2):

> I define precarious employment as work for remuneration characterized by uncertainty, low income and limited social benefits and statutory entitlements. Precarious employment is shaped by the relationship between *employment status* (i.e. self- or paid employment), *form of employment* (e.g. temporary or permanent, part-time or full-time) and *dimensions of labour market insecurity*.

This complex definition contributes to the lack of a regular and systematic set of indicators on precarious employment. Rather, it is usually statistically expressed by *proxies* such as the level of temporary employment and/or part-time employment and/or other employment situations. Due to these operational difficulties, precarious work is most frequently approached by means of qualitative studies (Molé 2010; Alves et al. 2011; Spyridakis 2013), contrary to studies that tend to measure the effect of a certain historical landmark as the current crisis.

Precariousness Is a Process with Long-term Effects

Precariousness usually starts early in young people's lives. Typically, it comes with the first attempts to find a job, irrespective of young people's professional or educational background. For people with a secondary education who want to enter the labour market, for those who seek a part-time job to pay for tertiary education and even for university graduates aiming to start on a professional career, a precarious position is generally the first experience of the labour market, and often of the subsequent offers obtained. But the current duration and repetition of precarious work in contexts of austerity and its widening to all educational strata give it a much more profound, longitudinal and structural character. Almost all our interviewees had been engaged in these non-standard labour relations, generally alternating precarious work with periods of unemployment, training or internship. All the examples below demonstrate this situation well, from Sara with informal earnings that barely hold her residential autonomy together, to Tatiana who is being 'held hostage' to a non-meritocratic and unregulated labour market, and Joana who is trying to compensate for lack of qualifications with a willingness to have three precarious and part-time jobs.

Living on the Edge

> Sara comes from a working class environment and has always been encouraged to help in the family business, gain her independence gradually and adapt to what the labour market had to offer (as a domestic worker, a waitress, etc.). These different involvements with the labour market and with the conquest of financial independence were an intermittent reality in Sara's life. At the same time she was encouraged by her family to invest in a higher education. So she did. When she finished her degree, she decided it was time to leave the parental home, regardless of the lack of stability of her job at the time, or the fact it had little to do with her degree course. This decision to leave home has prevented her ever since from being more daring in her professional career, because she just cannot afford to lose her job. She depends solely on her earnings, not because of her family's unwillingness to help financially, if necessary, but due to the work ethic shared by her whole family. Moreover, because her work in a shoe shop was supposed to be temporary, she has no contract, nor is she registered in the social security system. She has no social recognition for her financial-and housing-related autonomy.

Held Hostage to a Senseless Mobility

Tatiana is 24, and a social work graduate who is currently finishing her master's degree. She still lives with her parents, a working class couple from Oporto. She works as a social worker for a charity, the employer with which she started her professional career with a state-sponsored internship. But this internship ended and she was offered a part-time job as a self-employed worker, with the same workload but half the previous wage. With nothing else on offer and no entitlement to unemployment benefit, she accepted, despite the consequence of having to shrink her contribution to the family's expenses. Fortunately, or evidently, she has no immediate plans to live alone.

Stuck in an Semi-autonomy

Joana is 33, lives in Porto and comes from a working class family. She left school without completing the 10th grade. She lives alone during part of the week and the other with her parents because she feels that they need her assistance. She is a part-timer in a supermarket, but also works two days a week in a cosmetics store and is a filing worker for another company in the weekends. She has a tenured job in the supermarket and is self-employed in the other activities. With these three jobs she earns almost 600 euros per month after taxes. An amount that she divides between her own expenses (rent, utilities, transportation and food), and the goods she provides to her parents' household. Joana maintains a kind of assisted autonomy. She does some of the shopping for her parents in exchange for some meals and laundry services in the nights she stays at her parents. Joana doesn't think about the future. She has a boyfriend but has no plans to have a family. She is not happy with her currant accumulation of part-time jobs but she is afraid of losing any of them.

Precariousness as a Socially Stratified Phenomena

Precariousness is widespread and heavily stratified from a social point of view. It is age-specific, in the sense that young people all over Europe are especially vulnerable to it. Although it is also a country-specific phenomenon in the sense that the reasons for the fragile links with the labour market are very different between countries. Age and the national context interact to produce a precarious 'starting point' for young people in their struggle to break into the labour market in Portugal. Even so, not everyone is subject to the same 'starting point'. Educational attainment used here as a *proxy* for both social origin and destination is a strong predictor of when, how, at what pace and under which conditions integration into the labour market occurs (if at all). The patterns of integration in the labour market seem to be more or less determined by educational attainment, which, to a degree, contributes to the debate on the influence of education on the processes of social mobility and acts as a negative predictor for poverty. We state 'to a degree', as the relationship is far from 'linear'. We cannot sustain the argument that the higher the educational level the lower the 'level' and reiteration of precariousness. What is evident is that having or not having a degree/higher education qualification dramatically determines the characteristics of precariousness.

In the lower educational attainment pattern, the entry into the labour market is through full-time jobs and happens earlier with fewer interruptions lasting more than a year or longer and more formal employment contracts (see Table 6.1). Nonetheless, this is the group with the most frequent episodes of unemployment, though most of them are covered by the social security system. The precariousness in these cases lies most of all in the low work quality felt in the activity, the working environment itself and the earning levels. The pattern of the second group is characteristic of higher educational attainment, with the consequent later entry into the labour market and then a much more fragile link with the labour market.

Precariousness as Multi-Effect Experience

The inevitable consequence of this mode of labour market 'integration' is the spread of precariousness into other dimensions of these individuals' lives, namely by postponing residential or family transitions. This turns the idea of leaving the parental home into an ever delayed decision and, when accomplished, made possible predominantly by young people sharing a flat with friends and/or a partner. In combination with the endlessly delayed decision to have the first—as is the case of Ana below—or more children, the circumstances shared by these individuals put them at the heart of the issues involving the transition to adulthood, and simultaneously the

Table 6.1. Professional trajectories over time and by educational attainment (*n* = 52)

	Entry into the labour market	Link to the labour market	Trajectory in the labour market	Episodes of lack of job	Leaving home
Lower educational attainment	Sooner, standardised	Contract and temporary contract, full-time	Ascending or stable	Frequent official unemployment with benefits	Earlier, towards conjugality
Higher educational attainment	Later, high standard deviation	All atypical and precarious kinds of links	Instable, interrupted, unpredictable	Frequent situations of non-official unemployment	Early to study or late to consensual union

Source: adapted from Nico, 2014a

demographic problem: namely, the coincidence of an ageing population with a dramatic decrease of new births, together with the later transitions into adulthood and the self-limitation of childbearing due to financial restrictions that is severely affecting the whole of Southern Europe.

In this way, precarious labour easily turns into a precarious life. This happens through a dual—material and psychological—process. The material situation arises from the low wages, which are not enough to make ends meet, let alone to start planning for the future. This material restriction reinforces the psychological burden of young people's precarious condition: the constant fear of being dismissed without any kind of unemployment benefit, the long hard search for a new (even more precarious and low-paid) job, the possible return to the parental home and the feeling of failure that comes with the latter.

No-Win Situation, No Agency

Coming from a working-class background, Ana is suffering from hyper-reflexivity regarding her own life and from the incapacity to choose between two situations. Having lived alone for a few years, though recently joined by her boyfriend, Ana wants to leave her job (in her words, a very stressful one, marked by unpleasant hierarchical relations). She also wants to get married and pregnant. Knowing that one decision will exclude the other, she feels incapable of making a choice and is becoming more and more anxious, to the point that the only decision she seems able to make is to return to psychotherapy. A second nervous breakdown, again hidden from her family and friends, is the most predictable situation in the short term: from her family, there is the pressure to marry and have children; from her partner, there is the pressure to maintain a good salary. According to the statistics, she is doing fine: she has a permanent contract.

Waiting for Godot

Francisco is 27, lives in Lisbon and comes from a middle-class family. He is a Media Studies graduate but chose not to follow a journalist's path. He preferred to pursue post-graduate studies and to find a job in order to pay for his expenses. The only offer available was as a self-employed part-time worker doing extra-curricular activities with young children, a job that he had to accommodate for several years with several other jobs. Due to his low wage he only has accomplished one of his main objectives, leaving his parents' home and moving in with a friend some months ago. Francisco establishes this stage as a preparatory one, before being (financially) able to move in with his girlfriend and her children. On his worst months, he earns about 500 euros with an average of 700 euros after taxes. His salary is basically spent on gas to go to work and in-house expenses leaving little to help his girlfriend's expenses (who was an unemployed architect at the time of the interview). His chief objective is to move in with his girlfriend and children, after raising the financial conditions necessary to accomplish that aim. This has resulted in a wait that has been long, and that is not going to end in the foreseeable future.

Invisible Sacrifices

Luís is the first in his generation (of cousins) who did not go on to higher education and therefore does not have a degree. His choice of a technical course was received with some disappointment by his parents and family. Even greater was the concern at his decision to become a father at 24. As Luís said, with everything against him—the very small rented house, the lack of money for day-care—he still wanted to be a father at that point in his life. In order to attain that, he has had to make sacrifices. For the first two years of his daughter's life, he worked day and night shifts in a part-time job, alternating with those of his partner, just to guarantee that one of them was with their child at all times. There was simply no money for private day-care institutions. The media often needs to label generations, and the cohort included in this research has already been called the 'neither-nor generation'. Nonetheless, cases such as Luís' call attention to a different group of individuals, also invisible but probably quantitatively more significant, who belong to a struggling 'and-and generation', that try to reconcile important family, school and economic goals in a very short period of their lives.

Conclusions

Following a realist and qualitative approach, our aim has been to demonstrate the erosive and longitudinal effects of a declining welfare state, combined with an economic crisis and the austerity measures taken on its behalf, in the lives of individuals—especially for young people who, due to their position in the life span, are most vulnerable to interrupted or unlaunched lives and professional careers. By presenting complex and real-life stories, we aimed to highlight three aspects of a 'precarious well-being'. First, that precariousness is a process that leaves significant traces on individuals' biographies. The association between young people and precarious employment was a feature of Portuguese society long before the GFC and current austerity began, though it has definitely become more widespread as a result of current austerity measures. Prolonged precarious employment in its multiple forms is the main obstacle to the transition of young people to adulthood, since it seriously compromises the material basis for other stages such as 'leaving home' and starting their own family, independently of the order in which these processes are carried out. Precarious employment easily turns into a precarious life, a precarious transition to adulthood and a precarious future. Second, these traces are socially stratified. The nature and depth of these traces depends on the individual volume of economic, educational and social resources. Owing to the diverse nature of their origins and the course of their trajectories, the different groups of young people analysed here have been marked differently by the period of austerity in Portugal. Nevertheless, it is reasonable to argue that all of them have been—more deeply or more superficially—scarred by the crisis. And finally, it is a multi-effect phenomenon. Material stability and predictability are significant components (generally understood as basilar) of young people's lives and their notions of well-being, both objective and subjective, both current and projected into the future. Furthermore, these factors have the power to compromise or unbalance all other spheres of life.

After years of high unemployment accompanied by higher taxes and budget cuts in social expenditure, the material structure of a significant proportion of Portuguese families has been affected. The fulfilment of basic needs has become the priority and has made all other expenses secondary or even superfluous. This mindset has become deeply entrenched in young peoples' minds. But to what expense? Is ambition, is meritocracy, is *locus of control* compromised for the generations to come? Or, is a silent revolution taking place? Although the conjoint effects of a 'poor' and declining welfare state with a specific and pivotal timing of lives are undeniable and palpable, their longitudinal and subjective nature makes it a social time bomb, where timing and damage are hard to predict. The extent to which this may socially re-stratify economic and meritocracy values and beliefs may depend on the pace to which a 'generation for itself'—to combine Marx and Manheim's concepts—is developed, and how it is affected by economic rebound, media coverage and collective identity. In the short run, a 'generation in itself', conscious of sharing the unfortunate historical coincidence of growing up and entering adulthood in a specific economic and political environment, is the most likely. But at a second phase, it might ideologically divide the 'winners from the losers' of the crisis, the ones that succeeded, immigrated and/or maintained their plans from the ones that succumbed to the context. It might thus reify social inequalities that were there to begin with. The question remains, then, if there will be time to set the record straight, to develop a 'generation for itself', collectively conscious of themselves as forming a group that was—like no other in its time—exposed to extreme inequality and social injustice, and collectively determined to live and transmit to the next generations values of individual character, ambition and meritocracy, but on behalf of a better society.

References

Abbott, A. 2005. The historicality of individuals. *Social Science History* 29(1): 1–3.

Alves, N. de A., F. Cantante, I. Baptista, and R.M. do Carmo. 2011. *Jovens em Transições Precárias*. Lisboa: Mundos Sociais.

Carmo, R.M., F. Cantante, and N.A. Alves. 2014. Time projections: Youth and precarious employment. *Time & Society* 23(3): 337–357.

Dannefer, D. 2002. Toward a Global Geography of the Life Course: Challenges of Late Modernity for Life Course Theory. In *Handbook of the Life Course*, eds. J.T. Mortimer and M.J. Shanahan. New York: Kluwer Academic Publications.

Elder, G.H., M.K. Johnson, and R. Crosnoe. 2002. The Emergence and Development of Life Course Theory. In *Handbook of the Life Course*, eds. J.T. Mortimer and M.J. Shanahan. New York: Kluwer Academic Publications.

Elder, G. Jr. 1974. *Children of the Great Depression*. Chicago: Chicago press.

Mason, J. 2006. Six strategies for mixing methods and linking data in social science research. *NCRM Working Paper Series*. 4/2006.

Molé, N.J. 2010. Precarious Subjects: Anticipating Neoliberalism in Northern Italy's Workplaces'. *American Anthropologist* 112(1): 18–53.

Nico, M. 2011. *Transição Biográfica Inacabada. Transições para a Vida Adulta em Portugal e na Europa na Perspectiva do Curso de Vida*, Ph.D. Thesis. Departamento de Sociologia, Instituto Universitário de Lisboa.

———. 2014a. Variability of the Transitions to Adulthood in Europe: A Critical Approach to De-standardization of the Life Course. *Journal of Youth Studies* 17(2): 166–182.

———. 2014b. Generational Changes, Gaps and Conflicts: a View from the South. *Perspectives on Youth: European Youth Partnership Series*, 1st Issue '2020—what do we see?'. Luxembourg: Council of Europe and European Commission Publications.

———. 2015. Beyond 'Biographical' and 'Cultural Illusions' in European Youth Studies: Temporality and Critical Youth Studies. In *A Critical Youth Studies for the 21st Century*, eds. P. Kelly and A. Kamp, 53–69. Leiden: Brill.

O'Rand, A. 2009. Cumulative Processes in the Life Course. In *The Craft of the Life Course Research*, eds. G.H. Elder and J.Z. Giele. New York: The Guilford Press.

Spyridakis, M. 2013. *The Liminal Worker: An Ethnography of Work, Unemployment and Precariousness in Contemporary Greece*. Farnham: Ashgate.

Vosko, L.F. 2010. *Managing the Margins. Gender, Citizenship and the International Regulation of Precarious Employment*. Oxford: Oxford University Press.

Walther, A. 2006. Regulating Youth Transitions: trends, dilemmas and variations across different 'regimes' in Europe. In *Participation in Transition. Motivation of Young Adults in Europe for Learning and Working*, eds. A. Walther, M. du-Bois-Reymond, and A. Biggart. Frankfurt: Peter Lang European Academic Publishers.

7

Childhood and Juvenile Obesity in Italy: Health Promotion in an Era of Austerity

Giuseppina Cersosimo and Maurizio Merico

Introduction

Over the last decade, Italy has witnessed a significant increase in the prevalence of childhood and juvenile obesity. The prevalence of childhood and juvenile obesity, common to most Western and European countries, produces important effects in the lives of today's younger generations and can engender, in a medium- to long-term perspective, serious consequences for the physical health and well-being of future generations. Since 2008, the Global Financial Crisis (GFC) has accentuated an already existing process, by contributing to a decline in food quality, a

---

While the chapter is the result of collaborative work by the authors, Giuseppina Cersosimo took the lead in drafting the following parts: 'Exploring a social epidemiological framework for obesity' and 'The challenges of obesity and health promotion in Italy'; Maurizio Merico took the lead in drafting the following parts: 'Introduction', 'A renovated, post-GFC role for the family and the school in health promotion' and 'Conclusion'.

G. Cersosimo (✉) • M. Merico
University of Salerno, Salerno, Italy

deterioration in eating habits and an evident decrease in investments in healthcare. In Italy, these developments bring new and unfamiliar challenges for health promotion.

Research clearly demonstrates the deficiency of approaches that consider the increase in childhood obesity from only one perspective—particularly when that perspective emphasises medical or biological causes, which are often considered unsatisfactory and ultimately inadequate (Bona et al. 2009). Instead, the factors that have influenced the increase in childhood obesity are inextricably bound up with a range of social and cultural factors including gender, age, social stratification, local contexts and so on.

In this chapter, we argue for the adoption of a more comprehensive and holistic perspective to further extend the discussion, by connecting a social epidemiological framework for obesity, together with an analysis of the transformations in the process of socialisation of children and young people. This kind of approach opens up the possibility of identifying unexplored scenarios for understanding the increase of children and juvenile obesity. At the same time, it offers crucial insights for the development of preventive interventions and for health promotion. Indeed, this approach compels us to take into consideration the need for a new relationship and a mutual support between the different actors and agencies engaged at different levels and with different roles in addressing this complex issue (parents, school, media, health institutions and so on). Such an approach also highlights the pivotal role of the individual in the (re)definition of cultural patterns and lifestyles.

Karl Mannheim (1944, 1952) suggests that in times of crisis, the relationship between generation and education becomes at once a key issue to catch the changes that are taking place, and a vital context for transforming 'the direction in which modern society can develop' (Mannheim 1944, p.4). In other words, if the analysis of obesity is included in the transformation of educational processes and lifestyles, this can also contribute to the (re)definition of models of health promotion and reduction of risk behaviours in young people. As Hall et al. (2013, p.8) suggest, the crises of austerity and debates about welfare state futures present a 'moment of potential rupture'.

Exploring a Social Epidemiological Framework for Obesity: The Italian Case During Recent Years of Economic Crisis

In 2008, the world economy entered one of the most severe crises ever witnessed. In many Europeans countries, especially in the Mediterranean area, fruit and vegetable consumption decreased, while salaries were increasingly insufficient for families' monthly basic needs. Many families reduced their food consumption, choosing low-priced and less wholesome products. Indeed, 'the most vulnerable groups may have reduced their consumption by as much as 20 %' (Dave and Kelly 2012, p.254). This helps us to understand, together with our wider reasoning, the popular preference for less expensive junk foods.

In Italy, this lower economic disposal brought, at the same time, an increase in private savings and a decrease of consumption: in particular, −7 % in the consumption of milk, −5 % for oil, −3.4 % for bread, −2.1 % for fish and −1.5 % for fruits. On the other hand, Italians consume more pasta (+1.1 %) and eggs (+0.4 %). Thus, less healthy dietary habits are increasingly replacing the very celebrated Mediterranean diet, contributing to growing obesity levels (Sgabra and Erba 2012).

The World Health Organization (WHO) argues that obesity is currently one of the major global health problems. An Australian study found that people who experienced financial distress in 2008–2009 had a 20 % higher risk of becoming obese than those who did not (Siahpush et al. 2014). American children in families experiencing food insecurity are 22 % more likely to become obese than children growing in other families (Metallinos-Katsaras et al. 2012). In Italy, the percentage of obese people has increased from 8.6 % in 2000 to 10.4 % in 2012 (OECD 2014).

Childhood obesity has become increasingly widespread across different countries. Indeed, many developed and developing countries are facing the two competing health priorities of obesity and under-nutrition. However, it is often difficult to compare the prevalence of childhood overweight and obesity in different countries since the existing studies are often conducted over different time frames that are rarely comparable. Studies are also often focused on different age groups and using a variety of sampling and data collecting methods. In some studies, the prevalence of childhood overweight and obesity in Europe is higher in the Mediterranean areas with some 36–44 % children affected by these conditions compared with 15–29 % in North European countries (Kumanyika 2013, p. 4).

In Italy, the situation is similar to other industrialised countries, although in some surveys, and in much public health commentary and policy, it has recently become one of the most troubling contexts in Europe. According to the 2013 WHO report on nutritional and health conditions in Italy, 'up to 35 % of boys and 22 % of girls among 11-year-olds were overweight'; for 13-year-olds some '27 % for boys and 17 % for girls' were overweight, and among 15-year-olds, 26 % and 12 %' (WHO 2013, p.2). In 2010, Italy took part in the *Health Behaviour in School-Aged Children* (Currie et al. 2012) project, an international multi-centred study, which aimed to investigate the health awareness of children aged 11, 13 and 15 years. The study underlined how Italian adolescents tend to lose weight as they get older. Among 11-year-olds, one boy out of three and one girl out of four, respectively, 29.3 % and 19.5 %, are overweight (Currie et al. 2012), but among 15-year-olds, the percentage decreases to 25.6 % for boys and 12.3 % for girls. Obesity related complications such as Type 2 diabetes and arterial hypertension are increasing among children 'with an early outbreak of the disease and negative effects on the state of health of the entire population'. Furthermore, it should be noted that '2.8 % of health expenditure is estimated to be due to obesity' (Bona et al. 2009, p. 240).

It should be underlined, as the *'Okkio alla Salute'* and *'Zoom 8'* projects launched by the Ministry for Health (2012) pointed out, that geography plays a critical role in the prevalence of obesity. Indeed, the cases of overweight and obesity are more concentrated in the Southern regions of Italy, where some 15.2 % of children are obese, compared with 9.3 % in Central Italy and 8.2 % in Northern Italy. Campania is the most affected region where half the children attending the third primary class are obese or overweight, followed by Apulia, Molise, Abruzzi and Basilicata with percentages exceeding 40 % and differences related to socio-economic conditions (Censi et al. 2012).

In 2007, the Italian National Center for Preventing and Controlling Diseases supported a project entitled 'Enquiry system on behavioural risks among children and adolescents aged between 4 and 17 years', coordinated by the CNESPS-Iss (National Institute of Health—Epidemiology, Surveillance and Health Promotion), consisting of three different strands: the monitoring system '*Okkio alla Salute*', part of the *Childhood Obesity Surveillance Initiative*; '*Zoom 8*', a study on food habits; and the HBSC-Italy project on health behaviours. These different projects collected data from different populations and used different sampling methods, so the data are not comparable. '*Zoom 8*' was carried out in 2009 and 2010 and involved 2193 child–parent pairs from six regions (Friuli Venezia Giulia, Liguria, Marche, Lazio, Calabria and Sicily). The researchers measured children's height and weight and invited parents to answer two questionnaires concerning their children's food habits. The study revealed that fruit and vegetables are scarcely consumed by children: 23 % of parents declared that their children eat them less than once in a day, well below the recommended five times a day. Legumes too were rarely consumed: 53.7 % of children did not eat them at all and only 19.4 % ate them twice or three times a week. Fish was another food that children and young people seldom ate: around one-third of the sample was found not to eat fresh fish, half never ate fried fish and more than two-thirds did not eat preserved fish, such as tuna in oil (Censi et al. 2012).

Furthermore, the results showed that children were unlikely to drink milk frequently. Conversely, some types of food were over-consumed with potential negative health effects. Around 14 % of children, for example, ate more cured meats in a day than recommended by the Italian Society for Human Nutrition's guidelines. This consumption contributed to unhealthy intakes of fats and salt. Sugary drinks are recognised as one of the greatest 'culprits' in contributing to obesity. In Italy, 24 % of children drink them once a day and 17 % more than once a day. Biscuits and sweet snacks such as chocolate and cakes follow a similar trend. One-third of children eat at least one sugary snack once a day. '*Zoom 8*' findings suggested reducing the consumption of cured meats, sweets, drinks and increasing the consumption of legumes, fruit and vegetables which would result in more balanced diets with fewer calories and more vitamins, minerals and fibre.

The 2012 project 'Okkio alla Salute' involved 46,000 children attending the third class of primary school and 48,000 parents from all regions of Italy. Results suggested that few children seldom had what might be called a 'healthy' breakfast: 9 % of them did not eat breakfast at all, and 31 % ate an inadequate breakfast with too many proteins and carbohydrates. These food habits are identified as triggers of children's overweight and obesity. Furthermore, 22 % of parents declared that their children do not eat fruit and vegetables and that 44 % drink fizzy or sugary drinks. As for physical exercise, 17 % of children did none the day before the interview. 18 % played sport no longer than one hour a week. Moreover, results showed that 44 % of children have a television in their bedrooms and 36 % watch it and play videogames more than two hours a day. Only one child out of four goes to school on foot or by bicycle. It should be recognised that physical exercise is limited also because towns in these regions often do not have enough dedicated spaces and areas meant to facilitate and boost activity among children.

Regular physical exercise and healthy diets are less prevalent among people from lower socio-economic backgrounds and many empirical studies confirm that social factors have an impact on sedentary lifestyles (Lawman and Wilson 2014; Vilchis-Gil et al. 2015). Physical environment is thought to play a key role in determining activity patterns. That is why the European Union (EU) warned the many communities 'offering little or no safe spaces for children and young people to be physically active' (European Union 2014, 4).

Interestingly, some studies suggest that women are better able to maintain a healthy weight (Mancino et al. 2004, 2009; Sigmundová et al. 2011) and maintain their consumption of fruit and vegetables during periods of economic crisis (Agudo et al. 2002; Gwatkin et al. 2007; Roos et al. 2008). This can be explained from the standpoint of the results of a research conducted in 2012 in Southern Italy, which show that women consider, unlike men, eating as a desire, a pleasure rather than a need. They believe it is important to cut the caloric intake because for them there is no connection with the metaphor of the 'car-like' body, but rather with the body as a 'project', a representation of one's own self. So the body was, for each respondent, a presupposition that provides the basis for defining oneself as a subject in good shape and presentable, according to an individual (and collective) project linked to one's own physical and social well-being. For young women, such a project translates into a total adherence to the indications received by their education (ranging from such issues as healthy food to risky behaviours), as they believe they can prevent the onset of diseases (Cersosimo 2012).

The body must be considered instrumental for the optimal achievement of one's own performance along the biological and organic developmental process that leads to maturity; it is affected by many social factors penetrating into daily life actions (Goffman 1969). The relatively easy and smooth social interaction that 'nice looks' can provide suggests that the body is a form of 'capital', an expression of power and status, a form of symbolic distinction and capital that can be reinvested onto other forms. The body tends to be increasingly considered as a project and an integral part of the sense of self (Bourdieu 1980), an incomplete reality that by following a specific pathway can be converted into a social entity (Cersosimo 2012).

However, it is important to recall that this idea of the body project is realised by girls in particular through the influence of 'primary socialisation', in which mothers play a central role, and 'secondary socialization' in peer groups, fashion and the media. So as 'Zoom 8' maintained, children's lifestyles are socially, genetically and biologically influenced by their family environment and by social context.

In addition to hereditary predispositions to obesity, several biological mechanisms that could influence the risk of childhood (and adulthood) obesity are already present during pregnancy (Carter 2010). Family environment shapes children's food habits. First, parents often determine which kinds of food are eaten by children, in turn shaping some of their future food preferences. Some argue that the level of acceptance of a particular type of food is proportional to the exposure to it and can be fostered by watching others eating the same type of food (Savage et al. 2007). Unfortunately, it seems that less than half of Italian parents (44.7 %) have a good level of awareness of 'healthy diets' (Censi et al. 2012), and that this percentage is higher across Northern regions and among better educated people. Moreover, children are embedded in neighbourhoods, peer groups, schools and childcare facilities in which others influence their food preferences and practices:

by transposing their social norms and attitudes, food likes and dislikes, and consumption practices and affect their food habits through exposure and learning processes. (Reisch et al. 2013, 409)

Reisch et al. (2013, p.409) continue, 'These social groups also act as "communication buffers" between the children and the advertising and media messages that group members filter and evaluate'. These concerns will be discussed in the following sections.

The Challenges for Obesity and Health Promotion in Italy

The concept of *Globesity* is increasingly central to health promotion debates. *Globesity* indicates that obesity affects a large percentage of the world population. Obesity is increasingly understood as a worldwide social problem that constitutes a global public health crisis. It should be recognised that 'halting and reversing current trends is (…) a broader societal challenge that has become an explicit goal of sustainability strategies worldwide' (Reisch et al. 2013, p. 409). This is true also for Italy, because Italy is second only to Greece for overweight (including obesity) among children aged 5–17 (Kumanyika 2013).

Given the escalating concern over obesity-related diseases, the EU Action Plan on Childhood Obesity underlines that this 'issue threatens to have a highly negative impact on health and quality of life and may overwhelm our healthcare systems in the near future' (European Union 2014, p.3). In this sense, it is important to promote healthy lifestyles and behaviours among children and—as the EU Action Plan suggests—'to address risk factors for chronic disease in order to reduce premature death and disability at all ages, and to tackle health inequalities' (European Union 2014, p. 7).

The European Action Plan on Childhood Obesity points out that 'around 7 % of national health budgets across the EU are spent on diseases linked to obesity each year'. Lost productivity 'due to health problems and premature death' entails further indirect costs. According to estimates, 'around 2.8 million deaths per year in the EU result from causes associated with overweight and obesity' (European Union 2014, p.2). The Italian Ministry for Health estimates that:

> 44 % of patients affected by Diabetes Type II, 23 % of patients affected by ischemic heart disease and up to 41 % of patients affected by cancer developed these pathologies because of obesity and overweight. (Ministero della Salute 2014a)

Obesity in Italy has an impact on health expenditure in terms of direct and indirect costs due to its metabolic, cardiovascular and systemic complications, side effects on organs, and various social relational consequences in childhood such as low levels of self-confidence, social exclusion and depression that cost the Italian National Health System about 8.3 billion euros, or 6.7 % of the entire health expenditure (Ministero della Salute 2014b).

Obesity triggers to which children, and adults, are exposed, including food and/or 'lifestyle' advertisements, and physical inactivity, are often underestimated. Some suggest that this has already translated into the failure of several strategies to reduce child and adolescent obesity (Reisch et al. 2013). For example, some studies suggest that students attending schools with a fast-food outlet within 1 kilometre consume fewer fruit and vegetables, and drink more sugary drinks. They register a 6 % increase in overweight and a 7 % increase in obesity in comparison with students attending schools located further from fast-food outlets (Davis and Carpenter 2009).

Primary prevention strategies that aim to promote healthy dietary behaviours during a child's academic career are often ineffective. Some strategies suggest that schools, children and parents should be involved by paediatricians and General Practitioners who, because of their expertise on the subject, can promote better health education, increased awareness and more appropriate solutions for obesity-related diseases by improving lifestyles and healthy eating behaviours. Schools can be an effective space for early health promotion, and for combating children's reluctance to accept healthy food such as fruit and vegetables that are high in fibre and low in calories (Kontopodis 2015). Health promotion among adolescents also represents a priority in education and health in terms of present and future cost reductions. Health education in schools or youth centres has the potential to be effective since it involves those actors of the educational process who are able to seize and embrace the idea of health promotion. The WHO, for example, argues that overweight and obesity are preventable and that 'supportive environments and communities are fundamental in shaping people's choices, making the healthier choice (…) the easiest choice'. This choice should be 'accessible, available and affordable' (WHO 2015).

Some have suggested that children and young people should be encouraged to think that health is part of the economic and social development of their country to which they can—and should—contribute (Latouche 2006). In this view, health promotion and primary, secondary and tertiary prevention are neither effective nor efficient if they are considered only in terms of health. In a post-GFC environment, the risk is to further downsize prevention in terms of costs and personal engagement. The failure of various prevention and food education programmes in primary and secondary schools may be due to their partial or untimely implementation, since children have often already developed unhealthy lifestyles and eating behaviours in their families with their parents or their peer groups.

The European Commission strategy on Nutrition, Overweight and Obesity-related health issues identified six priority areas: 'better informed consumers', 'making the healthy option available', 'encouraging physical activity', developing evidence-based policy making, 'developing monitoring systems', focusing on children, young people and low socio-economic groups (European Union 2014, pp. 5–6). Health education and prevention are explicit in their promotion of healthy diets, the encouragement to consume fruit and vegetables rather than junk food, and the promotion of less sedentary lifestyles. Actions of prevention should be focused on the very first years of life when some family and individual factors can turn to risk factors for child obesity. Family factors such as parents' obesity and unhealthy lifestyles, and individual factors such as unhealthy diets and low levels of physical activity can increase the likelihood of children developing obesity and overweight.

In Italy, health promotion programmes targeting children's obesity have been largely unsuccessful for a number of reasons. In the first instance, all Italian regions have different prevention and nutrition education programmes. Furthermore, primary and secondary schools have their own autonomy on how to develop and deliver their health promotion programmes. Finally, there is very limited knowledge of the different actors involved in these projects because of a limited process of monitoring and evaluation of projects undertaken. Overall, this means that in Italy—in schools, in particular—there are few models for fostering the participation of different social actors in the health promotion processes.

A Renovated, Post-GFC Role for the Family and the School in Health Promotion

Given these challenges, we now proceed to consider the transformation of the roles of agencies of socialisation, with particular attention to the family and the school—the two institutions usually more closely involved in health education and health promotion. Our discussion is located in a changing socio-cultural context where stable and shared sets of beliefs, values and practices are no longer transmitted to younger generations, but instead is characterised by features such as autonomy, selectivity and fluidity (Besozzi 2012). More broadly, the transformations that have taken place in Italy (as well as in other Western countries) over the last decades have brought a *pluralisation* of agencies, contexts and actors involved in the education of children and young people (Giovannini 1987). This pluralisation has not only increased educational opportunities, but also restructured the overall educational process with an increasing interaction between formal and informal processes of education. In this sense, it can be argued that a model of 'flexible socialisation' has appeared, in which the expectations, contents and outcomes offered by the different agencies to children and young people are heterogeneous and often contradictory (Garelli, Palmonari and Sciolla 2006). In a context characterised by complexity, differentiation and contingency, the individual becomes the new centre of his/her socialisation (Chisholm and Deliyanni-Kouimtzis 2014), being charged with the responsibility for negotiating a balance between chances and choices (Merico 2011). Within the process of socialisation, young people are required to reflexively (re)arrange their understandings in order to continuously (re)define a sense of sharing and stability that can no longer be taken for granted (Besozzi 2006; Colombo 2011).

At the same time, there continues to be an emphasis placed upon the 'restricted sociality' (family, friends and affections) (Buzzi et al. 1997, 2002, 2007) that is often meant as a safe haven against diffuse uncertainty and on which young Italians rely for a prolonged time (Scabini and Rossi 2006; Besozzi 2009). It is worth considering also that among families, there is some research that suggests that the relationship between children and parents in Italy has generally shifted from a situation of (explicit) conflict, towards one of empathy and negotiation, designating a context where dialogue and reciprocity seem to prevail (Garelli et al. 2006). However, this new connection between generations produces relationships that do not necessarily entail shared meanings and choices (Besozzi 2012).

In other words, while still playing a relevant role in the education of children, the family is no longer the centre of young people's everyday life (Chisholm and Deliyianni-Kouimtzis 2014), and becomes only one of the spaces in which food and activity practices are formed. At the same time, the family seems more and more fearful and powerless in dealing with children's problems, particularly when these concern eating disorders such as anorexia nervosa. These changes become crucial for our discussion because, together with other actors involved in primary socialisation (Berger and Luckmann 1966), the family has a basic influence upon quantitative and qualitative aspects of children's eating attitudes and behaviour (Censi et al. 2012). In particular, parents are still considered as 'the primary individuals responsible (...) for shaping their children's first food choices' and, consequently, as having a critical role 'in the formation of eating and activity habits' (European Union 2014, 16). The challenge, then, is how to reconcile and revitalise this function in connection with the challenges of overweight and obesity. How can the role of the family in the process of health education, and the definition of dietary habits, be redefined in connection with the contribution of the other agencies of socialisation, and the growing centrality of the individual?

At the same time, the school is increasingly losing its authority as a space of socialisation, alongside a growing attention paid from students (and their parents) towards its instrumental role rather than its expressive function (Buzzi et al. 2002). Here the question does not simply involve the declining level of trust in teachers and formal instructors. Rather, it deals with the fact that the school seems no longer able to address children and young people's orientations, values and behaviours (Besozzi 2009). And, as already seen for the family, this sets a new and not yet fully acknowledged challenge for our discussion, because schools have been usually (and are still) considered an 'essential environment (…) for tackling overweight and obesity in children and young people' (European Union 2014, 12), both in relation to the promotion of dietary habits and the encouragement of healthy lifestyles.

In this context, it is vital to briefly discuss the contribution of (old and new) media (Morcellini 1992) to the definition, sedimentation and diffusion of lifestyles and dietary habits. First, there is a need to consider these media as major channels of 'messages that may lead to the development of unhealthy dietary preferences' (European Union 2014, 15), as well as 'smart' (and often 'unhealthy') food habits (Lewis and Hill 1998). Second, as clearly shown by the 'Zoom 8' project, after 'doctors, nutritionists and pediatricians', the mass media are the second most important source of information (even for parents) in relation to (healthy) dietary advice and guidance. Third, we ought to take into account the correlation between the exposure to media such as TV, video and computers—as indicators of increasingly sedentary lifestyles—and the proportion of overweight and obese children and young people (Censi et al. 2012).

More generally, we need to take into account that—as for other spheres—the definition and sedimentation of attitudes, practices and behaviours dealing with health, self representations and dietary lifestyles, generally occur well before the period in which educational institutions are able to intervene with their plans and projects. Therefore, the latter often become ineffective, because interventions usually occur when lifestyles and dietary habits are already firmly developed. It follows that, without an adequate and timely guidance, children and young people risk being socialised towards unhealthy eating behaviours and habits in terms of what, how much and where they eat, with implications for their physical development and their perceptions of a healthy and socially accepted body (European Union 2014).

In this context, we can argue that any actions aimed at promoting health or preventing obesity need to be based on a 'new pact' in a post-GFC environment characterised by a 'de-generation' of the generation pact with important consequences for the present and future of policies and interventions for children and young people (Sgritta 2014). Any 'new pact' should be grounded in the overt mutual engagement of different educational agencies, as well as on a growing connection and mutual support among different actors (individuals and institutions) and contexts (Fornari 2014). Paediatricians and health institutions must be involved together with other formal and informal educational agencies. However, we suggest that this 'new pact' needs to explicitly involve, once again, the family and the school, because eating habits acquired in childhood and youth are more likely to be kept during adulthood (Censi et al. 2012).

Rather than reducing the role of the family and the school, the changes we describe have deeply transformed their contribution and presented them with new challenges. This is not only due to the fact that they are the institutions primarily related to food supply (meals, canteens, etc.). Indeed, it has been highlighted that their contribution to influencing eating styles tend to sediment and persist over time, especially when the peer group is involved (Jelalian and Steele 2008; Bell et al. 2014). However, as we have tried to explain, they can reach the hoped-for goals of addressing obesity (European Union 2014) only if incorporated in a larger network of actors. And, above all, if future interventions are based on new forms of dialogue between, and engagement of, generations and institutions, which also need to be considered as targets of health education and promotion. In other words, a breakthrough in health promotion is needed to ameliorate the effects of austerity on health conditions and particularly on childhood obesity. However, its effectiveness will depend not only upon increased financial support, but also upon the ways in which major changes in intergenerational relationships and in educational patterns are taken into account.

Conclusion

Our analysis draws attention to at least two issues. In the first instance, as in other Western countries, obesity in Italy affects a growing proportion of children and young people, and assumes particular characteristics in relation to regional, educational and economic factors. This reflects a lack of awareness from adults, parents and teachers in particular, and a more general carelessness on the part of institutions. On the other hand, this phenomenon should be examined according to the perspective assumed in this chapter, within the more general transformation of educational processes. These involve, at the same time, the pluralisation of educational agencies and the emergence of new challenges in the relationship between young people, adults and institutions that reduce the possibility of properly influencing children's food and dietary habits. These issues indicate a gap that is difficult to bridge if we take into consideration the relationships between adult generations and their children. This gap results in a lack of support, and of food and health education, for children. The agencies that could further affect eating behaviours do not seem significantly capable and equipped in order to encourage appropriate lifestyles. In an age of austerity, effective health promotion aimed at addressing the increase of obesity must be grounded in the recognition that educating children entails, at the same time, educating significant adults and agencies to adopt and promote healthy lifestyles.

In the end, health promotion needs to broaden—as we have tried to do in this chapter—the horizon of the issues and perspectives taken into account, as well as to involve, together with children and young people, the generation of their educators (Cersosimo 2005). Furthermore, at its base, there should be a process of mutual engagement that might generate preventive programmes capable of involving all the actors that contribute to the definition of dietary habits. Only in this way can health promotion engender a process that can have a positive impact on the life chances of present and future generations.

References

Aagudo, A., N. Slimani, M.C. Ocke, A. Naska, and EPIC Working Group on Dietary Patterns. 2002. Vegetable and fruit consumption in the EPIC cohorts from 10 European countries. *IARC Scientific Publications Series* 156: 99–103.

Bell, S.L., S. Audrey, A.R. Cooper, S. Noble, and R. Campbell. 2014. Lessons from a peer-led obesity prevention programme in English schools. *Health Promotion International*. First published online April 6, 2014 [online]. Available from: http://heapro.oxfordjournals.org/content/early/2014/04/05/heapro.dau008.full. Accessed 1 Oct 2015.

Berger, P.L., and T. Luckmann. 1966. *The Social Construction of Reality: A Treatise in the Sociology of Knowledge*. New York: Anchor Books.

Besozzi, E. 2006. *Società, cultura, educazione*. Rome: Carocci.

———. ed. 2009. *Tra sogni e realtà: gli adolescenti e la transizione alla vita adulta*. Rome: Carocci.

———. 2012. Tra bisogni di appartenenza e voglia di trasgressione. In *Il confine sottile. Culture giovanili, legalità, educazione*, ed. L. Caimi. Milan: Vita e Pensiero.

Bona, G., A. Busti, F. Prodam, and S. Bellone. 2009. Obesità e sindrome metabolica in età pediatrica. *Prospettive in Pediatria* 39(156): 239–245.

Bourdieu, P. 1980. Le capital social. Notes provisoires. *Actes de la Recherche en Sciences Sociales* 3: 31–42.

Buzzi, C., A. Cavalli, and A. de Lillo, eds. 1997. *Giovani verso il Duemila. Quarto rapporto IARD sulla condizione giovanile in Italia*. Bologna: Il Mulino.

———. eds. 2002. *Giovani del nuovo secolo. Quinto rapporto IARD sulla condizione giovanile in Italia*. Bologna: Il Mulino.

———. eds. 2007. *Rapporto giovani. Sesta indagine IARD sulla condizione giovanile in Italia*. Bologna: Il Mulino.

Carter, S.K. 2010. Beyond control: Body and self in women's childbearing narratives. *Sociology of Health & Illness* 32(7): 993–1009.

Censi, L., D. D'addesa, D. Galeone, S. Andreozzi, and A. Spinelli. 2012. *Studio ZOOM8: l'alimentazione e l'attività fisica dei bambini della scuola primaria*. Rome: Istituto Superiore di Sanità (Rapporti ISTISAN 12/42).

Cersosimo, G. 2005. *La costruzione della Salute. Percorsi di sviluppo dell'educazione sanitaria in Italia*. Bologna: Clueb.

————. 2012. Women and Alcohol: a Study in the South of Italy. *Bulletin of the Transilvania University of Brasov. Series VII: Social Sciences and Law* 5(1): 9–24.

Chisholm, L., and V. Deliyianni-Kouimtzis, eds. 2014. *Changing Landscapes for Childhood and Youth in Europe.* Newcastle upon Tyn: Cambridge Scholars Publishing.

Colombo, M. 2011. Educational choices in action: young Italians as reflexive agents and the role of significant adults. *Italian Journal of Sociology of Education* 3(1): 14–48.

Currie, C., C. Zanotti, A. Morgan, D. Currie, M. de Looze, C. Roberts, and O. Samdal, eds. 2012. *Social determinants of health and well-being among young people. Health Behaviour in School-aged Children (HBSC) study: international report from the 2009/2010 survey.* Copenhagen: WHO Regional Office for Europe.

Dave, D.M., and I.R. Kelly. 2012. How does the business cycle affect eating habits? *Social Science & Medicine* 74(2): 254–262.

Davis, B., and C. Carpenter. 2009. Proximity of Fast-Food Restaurants to Schools and Adolescent Obesity. *American Journal of Public Health* 99(3): 505–510.

European Union. 2014. *EU Action Plan on Childhood Obesity 2014–2020* [online]. Available from: http://ec.europa.eu/health/nutrition_physical_activity/docs/childhoodobesity_actionplan_2014_2020_en.pdf. Accessed 1 Oct 2015.

Fornari, S. 2014. Socializzazione. In *Intersezioni tra discipline. Elaborare concetti per la ricerca sociale*, ed. R. Memoli. Milan: Franco Angeli.

Garelli, F., A. Palmonari, and L. Sciolla, eds. 2006. *La socializzazione flessibile. Identità e trasmissione dei valori tra i giovani.* Bologna: Il Mulino.

Giovannini, G. 1987. I molti luoghi, tempi, attori della formazione: un'analisi del policentrismo a partire dall'offerta. *Studi di sociologia* 25(1): 3–17.

Goffman, E. 1969. *Where the action is. Three essays.* London: The Penguin Press.

Gwatkin, D.R., S. Rutstein, K. Johnson, E. Suliman, A. Wagstaff, and A. Amouzou. 2007. Socio-economic differences in health, nutrition, and population within developing countries: an overview. *Niger Journal Clinical Practice* 10(4): 272–282.

Hall, S., D. Massey, and M. Rustin, eds. 2013. *After neoliberalism? The Kilburn manifesto.* London: Lawrence & Wishart.

Jelalian, E., and R.G. Steele, eds. 2008. *Handbook of Childhood and Adolescent Obesity.* New York: Springer.

Kontopodis, M. 2015. How and why should children eat fruit and vegetables? Ethnographic insights into diverse body pedagogies. *Social Science & Medicine* 143: 297–303.

Kumanyika, S. 2013. INFORMAS (International Network for Food and Obesity/non-communicable diseases Research, Monitoring and Action Support): Summary and future directions. Obesity reviews. *International Association for the Study of Obesity* 14(1): 1–54.

Latouche, S. 2006. *Le pari de la décroissance*. Paris: Fayard.

Lawman, H.G., and D.K. Wilson. 2014. Associations of social and environmental supports with sedentary behavior, light and moderate-to-vigorous physical activity in obese underserved adolescents. *Journal of Behavioral Nutrition and Physical Activity* 11(1) [online]. Available from: http://www.ijbnpa.org/content/pdf/s12966-014-0092-1.pdf. Accessed 15 Oct 2015.

Lewis, M.K., and A.J. Hill. 1998. Food advertising on British children's television: A content analysis and experimental study with nine-year olds. *International Journal of Obesity and Related Metabolic Disorders* 22(3): 206–214.

Mancino, L., B.-H. Lin, and N. Ballenger. 2004. *The Role of Economics in Eating Choices and Weight Outcomes. Agriculture Information Bulletin. 791.* Washington, DC: Economic Research Service (ERS), U.S. Department of Agriculture (USDA).

Mancino, L., J. Todd, and B.-H. Lin. 2009. Separating what we eat from where: Measuring the effect of food away from home on diet quality. *Food Policy* 34(6): 557–562.

Mannheim, K. 1944. *Diagnosis of Our Time: Wartime Essays of a Sociologist.* New York: Oxford University Press.

———. 1952. The problem of generations. In *Essays on the Sociology of Knowledge*, ed. K. Mannheim. New York: Oxford University Press.

Merico, M. 2011. Chances and choices: Patterns of life planning and future orientations among Italian young people. *Italian Journal of Sociology of Education* 3(1): 97–114.

Metallinos-Katsaras, E., A. Must, and K. Gorman. 2012. A Longitudinal Study of Food Insecurity on Obesity in Preschool Children. *Journal of the Academy of Nutrition and Dietetics* 112(12): 1949–1958.

Ministero Della Salute. 2014a. Obesità [online]. Available from: http://www.salute.gov.it/portale/salute/p1_5.jsp?lingua=italiano&id=175&area=Malattie_endocrine_e_metaboliche. Accessed 14 Oct 2015.

———. 2014b. Piano Nazionale della Prevenzione 2014–2018 [online]. Available from http://www.salute.gov.it/imgs/C_17_pubblicazioni_2285_allegato.pdf. Accessed 14 Oct 2015.

Morcellini, M. 1992. *Passaggio al futuro. Formazione e socializzazione tra vecchi e nuovi media*. Milan: Franco Angeli.

OECD. 2014. Obesity Update. Paris: OECD Publishing [online]. Available from www.oecd.org/els/health-systems/Obesity-Update-2014.pdf. Accessed 1 Feb 2016.

Reisch, L.A., W. Gwozdz, G. Barba, S. de Henauw, N. Lascorz, and I. Pigeot. 2013. Experimental evidence on the impact of food advertising on children's knowledge about and preferences for healthful food. *Journal of Obesity* 2013: 13 [online]. Available from http://www.hindawi.com/journals/jobe/2013/408582/cta/. . Accessed 14 Oct 2015.

Roos, E., K. Talala, M. Laaksonen, S. Helakorpi, O. Rahkonen, A. Uutela, and R. Prättälä. 2008. Trends of socioeconomic differences in daily vegetable consumption: 1979–2002. *European Journal of Clinical Nutrition* 62(7): 823–833.

Savage, J.S., J. Fisher, and L.L. Birch. 2007. Parental influence on eating behavior: conception to adolescence. *The Journal of Law, Medicine & Ethics* 35(1): 22–34.

Scabini, E., and G. Rossi, eds. 2006. *Le parole della famiglia*. Milan: Vita & Pensiero.

Sbraga, L., and G.R. Erba. 2012. *La crisi nel piatto: come cambiano i consumi degli italiani*. Rome: Ufficio Studi Confcommercio.

Sgritta, G.B. 2014. De-generazione: il patto violato. *Sociologia del lavoro* 136: 279–294.

Siahpush, M., T. Huang, A. Sikora, M. Tibbits, R. Shaikh, and G. Singh. 2014. Prolonged financial stress predicts subsequent obesity: Results from a prospective study of an Australian national sample. *Obesity* 22: 616–621.

Sigmundová, D., E. Sigmund, K. Frömel, and A. Suchomel. 2011. Gender Differences in Physical Activity, Sedentary Behavior and BMI in the Liberec Region: the IPAQ Study in 2002–2009. *Journal of Human Kinetic* 28: 123–131.

Vilchis-Gil, J., M. Galván-Portillo, M. Klünder-Klünder, M. Cruz, and S. Flores-Huerta. 2015. Food habits, physical activities and sedentary lifestyles of eutrophic and obese school children: a case–control study. *BMC Public Health* 15: 124 [online]. Available from: http://www.biomedcentral.com/1471-2458/15/124. Accessed 15 Oct 2015.

WHO (World Health Organization). 2013. *Nutrition, Physical Activity and Obesity—Italy* [online]. Available from: http://www.euro.who.int/__data/assets/pdf_file/0018/243306/Italy-WHO-Country-Profile.pdf. Accessed 14 Sept 2015.

———. 2015. Obesity and overweight Fact sheet N°311. Available from: http://www.who.int/mediacentre/factsheets/fs311/en/. Accessed 15 Oct 2015.

8

Negotiating the Interface: The Complexities of Exercising Road Safety 'Responsibility and Choice' on Melbourne's Fringe

Kerry Montero

'Poor People Don't Drive Cars'

The Australian Federal Treasurer Joe Hockey is being interviewed on radio and is billowing in his own wind, defending his government's proposed increase in fuel excise: *'The poorest people'*, he blusters, *'either don't have cars or actually don't drive very far in many cases'* (ABC Radio 2014).

The pronouncement made by the then Liberal (Conservative) Government Treasurer just under a year into his tenure failed to convince his critics that the proposed increase was a progressive tax that would, in fact, disadvantage higher income earners, and, by implication, advantage low-income people. Nor did it do anything to improve his image as an unsympathetic, out-of-touch and incompetent politician committed to relentlessly push through the new government's ramped-up neo-Liberal agenda of spending cuts,

K. Montero (✉)
RMIT University, Melbourne, VIC, Australia

taxation changes and support of the 'lifters', rather than the 'leaners', in Australian society. The statement reverberated for many weeks, as fodder for numerous satirical cartoons and comedy skits, as the subject of a flurry of opinion pieces and fact checks, and became another nail in the coffin of a government leadership that seriously lacked credibility and gravitas (the Treasurer would lose his job following a successful leadership 'coup' that replaced Tony Abbott as Australia's prime minister in late 2015).

Why did the issue resonate so strongly? Why the public outrage, in a country where the political landscape is as flat as its topography? Part of the answer to these questions resides in the unique place the car occupies in the Australian social and cultural landscape—one could almost say the Australian 'psyche'. The car has long been central to economic and social life in Australia. The issue of car ownership goes to the heart of commonly held assumptions and myth making of Australian life, for reasons that I will explore later in this chapter.

This love affair/dependence comes at a cost. Joe Hockey's cynical claim that wealthy people drive more, and therefore spend more on fuel, disguised the fact that those on lower incomes spend proportionately more on fuel and associated car-related costs and are in fact more dependent on the car than those with higher incomes (Dodson 2014). This is due to several interrelated factors and has far-reaching implications for many young people, particularly those living on the expanding urban–rural 'interface' of Australian cities. This chapter explores some of these factors and the implications for the ways that the 'responsibilisation' (Kelly 2001) of young people is enacted in relation to road use. These processes of responsibilisation reveal key dimensions of the choices made clear, or cut off, in the *moral economies* that shape young people's health and well-being at this interface.

'If You're Not Comfortable, Get Another form of Transport'

As the Treasurer was making his statement, around 120 11-year-old students in a government school in the municipality of Casey, on the south-eastern outskirts of Melbourne, were participating in small group discussion activities as part of the road safety programme *Fit to Drive*.

The 16- to 17-year-olds, most of whom already have their 'Learner's Permit',[1] and regularly travel as passengers in cars driven by their peers, are likely to be very familiar with the realities of a family on the fringes of Melbourne, coping with the necessity of maintaining a two- or three-car household on a low or fixed income.

On that day, they were learning about factors contributing to high crash rates among young people, and developing strategies to avoid dangerous situations and 'keep themselves safe' on the roads. They discussed and debated the influences of peers on a young person's driving, reflected on what makes them feel safe in a car, and what passengers can do to encourage and support safe driving. They analysed different—and for many, familiar—scenarios that young people find themselves in: a young driver with a rowdy carload of friends being egged on to 'floor it', or piling more people into an already overcrowded car; or the unlicensed young driver at the last minute replacing the designated driver because she had consumed a few drinks at the party after all. They devised strategies, and acted these out for each other, practising assertive behaviours in role plays. Despite the sobering moments in the morning's workshop, where they were presented with causes and consequences of car crashes and their impacts on whole communities, heard stories and analysed case studies, the students' feedback revealed that they found the workshop fun and engaging, echoing the feedback from other schools: 'the activities were interactive and a good way for us to learn'—as well as 'a valuable lesson and a MUST for teens' as one 17-year-old male advised (Groundwater Secondary College June 2013).

As a colleague and I (Montero and Kelly 2016) have discussed in greater detail elsewhere, *Fit to Drive* is just one of the wide-ranging road safety education and legislative initiatives that have been introduced over recent years in Australia to address the problem of young people's overrepresentation in road crash fatalities and serious injuries. A key message of population-based and targeted road safety promotion and education is the moral imperative of individual 'responsibility', and 'good choices'. These messages are a key focus of *Fit to Drive*, in which university

---

[1] In Victoria, Australia, young people may obtain their Learner's Permit at 16, and sit for their Driver's License at 18. As part of the Graduated Licensing System as learner drivers they are required to obtain 120 hours on road driving experience with a fully licensed driver. Once licensed they are subject to restrictions ('graduated' over two years) before becoming fully licensed.

undergraduates are employed as 'road safety ambassadors' (Spencer and Montero 2011) to facilitate the small group discussions and activities in the programme workshop. It is these interactive small group sessions with the 'near peer' role model-facilitators that students particularly highlight as engaging, thought-provoking and transformative.

The student evaluations at the end of the session indicate that they have absorbed the messages. Asked what they would do differently, their responses are models of assertiveness: *'Be more responsible as a passenger and speak up if I have to if there is a risk'; 'Voice my opinion and don't let peer pressure get to me when driving'; 'Speak up if I feel unsafe in a car with someone else driving'; 'Let the driver know if I feel uncomfortable or unsafe'.* And of prevention: *'Never ever consider getting into a car when they are overloading'; 'Pay more attention to how tired I am feeling and don't use phones when driving'* (a selection of comments taken from *Fit to Drive* evaluation forms).

These responses are in harmony with comments regularly encountered in the *Fit to Drive* workshops across the state. Research conducted on the programme reveals that young people consistently demonstrate a ready acceptance of the idea of individual responsibility for 'safe choices' in relation to driving and road use (Montero and Kelly 2016). One young woman is clear in her advice: *'If you're not comfortable, get another form of transport'.*

How realistic is this advice in the Australian context of growing populations on the expanding urban–rural 'interface' areas of large cities? What health and well-being choices are available to different groups of young people at this interface?

'Melbourne Today Is Greatly Dependent on the Motor Vehicle and Inevitably Will Continue to Be'[2]

The area where I grew up, in 1960s Melbourne, was typical of the working-class suburbs built around quarries and industry close to the city in the century following the European invasion of Australia in 1778.

---

[2] Country Roads Board News, No. 34 December 1976c

Nothing remained of the original grassy woodland, and the local creek where we played—one of the gentle waterways flowing down to the Yarra River that had become 'official or unofficial dumping grounds for suburban refuse' (Boyd 1968/2010, p. 94)—was clogged with effluent, rubbish, industrial waste. It was only the alert eye and ear that could still find traces of the way of life of the Aboriginal peoples who had lived and passed through the area for countless millennia.

Life for the new families that settled there developed its own rhythms. Workers walked to their jobs in the quarries, brickworks, textile and boot factories, or rode bicycles, or caught the trams that ran down any of the several lines that serviced the inner northern suburbs. School was a walk away, perhaps a tram or bus ride, as were sporting events, picture theatres, dances, community gatherings. Successive waves of migrants found a home there and transformed the culture as the post-war population grew.

Sometime in the late 1960s, my friends and peers started to disappear from our local school, their families leaving their rented houses, attracted by the lure of buying a home in the new suburbs that were growing up on the edges of the city, occupying land that had once been forest, or, latterly, farms and orchards—the 'food bowl' of the city. This was the start of what architect and social commentator Robin Boyd (1968/2010, p.93) calls the 'second period of pioneering' in Australia, a continuation of the 'Australian Ugliness'. The blueprint, and ethos, had been established for successive waves of encroachments on the land, which saw the 'subdividers arrive, and behind them the main wave of suburbia' when 'all the remaining native trees came crashing down before the bulldozers' (Boyd 1968/2010, p. 33). With this suburban 'sprawl' came a fundamental shift in the way people lived their lives.

The exodus to the outer fringes of the city coincided with the rise of the private motor vehicle as the dominant transport mode for people in Western societies and corresponding neglect of the public transport system by successive governments. The early years of the twentieth century had seen a rapid growth in the public transport network in Melbourne (Cannon 1967; Mees 2010). Tramways and government-operated railway systems competed with each other in extending to the boundaries of urban growth and beyond, 'leading rather than following urban development' (Mees 2010, p. 96). Easily accessible, reliable and regular services made getting around—travelling between work, school, social events and home—relatively easy. Over the past six decades or more, however, public transport has been systematically neglected by successive federal and state governments in favour of expansion of roads systems, and this has given rise to 'the car-dependent suburbanite' (Dodson and Sipe 2008, p.17).

A substantial body of research has revealed the problems created by dependence on the motor car, and presents strong evidence of significant improvements in the 'liveability' of cities, across a number of measures, where there is better access to efficient public transport (Dodson and Sipe 2008; Badland et al. 2015). Given this evidence, how do we account for the neglect of public transport and the promotion of car ownership? In this context, it is worth examining the role and power of the automotive industry in Australia.

There was early acceptance by the modern state on the central role of the car in the promotion of economic growth. Following an initial phase of government-imposed restrictions on the use of cars during the late nineteenth and early twentieth centuries, governments in the USA and Western Europe adopted policies that actively promoted the private motor vehicle. From the outset, the automotive industry was active in lobbying for the development of legislation, infrastructure and public works to promote the car. One key early focus for their lobbying efforts was for improvements in road quality (Paterson 2007, p.115). By this initiative, they achieved a shift in the burden of costs for development and maintenance of roads systems to the public (government) sector, thereby protecting the profits of car manufacturers. In Germany and Italy, an additional impetus for the extension and upgrade of roads systems was the military agenda. In other countries—notably the USA, but extending to other developed countries—the automotive and allied industries were successful in influencing successive governments to devote significant public monies to the expansion of road networks in the service of the private car (Paterson 2007, p. 117). Indeed, since World War II, '[T]he coalition of car, oil and construction companies, allied with highway and municipal engineers' has been described as the most powerful political lobby in the USA and UK (Paterson 2007, p.117).

The other factor promoting the dominance of the car has been the neglect of alternative transport by governments in those countries that have aligned their economic development to the motor car, where '[S] tate spending on transport since 1945 has systematically favoured roads' (Paterson 2007, p. 118). Freestone (2010, p. 149) has described the 'influence of American development trends' on urban planning in Melbourne and other Australian cities, particularly from the 1950s onwards. Post-World War II, transport planning privileged cars and motor transport, with emphasis on the development of roads systems, and reliance on technical expertise provided by American planning experts (Freestone 2010, p. 160). The beginning of the freeway era for Melbourne was characterised by the commitment to a future of freeways, with transport planners unilaterally 'catering for the motor car', often, it was argued, at the cost of communities and environment affected by these freeways (Freestone 2010, p. 162). By the 1970s, such was the negative feeling towards freeways in the community and some political circles that the Country Roads Board (CRB), which at that time was the Victorian state government agency that had responsibility for the rural and urban road network, apparently deemed it necessary to acknowledge and appease community opposition and to undertake concerted public relations exercises. CRB newsletters of this period—targeting the general public—contain articles about the necessity and desirability of freeways, even their 'environmental benefit', with titles such as 'Freeways an asset' and 'The ecology of transportation' (CRB Newsletter *No. 33* August 1976a, b).

Despite widespread opposition and a vocal and active anti-freeway movement involving community protest, blockades, negative media attention and 'green bans' by building unions (Dingle and Rasmussen 1991, p.318; Mees 2000, p. 54), road interests succeeded in lobbying for the expansion of freeways and, at the same time, advocated for reductions in public transport services. The development of an expansive freeway network was firmly embedded in planning policy by the early 1960s (Dingle and Rasmussen 1991). With planners largely eschewing meaningful consultation, radial road systems were built over waterways, suburbs were fractured and public transport degraded (and later privatised).

The new outer suburbs had not been provided with extended tram services or new rail infrastructure. Instead, grandiose freeway schemes, from an even more rapidly suburbanising and prosperous United States, were inveigling their way into state government metropolitan plans. Freeways gnawed into transport budgets, leaving little for new public transport links. Trams and cars came into conflict in crowded city streets. (Dodson and Sipe 2008, p. 17)

Inextricably linked to urban development, 'the car was aiding and abetting city spread between and beyond the main suburban rail corridors' (Freestone 2010, p. 149). By the early 1970s, it was clear that Australian cities had become 'primarily development-driven with their urban forms largely determined by increasing car dependence' (Freestone 2010, p. 164). By the beginning of the twenty-first century, it was estimated that 83 % of Melbourne's population lived outside the 'transit rich' areas of Melbourne (Cheal 2003, cited in Dodson et al. 2007).

The legacy of this planning history, at a time of major growth in outer-urban housing developments in Australian cities, was that there was little corresponding development in public transport in these areas (Dodson et al. 2006). Some accounts of the growth in the use of private motor vehicles, and a concurrent decline in investment in, and use of, public transport, have identified this shift as an inevitable development, a result of invisible, quasi-'natural' forces (see Mees 2010, p. 14 for discussion of this; see also Paterson 2007, p. 92). However, this view overlooks the role of government in policy and planning related to urban planning and infrastructure, and, from the 1980s and 1990s, the impact of neo-Liberal policies that oversaw the widespread privatisation of state-owned services that 'resulted in a retreat from proactive government involvement in economic development, infrastructure provision, and spatial planning' (Tonts and McKenzie 2005, citing Hardy et al. 1995). In Australia, the issue of public transport 'has largely disappeared from the policy agenda' with the Federal Government retaining 'no current interest in urban public transport infrastructure, policy or finance' (Dodson et al. 2006, p. 4).

For the students in the *Fit to Drive* workshop at Groundwater College, and indeed for many young people now living in Melbourne (let alone regional and rural Victoria), the practical difficulties of acting on the advice to 'get another form of transport' are manifold. Alternative options do not always exist and, where they do, are often inadequate. The high cost of public transport, problems of erratic and uncoordinated public transport schedules, routes and connections, and serious concerns about safety have all been cited as significant obstacles to getting around for young people who live in the rapidly expanding outer-urban areas of Australia's second largest city (YACVic 2004, p. 29; Currie 2007, p. 89). These factors have contributed to the structural disadvantage identified as a feature of these areas, with a growing recognition of 'the potential emergence of "two Melbournes": a successful and "choice rich" inner core, and a fringe with fewer choices' (Ministerial Advisory Committee Metropolitan Planning Strategy 2012, p. 16), where high transport costs contribute to the economic and social difficulties of people living in these areas (Dowling and Willingham 2012).

As the working-class families vacated the inner city suburbs, from the 1970s the by now familiar process of 'gentrification' occurred. The wealthy, many of them middle-class professionals, flowed in as the quarries and council rubbish tips were turned into parks, the creeks rehabilitated and reforested, the terrace houses and bungalows snapped up and renovated. The factories, brickworks and warehouses my family and their friends worked in were turned into high-priced apartments, with the industrial history promoted as a 'desirable' feature, and the new inhabitants waxed lyrical about the working class and 'ethnic' charm of the place. As Dodson and Sipe (2008, p. 51) note: 'Since the 1960s the wealthy have retaken the historic city cores, with their abundance of jobs, services and public transport links', while 'the outer suburbs have been the places where those on the lowest incomes have been directed by housing and labour markets'.

'The Great Australian Dream Gets Dreamier'[3]

As the suburbs of Australian cities expanded—as they continue to expand—house blocks got smaller, but houses got bigger, and were promoted with increasingly luxurious options for the consumer, a trend that was already noticeable by the early 1980s, when a prominent

---

[3] 1980s advertising poster for housing industry builder AV Jennings

house building company proclaimed in an advertising poster, 'The great Australian dream gets dreamier' (Edwards et al. 2013, p. 105).

Just how dreamy is it? What is the legacy of the planning policies that left populations on the fringes of Melbourne without real alternative transport options to the car? In the era of neo-Liberal policy agendas that have seen government retreat even further from a responsibility for urban planning and regulation in favour of free market economics (Cook and Ruming 2008), it has been argued that suburban developments have been occurring in an increasingly 'market-driven ad hoc' fashion, unencumbered by a process of 'careful and considered strategy-led planning' (Buxton and Goodman 2014, p. 140). In Victoria, the government, having 'radically deregulated its land use planning system', and 'largely given planning away to private interests' has ceded 'unprecedented power to developers to determine the shape and function of [the] city' (Buxton 2014). How has this market-driven development, alongside the privatisation of transport and road building, affected the lives and well-being of those who have been drawn to them?

There is clear evidence that the poorly planned expansion of low-density, low-cost housing has entrenched structural inequalities. Several authors highlight the importance of transport in day-to-day life and have analysed the ways in which inequality of access to convenient, flexible and affordable transport exacerbate social disadvantage (Dodson et al. 2007; Smyth 2007; Maher 1994). Factors identified as contributing to 'locational disadvantage' associated with living in these areas include problems of poor access to public transport, services and appropriate infrastructure (YACVic 2004; Dodson et al. 2006; Lowe et al. 2015; Maher 1994):

> Although initially cheaper to purchase, these developments often incur higher 'hidden' on-going costs, as the lower residential densities are unable to support local services, employment and public transport infrastructure. (Badland et al. 2014, p.68)

Poor access to a motor vehicle and public transport can result in 'social isolation, reduced opportunities for meaningful employment and skill development and a cycle of debt' (Badland 2015, p. 27).

While much research focuses on transport to work (with limited access to employment in local municipalities, it is often necessary for many people to travel long distances to work by car), the lack of viable transport options is also a serious issue for increasing numbers of tertiary students. With limited incomes, many young students are obliged to travel long distances to university. Their reliance on the car places an additional financial, health and time burden on them (Mees 2010; YACVic 2004, p.30).

A consideration of the impact of car dependence reveals other problems associated with unplanned and under-resourced growth in suburban housing developments in 'greenfield sites'. Urban environments have been identified as 'an important determinant of health behaviours and outcomes' (Lowe et al. 2015, p. 132), and car dependence has been identified as one of the contributing factors to deterioration in health (Dodson et al. 2006), dislocation of communities, growth in pollution levels and general environmental degradation (Paterson 2007; Younger et al. 2008; Department of Infrastructure and Transport Commonwealth of Australia 2011). Dependence on the motor car has been directly associated with higher rates of traffic fatalities and injuries in comparison with cities that are better serviced by public transport (Coalition for People's Transport 2004, p.11). Health and community service providers point to poor planning as a major contributor to the creation of an 'obesogenic' community in one new outer suburban development (Johnston 2015), while elsewhere a range of factors associated with poor urban design were identified as leading to an epidemic in chronic illnesses such as obesity, heart disease and diabetes along with a decline in general well-being, an issue that has given rise to public and media discussion (Johnston 2015):

In many new estates on Melbourne's fringes there is a paucity of public transport, parks and open space. Schools and services are too far to walk to, large houses have swallowed backyards, commuters sit for long periods in traffic and fast food is often the only offering at the local convenience store. (Perkins 2012)

More recently, concern has been expressed about the impacts on food production and supply for Melbourne, as the food growing areas are taken over for residential development (Buxton et al. 2011). Projections for future sustainability of cities have identified the continuation of current levels of car use as unsustainable, with serious social and environmental consequences (Banister 2005, p. 247).

Increased isolation and reduced independence caused by lack of access to affordable, reliable and safe public transport have been identified as major issues related to the disadvantage that is experienced among vulnerable population groups, such as the elderly, disabled, families with small children and the young. Young people are identified as one of the groups additionally disadvantaged by inadequate transport options. Research and consultation with young people in outer-urban areas of Melbourne consistently cite difficulties with transport as a major concern, with serious impact on quality of life, educational and work opportunities (Karapetkos and McLeod 1992; Chang et al. 2001; Estridge and Cornell 2003; YACVic 2004; Currie 2007). 'Poor public transport' was highlighted by young people interviewed in a Youth Affairs Council of Victoria (YACVic) study as the 'worst thing about living in their area and something they would ideally change in their community to make it a better place in which to live' (YACVic 2004, p. 32). Lack of access to transport restricts opportunities for social and community activities and impacts on community connectedness (YACVic 2010). The increasing proportion of young people who live in the outer-urban suburbs, located on the 'interface' of urban Melbourne and the surrounding regional areas (NLT Consulting 2006; YACVic 2004) include many of the young people who participate in *Fit to Drive* programmes held in those areas, and 'access to public transport' has been consistently raised as an urgent issue in the *Fit to Drive* community youth forums held regularly in the programme catchment areas.

'You Always Have Choices'[4]

In this chapter, I have argued that the character of urban expansion in Australian cities, and the subsequent dependence on the car, has been shaped by the substantial economic interests and formidable political influence of the automotive and allied industry. Road safety occupies an interesting place in this relationship. Paterson (2007, p. 41) argues, for instance, that at critical points in its history, road safety has represented a key means for both industry and state to secure the acceptance and status of the private motor vehicle:

---

[4] 16 year old female student, St Helena Secondary College.

[O]ne could suggest that safety has been the principal site around which states and firms have acted to legitimise car culture, seeing the threats to personal safety as the core issue which could serve to delegitimise automobility.

The automotive industry became involved early in its history in lobbying to ensure that responsibility for the building and maintenance of roads designed for safe traffic of the car was devolved to government. Improved attention to car safety was taken up in the wake of consumer pressure in the 1960s (Nader 1965). Car companies have been visibly involved in the promotion of safety values while at the same time promoting cars for their qualities of speed, power, dominance, even danger. The safety promotion activities of road safety authorities have historically been closely associated with car industry 'product'. Attention is given to the promotion of 'safe car choices' on road safety authority websites and other sites of education and promotion such as the Transport Accident Commission (TAC) and Royal Automobile Club of Victoria (RACV)[5] (Harris and Thompson 2010). A focus on 'safety features', such as air bags, automated braking systems and other technologies designed to ensure the legitimacy of the car as safe and dependable, are promoted as desirable or compulsory features of different car models. Some areas of the car industry have given support to road safety promotion in other ways. Ultimately, these are legitimating activities that work to shore up the hegemony of the private automobile and the neglect of public transport.

The responsibility for making 'safe choices' in relation to transport is constructed as an individualised one: the individual as a good, responsible consumer (of safety features), and as a driver or passenger who is risk-aware and exercises responsibility and restraint. Road safety programmes such as Fit to Drive are firmly embedded in the governmental project of the cultivation of 'practices of the self' to produce the healthy (young) citizen (Lupton 1995; Kelly 2001, 2013): an 'ideal self'—'a self that is autonomous, choice making, prudent, risk aware, and, above all, responsible' (Kelly 2013; Montero and Kelly 2016). However, as I have argued

---

[5] The TAC is the state government-owned body, which is responsible for payment of treatment and benefits to people who have been injured in transport accidents. The RACV is motor vehicle users' member association. A major focus of both these organisations is the promotion of road safety.

here, there are complexities and intransigent realities behind this seemingly self-evident proposition of individualised choice. Jo Pike and Peter Kelly (2014), drawing on the work of Lee and Smith (2004), employ the insights offered by an understanding of the 'moral geographies' at work in the formation, expression and enactment of moral positions with respect to individualised 'choices' (food, transport, leisure, cultural and social practices) to analyse the 'moral geographies' of young people and food. As Pike and Kelly (2014, p. 187) remind us,

> the geographies that shape choices, and in which choices are made, are also fundamentally shaped by privilege and disadvantage, by wealth and poverty, by inclusion and marginalisation, by justice and injustice, in all their complex ambiguities, permutations and combinations.

Clearly, the scope for exercising choice for those with fewer resources is severely restricted. The options for exercising 'safe choices' in transport are contingent on the existence of realistic alternatives such as safe transport options for young people commuting to work, study and social events, and most crucially, a reliable, realistically accessible, affordable and safe public transport system.

In the Australian context of growing populations on the expanding urban–rural 'interface' areas of large cities, areas that are notoriously transport- and infrastructure-poor, 'healthy', 'responsible' alternatives do not exist. 'Safe options' are fundamentally shaped by spatial geographies that are, in turn, linked to economic and social disadvantage. For the increasing proportion of young people living in the outer-urban suburbs of Australian cities and the surrounding regional areas, who have been identified as experiencing distinct 'locational disadvantage', lack of transport has a serious impact on educational and work opportunities, quality of life and health and well-being. This is the context in which the young people who participate in *Fit to Drive* programmes, many of which are held in 'interface' or outer-urban areas, must exercise their 'safe choices' and 'individual responsibility'. This raises moral/ethical consideration for practitioners working in this domain. As Pike and Kelly (2014, p. 7) observe, 'moral geographies' also refer to the 'theoretical, epistemological and methodological choices that geographers and social scientists [educators, health promotion and human service practitioners] make', as well as the 'social, economic, cultural and political practices and processes that shape the projects and work and objects of study that we become concerned with'. The uncritical deployment of technologies of governance in health promotion interventions may serve to reinforce, or at least mask, spatial/social inequalities. In the same way, practicing within a framework that recognises the moral geographies at work may open up a space for transformative practices.

While we remain in thrall to the private motor vehicle and committed to ever increasing expansion of cities that become in effect 'two cities', young people on the geographical and social–economic margins will continue to experience the effects on their health, well-being, economic and educational opportunities. Many young people are growing up in a 'perfect storm' of historical neglect of basic infrastructure and community amenities, and public policies driven by market forces indifferent to the needs of the population. This is a situation that is further exacerbated by the more recent neo-Liberal reforms that have overseen the acceleration of the shift to the privatisation of planning for development, and the promotion of corporate interests which benefit from unchecked, poorly resourced development. In a time of neo-Liberal reform agendas, incremental government withdrawal from support services and programmes, and measures to shift the burden of economic crisis onto those who are already struggling, young people who depend on these services and supports are further disadvantaged. Perhaps we need to pay more thoughtful attention to what we owe to the young people from whom we demand 'safe choices'.

References

Badland, H., C. Whitzman, M. Lowe, M. Daverne, L. Aye, I. Butterworth, D. Hes, and B. Giles-Corti. 2014. Urban liveability: Emerging lessons from Australia for exploring the potential for indicators to measure the social determinants of health. *Social Science & Medicine* 111(2014): 64–73.

Badland, H., R. Roberts, I. Butterworth, D. Hes, and B. Giles-Corti. 2015. *How liveable is Melbourne? Conceptualising and testing urban liveability indicators: Progress to date.* Melbourne: McCaughey-VicHealth Community Well-being Unit.

Banister, D. 2005. *Unsustainable transport. City transport in the new century*. Oxfordshire: Routledge.

Boyd, R. 2010. *The Australian Ugliness*. Melbourne: Text Publishing.

Buxton, M. 2014. This is not a plan. It is a hoax driven by money. *The Age*. Available from: http://www.theage.com.au/comment/this-is-not-a-plan-it-is-a-hoax-driven-by-money-20131009-2v8hi.html. Accessed 8 Oct 2015.

Buxton, M., and R. Goodman. 2014. The impact of planning 'reform' on the Victorian land use planning system. *Australian Planner* 51(2): 132–140.

Buxton, M., A. Butt, S. Farrell, and A. Alvarez. 2011. Future of the fringe: Scenarios for Melbourne's peri-urban growth. In Carolyn Whitzman. *State of Australian Cities Conference*, ed. Ruth Fincher, 1–9. Melbourne, Australia. 29 November-2 December 2011.

Cannon, M. 1967. *Land boomers*. London: Melbourne University Press.

Chang, E., K. Dixon, and K. Hancock. 2001. Factors associated with risk-taking behaviour in Western Sydney's young people. *Youth Studies Australia* 20(4): 21–25.

Coalition for People's Transport. 2004. *The place to be on PT: A vision for greater Melbourne's transport*. Melbourne: Victorian Council of Social Services.

Cook, N., and K. Ruming. 2008. On the Fringe of Neoliberalism: Residential development in outer suburban Sydney. *Australian Geographer* 39(2): 211–228.

Country Roads Board. 1976a. The ecology of transportation. *CRB News*, August, No. 33.

———. 1976b. Freeways an asset. *CRB News*, August, No. 33.

———. 1976c. Melbourne's road needs. *CRB News*, December, No. 34.

Currie, G. 2007. Young Australians: No way to go. In *No way to go: Transport and social disadvantage in Australian communities*, eds. G. Currie, J. Stanley, and J. Stanley. Australia: Monash University ePress.

Department of Infrastructure and Transport, Commonwealth of Australia. 2011. *Our Cities, Our Future A national urban policy for a productive, sustainable and liveable future*. Canberra Australia: Government of Australia.

Dingle, T., and C. Rasmussen. 1991. *Vital connections Melbourne and its Board of Works 1891–1991*. Melbourne: McPhee Gribble.

Dodson, J. 2014. Factcheck: Do poor people drive less? *The Conversation*. Available from: http://theconversation.com/factcheck-do-poor-people-drive-less-30509. Accessed 15 Sept 2015.

Dodson, J., and N. Sipe. 2008. *Shocking the Suburbs: Oil Vulnerability in the Australian City*. Sydney: UNSW Press.

Dodson, J., B. Gleeson, R. Evans, and N. Sipe. 2006. Transport disadvantage in the Australian metropolis: Towards new concepts and methods. Proceedings of the Second National Conference on the State of Australian Cities, 30 November—2 December 2005. Griffith University, Brisbane, [online]. Available from: http://www.griffith.edu.au/__data/assets/pdf_file/0008/81386/infrastructure-03-dodsonpdf. Accessed 25 June 2012.

Dodson, J., N. Buchanan, B. Gleeson, and N. Sipe. 2007. Investigating the social dimensions of transport disadvantage—1. Towards new concepts and methods. *Urban Policy and Research* 24(4): 433–453.

Dowling, J., and W. Willingham. 2012. Tale of two cities a happy story for inner suburbs. *The Age.* [online]. Available from: http://www.smh.com.au/business/property/tale-of-two-cities-a-happy-story-for-inner-suburbs-20121026-28b7t.html. Accessed 22 Nov 2012.

Edwards, R., V. Jennings, and D. Garden. 2013. *AV Jennings: Home builders to the nation.* North Melbourne: Arcadia.

Estridge, O., and N. Cornell. 2003. *Whittlesea Youth Network Youth Needs Analysis.* Melbourne: Praxis Consulting.

Freestone, R. 2010. *Urban nation: Australia's planning heritage.* Collingwood Victoria: CSIRO.

Hardy, S., M. Hart, L. Albrects, and A. Katos, eds. 1995. *An enlarged Europe: Regions in competition.* London: Jessica Kingsley.

Harris, A., and H. Thompson. 2010. *The First Step. Royal Auto August 2010.* Melbourne: Royal Automobile Club of Victoria.

Hockey, J. 2014. Australian Federal Treasurer Joe Hockey, *ABC Radio,* August 13. Available from: http://jbh.ministers.treasury.gov.au/transcript/075-2014/.

Johnston, C. 2015. *The Age* [online]. Available from: http://www.theage.com.au/victoria/wyndham-region-home-to-victorias-sickest-suburbs-20150527-ghb05g.html. Accessed 15 Sept 2015.

Karapetkos, A., and J. Mcleod. 1992. *Too Far From Civilisation: Young People's Perceptions of Living in a Growth Corridor.* Melbourne: Youth Affairs Council of Victoria.

Kelly, P. 2001. Youth at Risk: Processes of individualisation and responsibilisation in the risk society. *Discourse: Studies in the Cultural Politics of Education* 22(1): 23–33.

———. 2013. *The self as enterprise: Foucault and the 'spirit' of 21st century capitalism.* Aldershot: Ashgate/Gower.

Lee, R., and D.M. Smith. 2004. *Geographies and moralities: International perspectives on development, justice and place.* Malden MA: Blackwell Publishing.

Lowe, M., C. Whitzman, H. Badland, M. Daverne, L. Aye, D. Hes, I. Butterworth, and B. Giles-Corti. 2015. Planning healthy, liveable and sustainable cities: How can indicators inform policy? *Urban Policy and Research* 33(2): 131—1144.

Lupton, D. 1995. *The imperative of health: public health and the regulated body.* London/Thousand Oaks. Sage Publications.

Maher, C. 1994. Residential mobility, locational disadvantage and spatial inequality in Australian cities. *Urban Policy and Research* 12(3): 185–191.

Mees, P. 2000. *A very public solution: Transport in the dispersed city.* Melbourne: Melbourne University Press.

———. 2010. *Transport for suburbia: Beyond the automobile age.* London: Earthscan.

Ministerial Advisory Committee. 2012. *Metropolitan Planning Strategy 2012, Melbourne, let's talk about the future: Discussion Paper.* Melbourne: State Government Victoria.

Montero, K., and P. Kelly. 2016. *The aesthetics of health promotion. Beyond risk, reason and rationality.* London: Routledge.

Nader, R. 1965. *Unsafe at any speed: The designed-dangers of the American automobile.* New York: Grossman.

NLT Consulting PTY Ltd. 2006. *Staying connected. Solutions for addressing service gaps for young people living at the Interface. A report of the Melbourne Interface Councils.* Melbourne: Author.

Paterson, M. 2007. *Automobile politics, ecology and cultural political economy.* Cambridge: Cambridge University Press.

Perkins, M. 2012. *The Age* [online]. Available from: http://www.domain.com.au/news/health-fear-on-estates-20120314-1v3lw/. Accessed 15 Sept 2015.

Pike, J., and P. Kelly. 2014. *The moral geographies of children, young people and food. Beyond Jamie's school dinners.* Basingstoke: Palgrave Macmillan.

Smyth, P. 2007. Transport: A new frontier for social policy. In *No way to go: Transport and social disadvantage in Australian communities*, eds. G. Currie, J. Stanley, and J. Stanley. Australia: Monash University ePress.

Spencer, G., and K. Montero (2011). Empowering youth in schools to be safer road users; peer-led by undergraduates. *Australian Council of Road Safety Conference*, September 2011, Melbourne.

Tonts, M., and F.H. Mckenzie. 2005. Neoliberalism and changing regional policy in Australia. *International Planning Studies* 10(3–4): 183–200.

Younger, M., H. Morrow-Almeida, S. Vindigni, and A. Dannenberg. 2008. The built environment, climate change, and health: Opportunities and co-benefits. *American Journal of Preventative Medicine* 35: 517–526.

Youth Affairs Council of Victoria. 2004. *Snapshot from the edge. Young people and service providers on the urban fringe of Melbourne.* Melbourne: YacVic.

———. 2010. *A response to the Inquiry into the Extent and Nature of Disadvantage and Inequity in Rural and Regional Victoria.* Melbourne: YacVic.

9

Shame, Disgust and the Moral Economies of Young Women's Sexual Health in the North of England

Louise Laverty

Introduction

The range of austerity measures implemented in the UK following the Global Financial Crisis of 2008 has been accompanied by, and justified through, emotive and stigmatising discourses that recast blame on those suffering the greatest inequalities (Clayton et al. 2015; Tyler 2013). As a number of authors have noted, heightened stigmatisation in recent UK public and political discourse has created a division between the 'deserving' and 'undeserving' poor in society (Hancock and Mooney 2012; Tyler 2013; Wacquant 2009; Wacquant 2008). Most notably, as part of this shift in attitudes, poverty has been recast as the moral failure of the individual rather than the result of structural inequalities (Slater 2014; Valentine and Harris 2014; Wacquant 2008). This discourse is particularly evident

L. Laverty (✉)
University of Liverpool, Liverpool, UK

© The Editor(s) (if applicable) and The Author(s) 2017
P. Kelly, J. Pike (eds.), *Neoliberalism, Austerity, and the
Moral Economies of Young People's Health and Well-being*,
DOI 10.1057/978-1-137-58266-9_10

179

in the UK's Child Poverty Strategy (2011, p.4) where behavioural rather than structural causes are outlined. The cause of child poverty, according to this strategy, is 'a lack of opportunity, aspiration and stability' among children and their families, a lack that can be tackled by reducing criminality, teenage pregnancies and risky behaviour. To experience poverty, therefore, is to occupy a stigmatised social position (Ridge 2011; Ridge 2009; Sutton 2009) that people seek to distance and differentiate themselves from (Shildrick and MacDonald 2013).

Stigma, according to Goffman (1963), is often experienced through feelings of guilt and shame that arise from certain activities or discreditable social positions. It is important, then, to examine the role of emotions in the process of stigma (Lupton 2014; Sayer 2005). In exploring the use of emotions in policy, Lupton (2014, p.11) reports that certain campaigns are 'directed at arousing fear, shame, disgust as a means to promote the self-disciplined citizen'. In other words, emotions are used to create stigma with the aim of encouraging self-regulation and changing social norms (Bayer 2008). In this paper, I illustrate how stigma, enforced through shame and disgust, operates as a form of social control through the marking of moral boundaries around sexuality. Focusing on the experience of a young girl attending a youth club in a disadvantaged neighbourhood in the North of England, I explore how the social role of emotions affects who does, or does not, belong. Most importantly, I illustrate the very real consequences for young people experiencing shame and stigmatisation.

The Politics of Emotion

Sociological theories of emotion take a cultural approach that sees emotions both as embodied and social (Ahmed 2004; Hochschild 1979; Lutz and Abu-Lughod 1990). As such, emotions can be understood as involved in conveying socio-cultural messages (Geertz 1973) and signalling moral worth and value (Lutz 1990). In other words, emotions act as moral evaluations that 'come to articulate what are often unspoken sentiments in contemporary society about class, gender, sexuality, and ethnicity' (Nayak and Kehily 2014, p.1331). Emotions, therefore, do something; they are not simply the product of external disapproval (Sayer 2005). They create and reinforce boundaries that distinguish between those who are morally worthy and unworthy. Therefore, emotions are both relational and social, and in what follows, I briefly summarise the literature related to shame and disgust demonstrating how these emotions act as a form of social control.

Shame is defined as a bodily manifestation and social expression, a congruence of feeling, emotion and affects (Probyn 2004). It has been described as

a painful, sudden awareness of the self as less good than hoped for and expected, precipitated by the identification by others (imaginary or real) or simply by the ashamed self. (Manion 2003, p.21)

It differs from guilt in that shame involves the negative appraisal of self, while guilt results from a specific behaviour or action (Lewis 1992; Manion 2003). Shame is an emotion that is aroused by a crisis, drawing attention to a moral breach, which results in anticipated or felt stigma (Scambler 2004, 2009). This suggests that shame can act as a normalising gaze that makes it possible to classify and consequently punish those who transgress moral norms.

In a similar way to shame, disgust is embodied and is an emotion produced by social norms (Lupton 2014). Often viewed as a reflex because of the physical nature of the emotion, Kolnai (2004) argues that it is not only material objects that elicit disgust, but moral worth and character that also cause a reaction. Disgust acts by linking our senses and bodily experiences and often adheres to the object or person that is its cause (Kolnai et al. 2004). Importantly, like shame, it creates and maintains boundaries. It does so when there is shared revulsion at behaviours and people that betray social norms (Deigh 2006). In sum, shame and disgust demonstrate the link between the embodied physical experience and the social role of emotion that allows moral judgements and values to be felt, and therefore to become real.

The Governance of Respectable Sexuality

There is an abundance of literature examining the moral panics around women and girls' sexualities and how they are constructed as intrinsically problematic (Renold and Ringrose 2008, 2011, Ringrose and Barajas

2011; Ringrose and Renold 2012; Skeggs 2005; Walkerdine 2011). These moral panics are constructed and shaped by a complex range of intersecting social identities and positions including, but not limited to, gender, hetero-normativity, class, age and race (Karaian 2014; Mattis et al. 2008; McCall 2005; Skeggs 2005). Skeggs (1997) and Lawler (2005), for example, have described how white working-class women are constantly challenged to perform respectable forms of femininity in order to avoid shame. On the other hand, disadvantaged black women and girls are often hyper-sexualised (Mattis et al. 2008) in ways that can leave them more vulnerable to stigma when they fail to achieve acceptable femininity. This suggests that although there may be common outcomes of moral panics around sexuality, the designation of shame and disgust, for example, may be experienced differently. As Mattis et al. (2008, p.419) note, 'one is neither a singularly gendered, racialized nor classed being'.

The 'respectable femininity' that women are judged by, however, is likely to be based on a similar stereotype of whiteness, pureness and middle-class heterosexual femininity. Karaian (2014) suggests that this 'respectable femininity' is a neo-Liberal strategy of responsibilisation to govern women through shame. Within a neo-Liberal context, individuals are encouraged to be moderate, rational, decision makers in control of their bodies. Those who are constructed as responsible can be managed through self-governance while those who fail are subject to intervention (Adam 2005; Rose 1996). Young women, in particular, are said to be increasingly the focus of neo-Liberal regulation (Harris 2004) that encourages 'responsibility to choose good choices, second to take responsibility for the consequences of those choices, and third, being responsible for making those choices' (Graham 2007, p.205).

The Common: An Ethnography of an English Youth Club

This chapter draws on an ethnographic study of a youth club in the North of England conducted between June 2012 and September 2013. The study explored the conditions that enabled or constrained young people's ability to participate in their neighbourhood, focusing particularly on the role of welfare and wider cuts, and the practices that young people use to establish and maintain value and inclusion among their peers. This included, for example, moral economies of care in which food circulated among young people in the context of food poverty. The ethnography consisted of 14 months of participant-observation generated through more than 400 hours of data collection, alongside 15 photo elicitation and visual mapping interviews, 3 focus groups and numerous informal interviews with attendees.

The advantage of using ethnography with young people, as noted by other prominent authors in the field (Christensen 1993; Hammersley and Atkinson 1983; James et al. 1998; James and Prout 1997), is that it allows members' interests and priorities to emerge and direct the research, and 'emphasises working with people rather than treating them as objects' (Wolcott 1999, p.66). I consulted with the young people about what methods, if any, would be acceptable to them and I tried to remain adaptable in my approach.

The majority of my fieldwork occurred in the enclosed space of the youth centre, the Common. The Common is a youth and community centre situated in the neighbourhood of Sandyhill on the outskirts of a midsize town. The neighbourhood is one of the most deprived wards nationally in the Indices of Multiple Deprivation, which were used as a proxy to support the self-identification of the area as working class (Department for Communities and Local Government 2015). Furthermore, local statistics showed that the area reported lower-than-average life expectancies (compared with regional and national figures), worse rates of unemployment, and lower educational attainment than the UK average.

The Common was established four decades ago, as a boys' club. The commemorative sign from its opening as a boys' club is still displayed at the entrance to the building, and despite a few extensions over the years, the main hub of the centre is the original design. However, over the decades, the building has fallen into a state of disrepair due to a lack of funding. While the centre is independent of the council youth services that have been subject to intense cuts over the past few years, they are dependent on charitable donations which have become increasingly difficult to secure in a financial climate dominated by austerity and cuts to statutory funding.

The youth centre is open six days a week all year round and is open for younger children (5–10 years, the 'juniors') during the afternoons and for teenagers (11–25 years, the 'seniors') later in the evenings. The senior session runs from 6.30 to 9.30 pm, and until 11 pm during school holidays. It is free for young people to attend and the majority of the attendees live in the local area, often within a few minutes' walk. On a typical night, the centre can expect anywhere in the region of 30–80 young people, depending on the night of the week and the weather. The majority of the attendees are boys, who tend to arrive at the start of each session and stay until the end, joining in one of the activities in the main room, pool tables and table tennis, or go to play football or basketball in the gym. In contrast, the few girls that attend are likely to drop in periodically over the course of the evening. The girls never come into the centre unaccompanied and organise to meet with friends beforehand.

The managers of the youth club, recognising that girls were often reluctant to come into the Common and join in activities, decided to open up a girls' room. As a result, the girls were constantly encouraged out of the main room by staff and into the assigned girls' room to get 'peace from the boys'. In creating the girls' room, therefore, the staff unwittingly signalled that the rest of the youth club was the boys' space. As well as *how* space was assigned, *what* space was assigned is also important. No 'male space' was given up in order to make room for the girls. Instead, a disused room on the periphery of the building was opened. This disused room had no heating and faulty lighting. In other words, nothing valuable was given up.

Girls at the Common

During my time at the Common, the neighbourhood Sandyhill was the subject of public scrutiny that frequently labelled the area as a problematic 'ghetto'. In what Wacquant (2007, 2008) describes as 'place stigma', Sandyhill was characterised as a troubled, and thus undesirable, place internationally, nationally and locally. In particular, a spokesperson from the United Nations caused controversy by describing several areas in the North of England, similar to Sandyhill, as 'no-go areas' through drug and gang warfare, comparing them to Brazilian Favelas (Brown 2012). In response to the 2011 riots, the UK Prime Minister David Cameron lamented the 'slow-motion moral collapse' (Cabinet Office 2011) in such communities, seen as the fault of broken families, in order to justify interventions such as the Troubled Families Programme[1] (Fletcher et al. 2012). Closer to home, the young people at the Common were described as 'yobs' and 'gangs' in the local press.

While Sandyhill has a history of disadvantage and a lack of investment, the introduction of austerity measures has further exacerbated insecurity in the area. The range of cuts implemented after the election of the UK Coalition Government in 2010, such as abolition of the Education Maintenance Allowance[2] (Chowdry and Emmerson 2010) and the Welfare Reform Act (The UK Government 2012)[3], has affected young people living in Sandyhill. The ways in which these measures are experienced often varies by age, gender and ethnicity. For example, for boys and particularly non-white boys, increased surveillance and the use of Antisocial Behaviour Orders have meant displacement and exclusion in public spaces and often the neighbourhood. For girls, the introduction of the bedroom tax disrupted kinship care arrangements that had previously mitigated the experience of disadvantage. Kinship care refers to being under the care of an extended family member that helps avoid the involvement of the state and allows the young person to remain in a familiar place with familiar people (Leinaweaver 2013, 2014).

The role of kinship care was an essential and normal practice around the Common, and mainly affected the girls. There was fluidity in the girls' home lives, moving between kinship care, more commonly with female caregivers, homes and foster care. The availability of a spare room with an aunt or grandmother was a general resource that helped the girls mitigate potential conflicts with parents and was essential following the illness or death of a parent. Almost all of the young people I engaged with

---

[1] A compulsory family intervention programme

[2] This allowance helped young people to attend further post-16 education and was found to be particularly successful in getting young people from the poorest families to stay on in education (Chowdry and Emmerson 2010)

[3] Which includes the under-occupancy housing penalty also known as the bedroom tax

at the Common had experienced at least one significant loss prior to the age of 14: parents, grandparents, aunts and uncles, siblings and friends.

In addition to, and perhaps because of, unstable and precarious home lives, the girls' attendance at the Common was sporadic at best. The boys dominated the main space; they controlled the activities in that space and were the recipients of the majority of funding. For example, funding for sporting equipment disproportionately benefited the boys, and they were given priority to take part in any funded activities. The girls frequently commented on the lack of resources and interest from the youth centre that had only allocated a girls' room on the outskirts of the building. Furthermore, the girls were subject to hostility from the boys, particularly those girls perceived to be sexually active. The boys were rarely punished for this behaviour, instead the girls were told to move away into their periphery space. As a result, many of the girls, after being on the receiving end of this antagonism, chose to leave the Common.

The regional youth services manager, Carrie, described the girls at the Common as 'the most troubled'. In particular, she suggests that a number of the girls 'use sex as a way of getting attention and affection'. During my time at the Common, five girls were publicly vilified as 'sluts' or 'slags'. All of the girls were in the care system, moving between formal placements and informal kinship care. Two girls, Jade (14, White British) and Kayla (14, mixed-race) were not from Sandyhill and so were already marked as outsiders. Hailey (14, mixed-race), Kima (15, Black British) and Jordan (15, Black British) grew up in the area. The five girls, in different ways, were seen as responsible not only for their actions, but also for the consequences of their sexual reputation and activity. In what follows, I focus my discussion on one of the girls, Jade, to explore how shame manifests itself in the everyday experiences of young women.

Jade: An Abject Figure?

Jade was a girl that I had repeated contact with and that other young people at the Common talked to me about. I had heard about Jade, before I ever met her. Jade, I am told, is 14 and is named as a 'slag'. She is first mentioned by Asia (14, Black British), her boyfriend Reuben (13, mixed-race) and Raymond (11, Black British) sitting talking in the girls' room. They are questioning why Jade comes to the Common, and Reuben replies 'you know why'. They quickly start talking about the boys (and men) that Jade has reportedly slept with. Asia mentions that Jade always talks about sleeping with Black men, but says that Jade is a racist. Reuben calls her disgusting. Raymond comments that he had heard Jade had been raped in the past. Asia and Reuben scoff and Asia replies, 'It's not rape if you enjoy it'.

In this initial exchange, the stories about Jade that circulate at the Common are first exposed. Jade is regarded as wholly responsible for her behaviour. Even when there are reports that Jade has been raped, the blame is projected back on to her. This is evoked through the idea of pleasure. Jade is ultimately deemed responsible to maintain and manage the boundaries of her body and thus is responsible for her 'failures'. I first meet Jade a few weeks later when she comes into the Centre with Carolyn (16, mixed-race), who she lives with in foster care, and Shannon (14, White British). Jade wears a red baseball cap that she keeps pulling over her short cropped hair, but other than this detail her clothing resembles the 'uniform' of the other girls. Jade immediately draws attention, the gaze of others fixing on her as she walks though the centre, and later that night we are told she is pregnant.

A few weeks later, however, I hear a different story from Shannon and Carolyn. Shannon's phone keeps going off, and Carolyn seems agitated. I ask what is going on and they explain that they are having a fight online on Blackberry Messenger (BBM) with Jade. I ask why and they tell me that they are not friends with her any more as she is a liar and has been saying things about Carolyn's family. Shannon tells me 'Jade isn't pregnant'. 'Well...' says Carolyn, 'I heard she got jumped and she lost it'. Shannon says she also heard that Jade had an abortion; 'so who knows', she says going back to her phone. She shows me the last message they sent each other, which is filled with expletives and ends with 'you stupid slag'. Shannon and Carolyn cut all ties with Jade explaining that the only reason they were friends with Jade in the first place was because they felt sorry for her, referring to the death of her mother. The girls are very vocal about their disapproval of Jade, and work to publicly distance themselves from her. It was as if any association with Jade would taint or contaminate them.

The concept of contamination was a big issue with regards to Jade. Jade only had two consistent friendships at the Common, with Jess (16, mixed-race) and Ruthie (14, Black British). Jade tried to initiate a number of other friendships but they quickly dissolved once they got to know of Jade's reputation. Ruthie explains that she gets a hard time for being friends with Jade, with other people at school asking why she is friends with a 'slut'. She has become tainted with the same label and derision as Jade. Ruthie has to explain to them that just because Jade is 'a slut does not mean I am'. She also tells me that she has started to understand that it is Jade's body, and if that is what she want to do with it then 'that's fine'; it does not affect *her* [Ruthie's] body.

In a later discussion, Ruthie tells me she does not agree with how Jade is treated, but also confides that she thinks 'Jade likes the attention, even if it is bad'. As evidence of this, Ruthie gets out her phone, showing me Jade's BBM profile. Jade's profile picture is a selfie; she is wearing false eyelashes and red lipstick and is pouting towards the camera with her arms pushed against her chest. Ruthie says 'it's bad isn't it, wait you should see the older one, it is worse'. The style of Jade's older picture is the same except she is only wearing a bra. 'See?' Ruthie tells me, 'she likes the attention'. In showing me these pictures, Ruthie is suggesting that Jade is actively pursuing attention, refuting norms of girls as passive, through a specific unacceptable form of visibility. Ruthie sees the pictures as attention seeking, which transfers from online to offline behaviour. In the following months, there are a number of reports that there are explicit images of Jade circulating at the centre and although there are disputes about who circulated the pictures, Jade is ultimately blamed for them. The consensus at the Common is that by pursuing and enjoying attention, Jade is deserving of the consequences.

Indeed, there are consequences to Jade's behaviour. She is subject to abuse on a regular basis. From the girls this sometimes takes the form of refusing to acknowledge Jade's presence, or more explicitly by loudly shouting across the room 'eugh, what is she doing here, no one wants her here'. The boys, in contrast, are more likely to publicly shame Jade, shouting and sneering about her behaviour as she walks past, calling her 'fucking foul'. One evening, Tyler (15, Black British) repeatedly attempts to shame Jade. Throughout the evening he follows her around the Common taunting her: looking, sneering and calling her disgusting in front of an audience, behaviour that is designed to elicit a shame response. She chooses to ignore this, pretending she has not heard him. After receiving no response, Tyler tries again, in front of a different audience, escalating the volume and explicit content that Jade could not fail to miss. He is publicly displaying his disapproval for her behaviour. Jade is expected to respond to this shaming, perhaps to show remorse, but instead chooses to feign ignorance, which is misunderstood as bravado. However, it was not only verbal assaults and threats that faced Jade. On a number of occasions, while I was at the Common, Jade was physically assaulted. Her status as a 'slag' was explicitly linked to the assaults.

Some of the youth workers colluded in avoiding engaging with Jade, warning me 'don't let her drag you in; she has done it to all of us, getting attention, telling lies, getting sympathy. Don't get involved'. Youth worker Robin's words echo the other young people, 'I don't even know why she comes here. I went to her house, when she was in foster care, and she was so rude to me, so rude, and just lies upon lies, I want nothing to do with her'. The youth workers, by refusing to work with Jade, reinforce the moral boundaries around the centre and collude in her stigmatisation. Jade is treated as undeserving of their support, a contamination that must be avoided. Jade stops coming in regularly, but she continues to be discussed, almost serving as a cautionary tale. Shortly after I finish fieldwork, Jade is reported as missing.

Conclusion: The Moral Dimensions of Shaming

I have argued that Jade is punished for her alleged sexual activity, regarded as morally deviant, through shame and disgust. This moral condemnation is rationalised through positioning Jade as deserving of punishment. This is evident in the incident in which Jade's rape is dismissed, but also in the way that the boys talk about Jade with one boy telling me 'if she's a lady treat her like a lady, if she's a whore treat her like a whore'. In addition, Jade's unrespectable feminine behaviour is racialised and classed in the way that she is positioned as 'white trash' by other young people. This is particularly important given that within the ethnically diverse neighbourhood of Sandyhill, being white is a marker of being an outsider. The other girls at the Common, who come from different ethnic backgrounds, have different experiences of slut shaming. What they have in common, however, is the use of shame that categorises them as deserving to be treated according to their status and behaviour. Here, 'slut-shaming' is a form of neo-Liberal governance with other young people taking the role of intervening in Jade's behaviour due to her failure to manage and control her own risk and body. Indeed, as the boys are not punished for this behaviour, they could interpret their actions as acceptable and necessary. It is intended to bring Jade back in line. While this finding is not new, the role of emotion provides a new way of examining the disciplinary practices that impact on girls. Shame and disgust is a way of marking moral boundaries that determine acceptable and unacceptable behaviour.

At the Common, Jade's personal life is publicly owned and shared. In contrast, in my year of knowing Jade, I never hear her side of the story. She strictly refused to talk about the subject. Perhaps discussing her experiences would mean that she had to recognise and acknowledge the shame imposed on her, thus, her safety was in her silence. In addition, it is clear from the example above that there are consequences to what has been termed 'slut-shaming' (e.g. Ringrose and Renold 2012). Jade and the other girls at the Common suffer through the shame imposed by others. As well as the withdrawal of friendship from their peers, and withdrawal of care from youth workers, the girls are also physically punished. Jade and Hailey are physically assaulted, while some of the other girls, such as Kima and Jordan, self-harm as a result of their stigmatisation. Furthermore, the girls are 'adultified' as they are treated as responsible for their behaviour. As Mattis et al. (2008) and others have warned, the adultification of girls can result in the withdrawal of protection from abuse as they are seen as complicit. The very real consequences mean that we should regard the role of emotion and stigma as strategies of exclusion.

Although I am drawing on the specific case of the youth club, it is interesting to note that these findings are echoed in other work that demonstrates that girls and women become particularly visible as 'sexualised bodies' (Puwar 2006). The girls at the Common become visible when they are perceived to violate acceptable forms of feminine sexuality, leading to exclusion. It is important to consider that this exclusion draws on existing social norms. Looking at the Common and its gender norms, it is clear that the centre's prioritisation of the boys and marginalisation of the girls have much deeper impacts than simply confining the girls to the periphery. Opotow (1990, p.1) has argued that the 'morally excluded are perceived as non-entities, expendable or undeserving, consequently harming them appears acceptable, appropriate or just'. I would argue that the shaming of Jade does exactly this.

In conclusion, this chapter has explored the social role of emotions in generating and regulating stigma and creating exclusion. This is important to consider as stigma is increasingly utilised as an acceptable and necessary force to change behaviour in public policy (Bayer 2008; Burris 2008; Karaian 2014). 'Slut-shaming' is a tactic that tries to reinforce certain sexual norms and punish deviance through evoking shame, disgust and guilt. Instead, it leads to exclusion and blames the individual for their deviance or failure. In turn, as issues such as poverty are subject to similar moral discourses, such as 'welfare-shaming', we are likely to see similar experiences of exclusion and blame laid at the feet of individuals (Clayton et al. 2015; Tyler 2013). Perhaps we should be more concerned with questioning who is being shamed and stigmatised and by whom.

References

Adam, B.D. 2005. Constructing the neoliberal sexual actor: Responsibility and care of the self in the discourse of barebackers. *Culture, Health & Sexuality* 7: 333–346.

Ahmed, S. 2004. *The Cultural Politics of Emotions*. Edinburgh: Edinburgh University Press.

Bayer, R. 2008. Stigma and the ethics of public health: Not can we but should we. *Social Science & Medicine* 67: 463–472.

Brown, J. 2012. UN says Liverpool has drug-related 'no-go areas' like those in Brazilian favelas. *The Independent* [online]. Available from: http://www.independent.co.uk/news/uk/crime/un-says-liverpool-has-drug-related-no-go-areas-like-those-in-brazilian-favelas-7462654.html. Accessed 6 June 2014.

Burris, S. 2008. Stigma, ethics and policy: A commentary on Bayer's "Stigma and the ethics of public health: Not can we but should we". *Social Science & Medicine* 67: 473–475.

Cabinet Office. 2011. PM's speech on the fightback after the riots. Available from: https://www.gov.uk/government/speeches/pms-speech-on-the-fightback-after-the-riots. Accessed 12 Mar 2014

Chowdry, H., and C. Emmerson. 2010. *An Efficient Maintenance Allowance?* London: Institute for Fiscal Studies.

Christensen, P.H. 1993. The social construction of help among Danish children: The intentional act and the actual content. *Sociology of Health & Illness* 15: 488–502.

Clayton, J., C. Donovan, and J. Merchant. 2015. Emotions of austerity: Care and commitment in public service delivery in the North East of England. *Emotion, Space and Society* 14: 24–32.

Deigh, J. 2006. The politics of disgust and shame. *The Journal of Ethics* 10: 383–418.

Department for Communities and Local Government. 2015. *The English Indices of Deprivation 2015*. London: National Statistics.

Department for Work and Pensions & Department for Education. 2011. *A New Approach to Child Poverty: Tackling the Causes of Disadvantage and Transforming Families' Lives*. London: The Stationery Office.

Fletcher, A., F. Gardner, M. Mckee, and C. Bonell. 2012. The British Government's Troubled Families Programme. *BMJ* 344: e3403.

Geertz, C. 1973. *The Interpretation of Cultures: Selected Essays*. New York: Basic Books.

Goffman, E. 1963. *Stigma: Notes on the Management of Spoiled Identity*. Englewood Cliffs, NJ: Prentice Hall.

Graham, L.J. 2007. (Re)Visioning the Centre: Education reform and the 'ideal' citizen of the future. *Educational Philosophy and Theory* 39: 197–215.

Hammersley, M., and P. Atkinson. 1983. *Ethnography: Principles in practice*. London: Routledge.

Hancock, L., and G. Mooney. 2012. "Welfare Ghettos" and the "Broken Society": Territorial Stigmatization in the Contemporary UK. *Housing, Theory and Society* 30: 46–64.

Harris, A. 2004. *Future Girl*. In *Young women in the 21st Century*. New York, London: Routledge.

Hochschild, A.R. 1979. Emotion Work, Feeling Rules, and Social Structure. *American Journal of Sociology* 85: 551–575.

James, A., C. Jenks, and A. Prout. 1998. *Theorizing Childhood*. Cambridge, UK: Polity Press in association with Blackwell Publishers Ltd.

James, A., and A. Prout, eds. 1997. *Constructing and Reconstructing Childhood: Contemporary Issues in the Sociological Study of Childhood*. London, Washington: Falmer Press.

Karaian, L. 2014. Policing 'sexting': Responsibilization, respectability and sexual subjectivity in child protection/crime prevention responses to teenagers' digital sexual expression. *Theoretical Criminology* 18: 282–299.

Kolnai, A. 2004. *On Disgust*. Peru, Illinois: Open Court Publishing Company.

Kolnai, A., B. Smith, and C. Korsmeyer, eds. 2004. *On disgust*. Chicago, IL: Open Court.

Lawler, S. 2005. Disgusted subjects: The making of middle-class identities. *The Sociological Review* 53: 429–446.

Leinaweaver, J. 2014. Informal Kinship-Based Fostering Around the World: Anthropological Findings. *Child Development Perspectives* 8: 131–136.

Leinaweaver, J.B. 2013. Towards an Anthropology of Ingratitude: Notes from Andean Kinship. *Comparative Studies in Society and History* 55: 554–578.

Lewis, M. 1992. *Shame: The Exposed Self*. New York: The Free Press.

Lupton, D. 2014. The pedagogy of disgust: The ethical, moral and political implications of using disgust in public health campaigns. *Critical Public Health* 25: 4–14.

Lutz, C.A. 1990. Engendered emotion: Gender, power, and the rhetoric of emotional control in American discourse. In *Language and the politics of emotion*, eds. C.A. Lutz and L. Abu-Lughod. Cambridge: Cambridge University Press.

Lutz, C.A., and L. Abu-Lughod, eds. 1990. *Language and the politics of emotion*. Cambridge: Cambridge University Press.

Manion, J.C. 2003. Girls Blush, Sometimes: Gender, Moral Agency, and the Problem of Shame. *Hypatia* 18: 21–41.

Mattis, J.S., N.A. Grayman, S.-A. Cowie, C. Winston, C. Watson, and D. Jackson. 2008. Intersectional Identities and the Politics of Altruistic Care in a Low-Income, Urban Community. *Sex Roles* 59: 418–428.

Mccall, L. 2005. The Complexity of Intersectionality. *Signs* 30: 1771–1800.

Nayak, A., and M.J. Kehily. 2014. 'Chavs, chavettes and pramface girls': Teenage mothers, marginalised young men and the management of stigma. *Journal of Youth Studies* 17: 1330–1345.

Opotow, S. 1990. Moral Exclusion and Injustice: An Introduction. *Journal of Social Issues* 46: 1–20.

Probyn, E. 2004. *Blush: Faces of Shame*. Minneapolis: University of Minnesota.

Puwar, N. 2006. Im/possible Inhabitations. In *The Situated Politics of Belonging*, eds. N. Yuval-Davis, K. Kannabiran, and U. Vieten. London: Sage.

Renold, E., and J. Ringrose. 2008. Regulation and rupture: Mapping tween and teenage girls' resistance to the heterosexual matrix. *Feminist Theory* 9: 313–338.

————. 2011. Schizoid subjectivities?: Re-theorizing teen girls' sexual cultures in an era of 'sexualization'. *Journal of Sociology* 47: 389–409.

Ridge, T. 2009. *Living with poverty: A review of the literature on children's and families' experiences of poverty*. London: Department for Work and Pensions.

————. 2011. The Everyday Costs of Poverty in Childhood: A Review of Qualitative Research Exploring the Lives and Experiences of Low-Income Children in the UK. *Children & Society* 25: 73–84.

Ringrose, J., and K.E. Barajas. 2011. Gendered risks and opportunities? Exploring teen girls' digitized sexual identities in postfeminist media contexts. *International Journal of Media and Cultural Politics* 7: 121–138.

Ringrose, J., and E. Renold. 2012. Slut-shaming, girl power and 'sexualisation': Thinking through the politics of the international SlutWalks with teen girls. *Gender and Education* 24: 333–343.

Rose, N. 1996. The death of the social? Re-figuring the territory of government. *Economy and Society* 25: 327–356.

Sayer, A. 2005. Class, Moral Worth and Recognition. *Sociology* 39: 947–963.

Scambler, G. 2004. Re-framing Stigma: Felt and Enacted Stigma and Challenges to the Sociology of Chronic and Disabling Conditions. *Social Theory & Health* 2: 29–46.

————. 2009. Health-related stigma. *Sociology of Health & Illness* 31: 441–455.

Shildrick, T., and R. Macdonald. 2013. Poverty talk: How people experiencing poverty deny their poverty and why they blame 'the poor'. *The Sociological Review* 61: 285–303.

Skeggs, B. 1997. *Formations of Class and Gende: Becoming Respectable*. London: Sage.

Skeggs, B. 2005. The Making of Class and Gender through Visualizing Moral Subject Formation. *Sociology* 39: 965–982.

Slater, T. 2014. The Myth of "Broken Britain": Welfare Reform and the Production of Ignorance. *Antipode* 46: 948–969.

Sutton, L. 2009. 'They'd only call you a scally if you are poor': The impact of socio-economic status on children's identities. *Children's Geographies* 7: 277–290.

The UK Government. 2012. Welfare Reform Act 2012. The United Kingdom.

Tyler, I. 2013. The Riots of the Underclass?: Stigmatisation, Mediation and the Government of Poverty and Disadvantage in Neoliberal Britain. *Sociological Research Online* 18: 6.

Valentine, G., and C. Harris. 2014. Strivers vs skivers: Class prejudice and the demonisation of dependency in everyday life. *Geoforum* 53: 84–92.

Wacquant, L. 2007. Territorial Stigmatization in the Age of Advanced Marginality. *Thesis Eleven* 91: 66–77.

———. 2008. *Urban Outcasts: A Comparative Sociology of Advanced Marginality.* Cambridge: Polity Press.

———. 2009. *Punishing the Poor.* Durham, NC: Duke University Press.

Walkerdine, S. 2011. Shame on you! Intergenerational Trauma and Working Class Femininity on Reality TV. In *Reality Television and Class*, eds. H. Wood and B. Skeggs. London: Palgrave Macmillan on behalf of the London Film Institute.

Wolcott, H.F. 1999. *Ethnography: A Way of Seeing.* Oxford, UK: AltaMira Press.

10

We Need Child Poverty! Making Sense of Public Attitudes to Poverty in the Age of Austerity

John McKendrick

Deceptively Straightforward: Making Sense of Child Poverty in an Era of Neo-Liberal Austerity

Child poverty is about children not having enough. This is not contentious and seems not to be complicated. In advanced economies, we often first learn that ours is a world with child poverty in schools. Children are familiarised with the realities of life for those presented as less fortunate in other places (contemporary global geographies of poverty) and at other times (local histories of poverty). As adults, we are presented with imagery of children in poverty to induce charitable donations as part of international responses to natural or political disasters. Creating a sense of a comfortable 'us', with responsibilities to a needy 'them' generate resources

J. McKendrick (✉)
Glasgow Caledonian University, Glasgow, UK

© The Editor(s) (if applicable) and The Author(s) 2017   **197**
P. Kelly, J. Pike (eds.), *Neoliberalism, Austerity, and the
Moral Economies of Young People's Health and Well-being,*
DOI 10.1057/978-1-137-58266-9_11

that can be used to ameliorate problems and lay the foundations for solutions to poverty. Paradoxically, the terra firma of global poverty may inadvertently complicate the reaching of a shared understanding of poverty within advanced economies, particularly when layered with neo-Liberal thinking in times of austerity.

Adding further complexity at the current time, in the UK at least, is what Owen Jones (2014) described as a shift in the 'Overton window' of political possibility that had drifted to the right of the political spectrum on the crest of a wave of neo-Liberal consensus that dominates political thinking in the twenty-first century. The first challenge—or shift back to the left—comes from progressive nationalism in Scotland, as the devolved government of the Scottish Nationalist Party positions itself against the logic of austerity that was promulgated by all main parties in the UK Westminster parliament in response to the Global Financial Crisis (GFC). Second, it is challenged by the shift to the left of the political spectrum within the Labour Party in 2015, currently the main opposition party in Westminster, culminating with the election of Jeremy Corbyn as leader. This shift is not limited to the UK. Rather, it is mirrored across Europe with the rise, for example, of Podemos in Spain and Syriza in Greece. Even if this shift in the politically credible does not widen the range of anti-poverty tools deemed worthy of consideration, it has checked the swing towards neo-Liberal tools in the UK that were being presented by all mainstream political parties as necessities in response to the fiscal 'crisis'.

Based on the understanding that poverty is about not having enough of what the majority in a society are able to access (McKendrick 2016a), this chapter accepts the majority position shared by civil society and poverty analysts that the scale of poverty in the UK can be estimated by careful interpretation of data on how many people exist/live on an income below 60 % of median household income (equivalised). Without suggesting that poverty always impairs children's well-being, this chapter acknowledges that the dominant impact of childhood poverty is to impact negatively on children's lives as lived and to inhibit their future prospects. The aim of this paper is to focus on the unravelling of a consensus position that, while grounded in neo-Liberalism, aspired to eradicate child poverty within a generation. Austerity has provided the context within which, at first, a regressive neo-Liberalism dismantled this consensus, only to be itself challenged by a thinking that appears even more progressive than that which previously prevailed. The particular focus of this chapter is how people in the UK make sense of the complexities of contemporary child poverty. Having asserted the importance of paying attention to what people think about poverty, the factors that might be expected to have shaped attitudes in recent times are outlined. Thereafter, the nature of contemporary attitudes towards child poverty is explored. Specific attention is paid to whether attitudes have shifted in the age of austerity and indeed, whether they might shift again in the years ahead.

Stick and Stones May Break My Bones, But Names Will Really Hurt Me

Although not dismissing the effectiveness and worth of not responding to taunts and refraining from retaliation, in contrast to the message of the well-known English-language nursery rhyme (in which 'names will never hurt me'), words *can* convey hurt and harm. More generally, it might be argued that there are five reasons why those interested in understanding society should be concerned with social attitudes.

First, social attitudes are of academic interest in and of themselves, without needing to fulfil some ulterior purpose. Understanding how people make sense of the world in which they live, describing these rationalisations and identifying the drivers that shape them is a worthwhile pursuit for scholars of society. However, attitudes are also important for the secondary impact that they might exert on behaviours. Thus, a second concern reflects what the nursery rhyme overlooks: attitudes can have an impact on recipients' lives. When politicians and social commentators pedal notions of an undeserving poor, for example, this impacts directly to undermine the sense of worth of those deemed unworthy of support. Negative attitudes are often directed crassly to whole populations (e.g., lone parents) and the hidden costs can be potent in terms of withdrawal from social life, undermining self-confidence and promulgating guilt. Third, expressed attitudes can provide insight to the likely behaviour of the view holder, particularly important if these are attitudes that are widely shared. Fourth, beyond the realm of everyday life, an awareness of social attitudes is also thought to inform, if not determine, what is politically favourable or possible. In addition to canvassing public responses through focus groups, intelligence on social attitudes is often cited (or inferred) by politicians, when proposing or justifying policy interventions. On the other hand, identifying *problematic* attitudes on poverty can identify priorities for action for the anti-poverty sector. For example, the Autumn 2013 edition of the Child Poverty Action Group's *Poverty* magazine was devoted to the public attitudes towards poverty, reporting recent work to better understand attitudes, and considering how the wider poverty debate might be reframed in a more respectful and productive manner (CPAG 2013). Finally, the interplay of social attitudes, their underlying drivers and behavioural responses to them provides a fascinating dynamic for those tracking social change. All of these reasons for considering social attitudes provide impetus for the current chapter.

The British Social Attitudes Survey: What Should We Think?

Researching attitudes is well established in Great Britain. Since 1983, the British Social Attitudes Survey (BSA) has canvassed opinions on these matters. The BSA covers a wide range of topics, some of which pertain to poverty. As summarised by Park et al. (2007), the BSA canvasses opinion on (i) the meaning of poverty, (ii) the prevalence of poverty and (iii) the causes of poverty. The BSA also canvasses opinion on attitudes towards welfare and government responsibilities in relation to welfare, both of which shed insight into what Britons think about poverty.

Thirty years' worth of BSA data are now available. To this canon of knowledge can be added qualitative explorations of these social attitudes, going beyond the headline statistics and trends to explore the underlying causes of these social attitudes and the implications of these opinions for anti-poverty work (Castell and Thompson 2007; Wood et al. 2012).

The BSA interviews over 3000 people in Britain aged 18 and over every year. Utilising the Postcode Address File, a random probability approach is used to select postcode sectors for field interviewing. This ensures that everyone has a fair chance of taking part in the survey (which increases the likelihood of the results being representative of the British population, although surveying north of the Caledonian Canal in Scotland is excluded on grounds of cost). Although new questions are added to canvass opinion on current issues, questions are primarily designed to be repeatable in order to chart changes in attitudes through time. Different types of weighting are applied to the survey population (selection weights, non-response model weights and calibration weights) to ensure that the analysis is based on a sample that is representative of the British population in terms of age, sex and region.

The scale of the problem of child poverty in the UK, an understanding of the ways in which austerity might be considered to be generating social insecurities at the current time, the way in which austerity has been framed in contemporary political debates and an understanding of whom austerity impacts upon most severely might each be conceived as factors that shape contemporary public attitudes towards tackling child poverty. Each is considered in turn below.

Child Poverty in the UK: The New Labour Years and Beyond

The eradication of child poverty was both an opening gambit and a parting shot of the New Labour political project. The announcement of the goal to eradicate child poverty within a generation was made by Prime Minister Tony Blair at the annual Beveridge lecture in 1999, finally manifesting itself in legislation under the leadership of Prime Minister Gordon Brown with the passing of the Child Poverty Act 2010.

In the early years of New Labour, tax and benefit changes lifted 600,000 children out of poverty (Fig. 10.1). However, the latter years of Tony Blair's tenure as prime minister were characterised by increasing rates of child poverty, with two-thirds of the progress being lost by 2007–08. A return to falling rates of child poverty in the final years of New Labour under Gordon Brown's leadership saw child poverty fall to its lowest level since the late 1980s.

In recent years, the level of child poverty in the UK has remained static, with projections suggesting that poverty will increase dramatically from

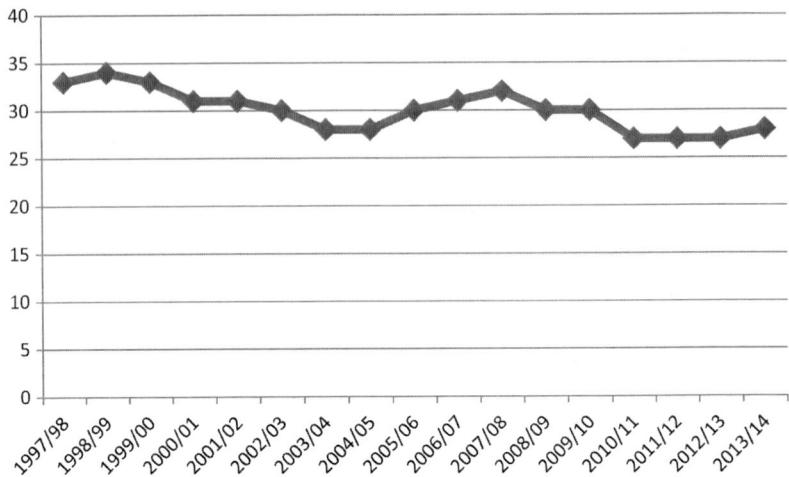

Fig. 10.1 Child Poverty in the UK, after-housing costs have been deducted, 1997–98 to 2013–14

2016 as a result of changes to levels of social security and entitlement to it. Using the after-housing costs measure of relative poverty favoured by those in civil society concerned with tackling poverty (McKendrick 2016b), it is currently estimated that 3.7 million children in the UK are living in poverty, equivalent to more than one in four children.

Austerity and Social Insecurity

Although the current UK government is a proponent of austerity (Cameron 2009), it has at its disposal and continues to utilise, four tools that provide social protection to the most vulnerable in society. It provides income (e.g., welfare payments), services to reduce demands on household income (e.g., the National Health Service), services to enable people to realise potential (e.g., Business Gateway) and protection against very low income and earnings (e.g., National Minimum Wage [NMW]). The UK government executes these functions by directly providing benefits and services, regulating both itself and others and discharging responsibility to various third-party providers. Inadequate use of these tools to promote social security is a means through which austerity is promulgated.

First, it is widely accepted that the NMW is an hourly rate that is currently set at a level that is insufficient to provide a 'living wage' (Scottish Living Wage Campaign 2014). The 2015 NMW is £6.50, compared to a living wage of £7.85 and a London living wage of £9.15 (Living Wage Foundation 2015). In effect, the UK government is permitting employers to remunerate workers at a level that is not sufficient to meet living costs. In a context where government has elected not to regulate the expansion of so-called zero hours contracts (Pennycook et al. 2013), this creates a labour market that offers low pay and insecurity for many workers. Although the UK Government has committed employers to pay workers aged 25 and over what it describes as a 'living wage' by 2020 (BBC 2015), in effect this is an enhanced NMW, rather than a full commitment to what is more commonly understood to be a 'living wage' (Veit Wilson 2015).

Second, since 2010, the UK government introduced a programme of spending cuts that reduced the funding available to the devolved and local governments. Budget cuts that go beyond the drive for efficiency savings are leading to significant service reconfiguration including service reduction, closure and transfer to other providers (Asenova et al. 2013). To date, most local authorities are cutting discretionary (preventative) rather than statutory (core) services while trying to protect essential services and front-line staff (Asenova et al. 2013; Asenova and Stein 2014). However, the largest cuts are anticipated to start in 2016, and will have multiple implications for both service providers and service users (Whittaker 2013; Scottish Government 2014). At a community level, this will affect large numbers of people—mainly those in poverty and in receipt of benefits (Taylor-Robinson and Gosling 2011; Lowndes and Squire 2012; Taylor-Gooby and Stoker 2011). Indeed, Asenova et al. (2013) already contend that the scale of these cuts has been even greater in deprived authorities, which are proportionately more grant-dependent.

Finally, the Welfare Reform Act 2012 introduced a number of changes to the tax and benefits system, mainly reducing entitlements and/or benefits (UK Government 2012), which impact upon claimants' financial security and social relationships. These changes include capping the total sum that individuals and households could receive in benefit, a reduction in housing subsidy for those considered to be under-occupying, a reduction in the level of Council Tax support, more conditionality for claimants and significant overall reductions in welfare spending.

Austerity implies the scaling back of government functions in response to budgetary pressures, rather than their outright withdrawal. In the UK, the state continues to provide social protection, although not at previous levels and not always as direct provision by the UK state.

Austerity as Neo-Liberal Opportunity

For the 2010–15 UK Coalition Government, austerity was presented as the *only* option available to deal with the UK's economic and fiscal condition. It served to legitimise huge reductions in public funding, in services, in benefits, as well as a range of 'reforms' to welfare, housing and education provision (the latter two primarily in England, much less so in the devolved countries of the UK). For the Coalition Government, there was no alternative—austerity was a necessity, a survival strategy that any responsible administration would have to pursue for the sake of the country. This notion of 'austerity' played a key role in both the 2010 and 2015 UK General Election campaigns. Others would contend that 'austerity' is a class-based strategy aimed at consolidating, defending and promoting the interests of the already affluent and wealthy against workers and the most disadvantaged in society (Atkinson et al. 2012; Harvey 2009; Mendoza 2015; O'Hara 2014). It follows that uncovering the political choices that form the basis of 'austerity' allows us to see it as a particular ideology and set of assumptions about the economy and wider society, and beliefs about how these ought to be structured.

Who Bears the Burden of Austerity?

To what extent has austerity impacted on the most disadvantaged in society? Data on income distribution trends add nuance to our understanding of impact. Figure 10.2 describes changes in household income in the UK since the GFC, indicating aggregate changes for the tenth of the

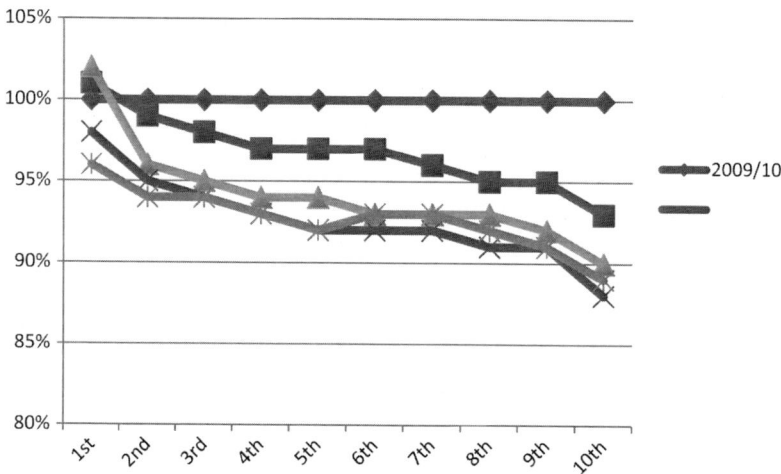

Fig. 10.2   Changes in household income in the UK, after-housing costs have been deducted, from 2009–10 to 2013–14, By Decile Group Medians (Income is equivalised for household composition and is set to 2013/14 prices to account for inflation)

population with the lowest income (1st), through to the tenth of the population with the highest income (10th). From the base year of 2009/10, the graph highlights how far income has fallen for each of the ten groups over the following four years (expressing income for each subsequent year as a proportion of household income in 2009/10).

It is apparent that income has fallen since 2009/10 across all groups. Indeed, all but the households with the very lowest incomes in the UK (decile 1) experienced three successive years of reduced household income from 2009/10 to 2012/13. Over this period, typical household income fell from £418 per week in 2009/10, to £404 in 2010/11, £389 in 2011/12 to reach £386 in 2012/13. Even so, the early years of austerity might be considered socially progressive in the (limited) sense that the income of the poorest households actually increased from 2009/10 levels for two years, while the most substantial drop in income was experienced by the most affluent. That is, by 2011/12, income at the 10th decile fell to 90 % of 2009/10 levels, whereas income at the 1st decile increased to 102 % of 2009/10 levels. It should be noted that this modest increase in household income among the lowest earners still represented a squeeze on household budgets as inflation at this time increased at a higher rate than household income: the annual rate of the Consumer Price Index was 3.3 % in 2010, 4.5 % in 2011 and 2.8 % in 2012 (ONS 2015). However, and notwithstanding the limitations of placing too much emphasis on data for a single year, between 2012/13 and 2013/14, changes in the distribution of household income (albeit modest in scale) have become regressive, with drops in income for the least affluent households, being contrasted with increases in income for the most affluent groups. So, while the median income at the 1st decile fell by £6 between 2011/12 and 2013/14, median income at the 10th decile increased by £4 between 2012/13 and 2013/14.

The claim, then, that austerity impacts most severely on the most vulnerable in society is oversimplistic. Rather, it is more accurate to assert that, in terms of household income, austerity in the UK initially impacted most on the least vulnerable, but that this 'progressive imbalance' has now been checked. Income trends and impending policy changes suggest that austerity is set to impact most severely on the most vulnerable in the years ahead.

What Should We Think?

Together the narrative of 'austerity as necessity', evidence that the UK Government was not maximising its use of tools for social protection, and evidence that the early years of austerity could be characterised as ones in which the highest earners saw the greatest falls in income, might encourage less sympathetic regard for social protection measures such as tackling poverty. At the same time, awareness of the adverse effect of austerity on vulnerable groups, and signs of an unravelling of the progressive adjustments that implied that the most able were most adversely affected, might encourage less support for measures designed to weaken social protection in the years ahead.

What Do We Think?

Before reflecting specifically on child poverty, it is useful to consider the broader contexts within which these attitudes are set, by reflecting on what Britons think about welfare and poverty in general.

Hardening of Attitudes Towards Welfare in the Twenty-First Century

BSA data suggest that although the majority of Britons agree that 'the welfare state is one of Britain's greatest achievements' (55 % in 2014), only a small minority of Britons can be characterised as being 'welfarist' in orientation (18 % in 2014, compared to 26 % who are anti-welfare and the majority who tend to adopt a centrist position). More significantly, a hardening of attitudes towards welfare can be observed in recent times (Fig. 10.3).

As we approached the GFC of 2009, and at the same time as rates of child poverty in the UK were falling, harsher attitudes towards welfare were expressed in terms of a shrinking of the small minority who were pro-welfarist in outlook (Fig. 10.3a); a collapse in less than a decade in the proportion of people who would support an increase in taxes in order to fund increased spending on health, education and social services (Fig. 10.3b); a similar scale of collapse over two decades in the proportion of Britons who would support increased spending on welfare benefits for the poor, even if it led to higher taxes (Fig. 10.3c); and a one-third reduction in the proportion who perceive that cutting welfare would damage people's lives (Fig. 10.3d).

Other than high levels of support for taxation to fund government spending on education, health and social benefits (Fig. 10.3b) coinciding with much of the first phase in the reduction in levels of child poverty in the UK (Fig. 10.1), there is little to suggest that attitudes towards welfare spending reflect the realities of child poverty. For example, falling support for government spending on welfare benefits for the poor (Fig. 10.3c) and growing disbelief that cutting welfare benefits would damage too many people's lives (Fig. 10.3b) characterise eras of both rising and falling levels of child poverty at the start of the twenty-first century (see Fig. 10.1).

Understanding the Problem of Poverty

Since 1986, a majority of Britons have consistently reported that there is 'quite a lot' of poverty in Britain (as opposed to reporting that 'there

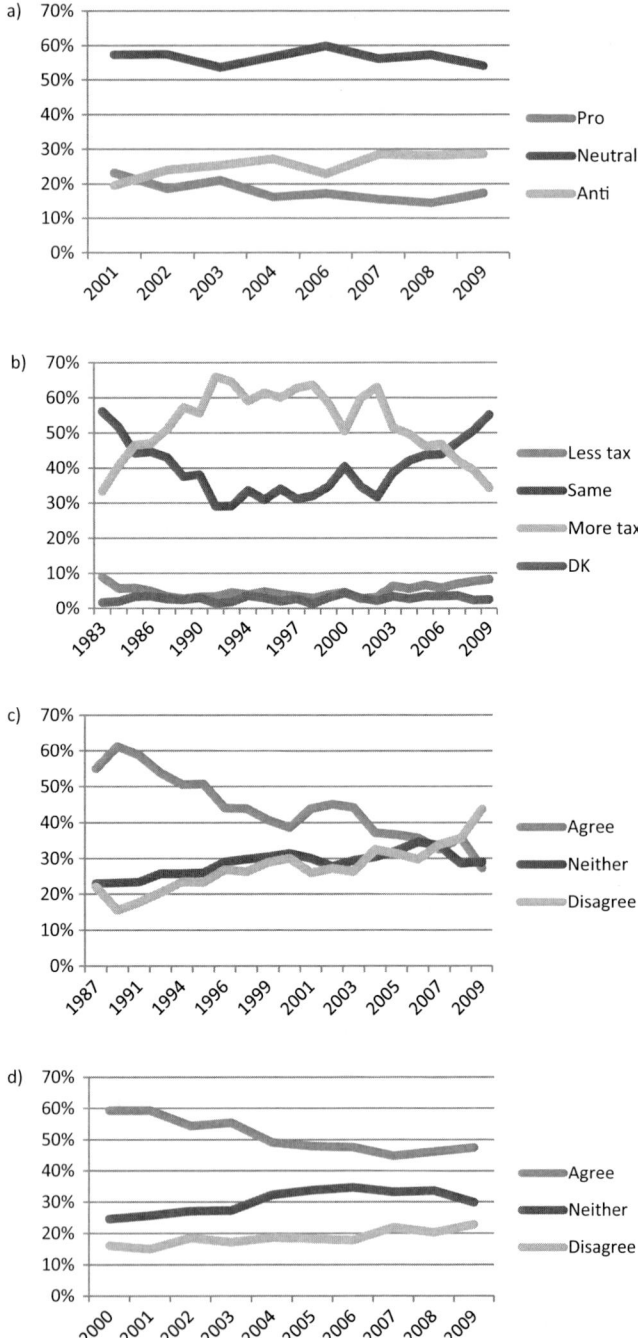

Fig. 10.3 Hardening of attitudes towards welfare in Britain

is very little real poverty'), although there is no consensus and opinions have fluctuated over time (Fig. 10.4a). Estimates for 2013 suggest that 64 % think that there is 'quite a lot' of poverty in the UK, not quite as high as the 72 % that held this opinion in the mid-1990s, but higher than the 53 % of 2006.

The trend for contemporary estimates of the amount of poverty (at that point in time) is broadly consistent with that for perceptions of recent trends and expectations of future trends. Thus, the proportion of Britons reporting that poverty was rising increased from the mid-1980s through to a peak in the mid-1990s (e.g., for past trends from 53 % in 1986 to 69 % in 1994), before falling to a low point in the middle of the first decade of the twenty-first century (e.g., for past trends from 69 % in 1994 to 34 % in 2006), before increasing once again in recent years (e.g., from 34 % in 2006 to 65 % in 2013) (Fig. 10.4b). Past and future estimates of poverty are the least stable of all attitudes towards poverty. Interestingly, there was also a tipping point at the millennium; thereafter, it became more common for Britons to think that poverty would increase more in the years ahead than it had in the years past. For example, in 1986, 53 % of Britons thought that poverty had increased in the last ten years, but only 48 % of Britons thought that poverty would increase in the next ten years; by 2010, the agreement with these perceptions were 50 % and 58 %, respectively (Figs. 10.4b and c). In 2013, although the percentage of Britons who expected poverty to increase was the highest ever recorded in the BSA, slightly more Britons perceived that poverty had increased in the last few years.

It is clear that the majority of Britons consider that poverty exists, that it has increased, and is expected to increase (Fig. 10.4).

Tackling Child Poverty as a Progressive Project and a Bulwark Against Neo-Liberalism

Tackling child poverty has almost universal public support, with 84 % considering it to be 'very important', and 15 % considering this to be 'quite important' in 2014. Although attitudes towards welfare may have wavered (Fig. 10.3), a clear majority of Britons consider that poverty

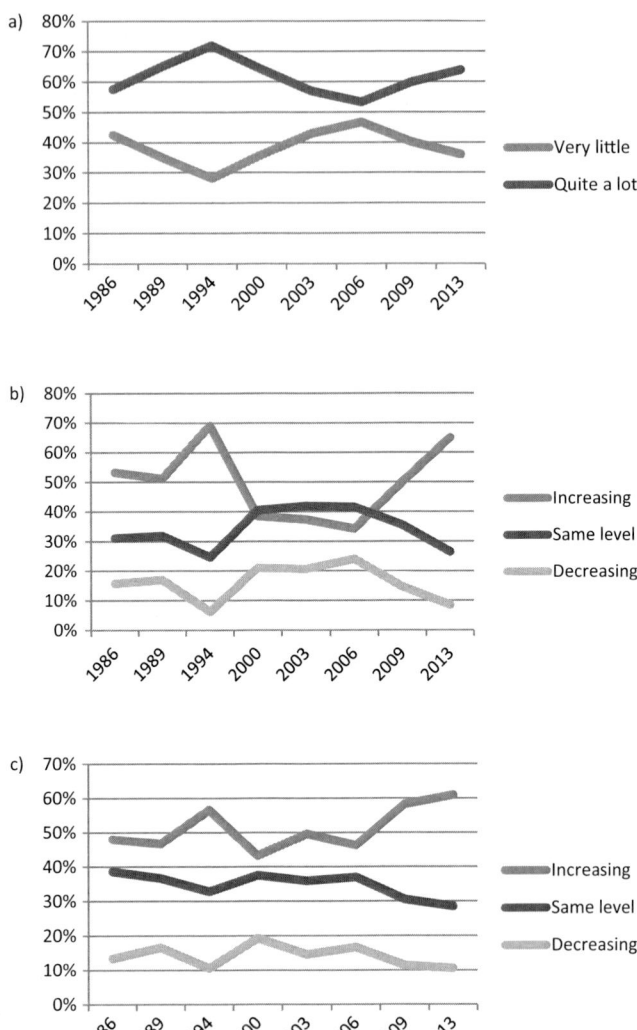

Fig. 10.4 Perceptions of poverty in Britain

exists (Fig. 10.4) and that it is important that child poverty is tackled. Neo-Liberal attacks on the affordability of social justice (discussed earlier in the paper) seem not to have undermined a sense of how important it is to tackle child poverty.

On the other hand, there are grounds for questioning the extent to which Britons conceive of tackling child poverty as a progressive project (Table 10.1). Foremost among perceived reasons for child poverty is parents' alcoholism, drug abuse or other addictions (a contributory reason according to 74 % of Britons in 2012, and the main reason according to 17 % in 2014). The tendency to seek explanation in the 'failings' of parents is also evident from the next two most common explanations offered for child poverty. Three in five (59 %) consider that 'parents not wanting to work' is a contributory reason (9 % considered this the main reason in 2014), and parents' lack of education is considered to be a contributory reason by 53 % of Britons (and the main reason according to 11 % in 2014). By way of contrast, far fewer Britons consider that inequalities in society (30 %), the low level of social benefits (19 %), and/or parental

Table 10.1 Perceptions of main (2014) and contributory (2012) reasons for child poverty in Britain

Reason	Main	All
Their parents suffer from alcoholism, drug abuse or other addictions	17.4 %	73.5 %
Their parents do not want to work	9.3 %	58.7 %
Their parents lack education	10.7 %	53.1 %
Their parents have been out of work for a long time	7.9 %	49.6 %
There has been a family break-up or loss of a family member	6.4 %	49.0 %
Their parents' work does not pay enough	11.4 %	46.1 %
There are too many children in the family	3.9 %	43.1 %
They live in a poor-quality area	6.4 %	41.9 %
They—or their parents—suffer from a long-term illness or disability	3.1 %	41.9 %
Because of inequalities in society	7.4 %	30.1 %
Their family cannot access affordable housing	2.1 %	28.7 %
Their grandparents were also poor: it has been passed down the generations	2.7 %	23.5 %
Their family suffers from discrimination, for example, ethnicity, age, disability	0.3 %	23.3 %
Social benefits for families with children are not high enough	5.9 %	18.5 %
Their parents do not work enough hours	0.9 %	18.0 %
Other reasons	3.5 %	1.3 %

Source: British Social Attitudes Survey

work not paying enough (46 %) are among the contributory reasons for child poverty.

Although there is support for tackling child poverty, the nature of the problem to be tackled is in many respects consistent with that neo-Liberal line of thought that finds fault in individuals and families for the problems that they experience.

Embracing Neo-Liberal Austerity Rhetoric?

The hardening of attitudes towards welfare in the years leading to the GFC (Fig. 10.3), and an understanding that the early years of austerity were not characterised by a growth in child poverty (Fig. 10.1), did not augur well for those promoting progressive policies at the onset of austerity. Although there is evidence that Britons are becoming more likely to acknowledge the growing risk of poverty through the austerity years (Fig. 10.4), there was no evidence that the incidence of child poverty is closely related to public attitudes towards it. Thus, at the onset of austerity, the context may have seemed conducive to neo-Liberal mantras, such as 'we are all in this together' and 'we cannot afford not to reduce public expenditure'.

However, as Fig. 10.5 demonstrates, austerity has not been characterised by a further hardening of attitudes towards welfare. Although it would be misleading to portray the British mindset as being wholly anti-austerity, the neo-Liberal rhetoric that has prevailed among political decision-makers has not garnered a groundswell of support among the wider public. Indeed, the fall in the proportion of those opining that the government should spend more money on welfare benefits for the poor, even if it means higher taxes (Fig. 10.3c), has been reversed to a degree in the austerity years (Fig. 10.5c).

Where to From Here?

Attitudes towards child poverty in the UK do not appear to be strongly coupled to either evidence of its incidence or the overarching character of policy responses to it. This logic that social attitudes determine the

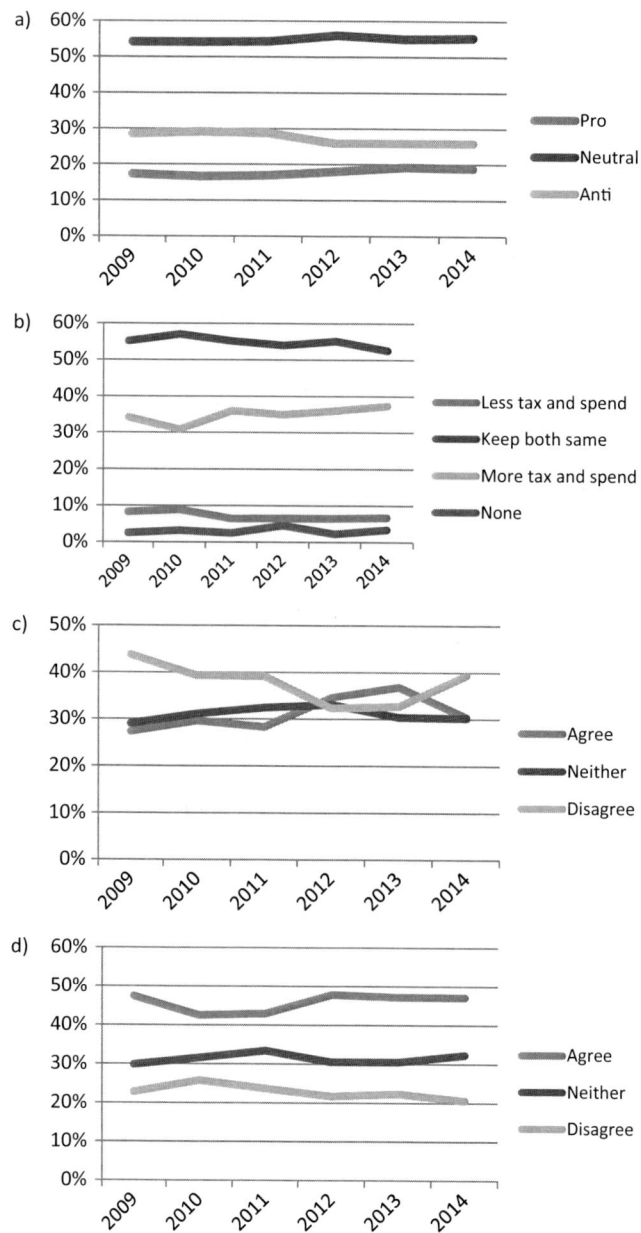

Fig. 10.5 Arresting the hardening of attitudes towards welfare in Britain in the austerity years

possibility of public policy appears not as strong as was expected. In the austerity years, this has worked to the advantage of those progressives concerned to tackle child poverty, in the sense that the absence of compelling evidence of an increase in child poverty and the neo-Liberal rhetoric of mainstream political policy has not undermined the dominant public opinion that it is important to tackle child poverty. What might be viewed as an attack on the most vulnerable in society through austerity and welfare reform has checked and, if anything, effected a reversal of the hardening of attitudes towards welfare that preceded the years leading to the GFC. Tackling child poverty remains on the agenda of citizens in the UK, even if the UK Government is proposing steps to alter the way in which this goal is articulated through the repealing of the Child Poverty Act 2010.

However, there is much in the British public's understanding of child poverty that resonates with neo-Liberal thinking. Underlying reasons for child poverty are primarily rationalised in terms of individual (rather than system) failings. One-half of the population do not agree that cutting welfare benefits would damage too many people. Only one-third consider that the government should spend more money on welfare benefits for the poor, even if this means higher taxes. It may be that Britons have become inured to child poverty or that the 'poverty porn' that often presents as current affairs/news is rallying opinion against a perceived undeserving poor, and it is clear that Britons are far from fully supportive or understanding towards those experiencing poverty.

All may not be lost to those concerned to challenge neo-Liberal thinking. Indeed, ironically, there is also evidence that suggests that austerity may be the nemesis of neo-Liberalism. Although the advent of austerity has not been accompanied by a strong reversal in outlook, the hardening of attitudes against the most vulnerable has been checked. While it cannot be assumed that the anticipated growth in the incidence of child poverty in the UK towards 2020 as welfare reforms are operationalised will lead to a reaction against the most regressive neo-Liberal tendencies, it is clear that social attitudes are malleable and that there is the basis for nurturing a moral economy of social justice. A moral economy of social justice may open the policy space for more progressive interventions to tackle child poverty in the UK.

References

Asenova, D., and B. Stein. 2014. *Assessing the social and community risks of council spending cuts In Scotland.* York: Joseph Rowntree Foundation.

Asenova, D., S. Bailey, and C. Mccann. 2013. *Managing the social risks of public spending cuts in Scotland.* York: Joseph Rowntree Foundation.

Atkinson, W., S. Roberts, and M. Savage, eds. 2012. *Class inequality in austerity Britain: power, difference and suffering.* Basingstoke: Palgrave Macmillan.

BBC. 2015. Budget 2015: Osborne unveils National Living Wage. *BBC Online* [online], July 8. Available from: http://www.bbc.co.uk/news/uk-politics-33437115. Accessed 29 Mar 2016.

Cameron, D. 2009. The age of Austerity. Speech at Spring Forum. *SayIt* [online], April 26. Available from: http://conservative-speeches.sayit.mysociety.org/speech/601367. Accessed 29 Mar 2016.

Castell, S., and J. Thompson. 2007. *Understanding attitudes to poverty in the UK.* York: Joseph Rowntree Foundation.

CPAG. 2013. Public attitudes to child poverty. *Poverty.* 146 (Autumn 2013). Available from: http://www.cpag.org.uk/content/public-attitudes-child-poverty. Accessed 29 Mar 2016.

Harvey, D. 2009. Their crisis our challenge: Interview with David Harvey. *Red Pepper*, March. Available from: http://www.redpepper.org.uk/Their-crisis-our-challenge/. Accessed 29 Mar 2016.

Jones, O. 2014. *The Establishment: and how they get away with it.* London: Penguin.

Lowndes, V., and S. Squire. 2012. 'Local governance under the coalition government: Austerity, localism and the "Big Society". *Local Government Studies* 38(1): 21–40.

Mckendrick, J.H. 2016a. What is poverty? In *Poverty in Scotland 2016: Tools for transformation*, eds. J.H. McKendrick, G. Mooney, G. Scott, J. Dickie, and F. McHardy, 29–40. London: Child Poverty Action Group.

——— 2016b. How do we measure poverty? In *Poverty in Scotland 2016: tools for transformation*, eds. J.H. McKendrick, G. Mooney, G. Scott, J. Dickie, and F. McHardy, 41–57. London: Child Poverty Action Group.

Mendoza, K.A. 2015. *Austerity: The Demolition of the Welfare State and the Rise of the Zombie Economy.* London: New Internationalist.

Office for National Statistics. 2015. Consumer Price Inflation. Statistical Bulletin. http://www.ons.gov.uk/economy/inflationandpriceindices/bulletins/consumerpriceinflation/previousReleases.

O'Hara, M. 2014. *Austerity bites: a journey to the sharp end of cuts in the UK.* Bristol: Policy Press.

Park, A., M. Phillips, and C. Robinson. 2007. Attitudes to poverty. York: Joseph Rowntree Foundation. Available from: https://www.jrf.org.uk/report/attitudes-poverty-findings-british-social-attitudes-survey. Accessed 29 Mar 2016.

Pennycook, M., G. Cory, and V. Alakeson. 2013. *A matter of time—the rise of zero-hours contracts.* London: The Resolution Foundation.

Scottish Government. 2014. *UK government cuts to welfare expenditure in Scotland—Budget 2014.* Edinburgh: Scottish Government.

Scottish Living Wage Campaign. 2014. *Living Wage Debate—Campaign Briefing.* Glasgow: Scottish Living Wage Campaign.

Taylor-Gooby, P., and G. Stoker. 2011. The coalition programme: A new vision for Britain or politics as usual? *The Political Quarterly* 82(1): 4–15.

Taylor-Robinson, D., and R. Gosling. 2011. English north–south divide. Local authority budget cuts and health inequalities. *BMJ* 342: d1487.

UK Government. 2012. *Welfare Reform Act (United Kingdom) (2012).* London: The Stationery Office.

Viet Wilson, J. 2015. Osborne's fictitious living wage. *Social Policy Blog* [online], July 10. Available from: https://paulspicker.wordpress.com/2015/07/10/john-veit-wilson-writes-osbornes-fictitious-living-wage/. Accessed 29 Mar 2016.

Whittaker, M. 2013. *Narrowed horizons: The fiscal choices at Spending Review 2013 and beyond.* London: Resolution Foundation.

Wood, C., J. Salter, G. Morrell, M. Barnes, A. Paget, and D. O'leary. 2012. *Poverty in perspective.* London: Demos.

11

Morality, Austerity and the Complexities of Sexual and Reproductive Health Services for Young People in South Africa

Kelley Moult and Alexandra Müller

Introduction

Healthcare service provision for young people in South Africa is a complex landscape—balancing youth and human rights, numerous laws, legally and professionally mandated obligations, and a tenuous and resource-strained implementation context, all set against the backdrop of a highly charged and morally contested area of state-based service provision. Sexual and reproductive health services (SRH) are therefore a far-from-settled arena—either for the healthcare workers who provide services, or for the young people who need to access them. In straddling the divide between official policies and client claims, front-line service providers, so-called street-level bureaucrats, often become disdainful of the 'ungrounded' directives from lawmakers and politicians who

K. Moult (✉) • A. Müller
University of Cape Town, Cape Town, South Africa

© The Editor(s) (if applicable) and The Author(s) 2017
P. Kelly, J. Pike (eds.), *Neoliberalism, Austerity, and the Moral Economies of Young People's Health and Well-being*,
DOI 10.1057/978-1-137-58266-9_12

217

are perceived as out of touch with implementation realities (Maynard-Moody and Musheno 2003). These conflicts are compounded in neo-Liberal environments of limited infrastructure and resources, such as the South African public health system.

This chapter will examine the decision-making processes of South African nurses providing SRH services to adolescents in health facilities in the public sector. Based on qualitative data from individual semi-structured interviews and workshop-based focus group discussions, the chapter will explore the impact of extremely limited financial and human resources on nurses' decisions around service provision, including the significant implementation gaps that exist in clinics, and the deleterious effects these have for the health and rights of young people. The chapter also explores nurses' feelings about and experiences of policy changes, and describes a number of structural obstacles to involving nurses in policy processes, including a lack of communication about existing policies, new policy initiatives from 'top' to 'bottom' level and workload pressure due to understaffing. Time for reflection on service provision, training, policy meetings and drafting committees is simply not within the reach of nurses in state-based clinical practice, and their voices are therefore not usually heard in these spaces.

The chapter argues that where policy is made that excludes the views of key implementing stakeholders, it is unsurprising that service provision at the 'coal face' often bears little resemblance to the intention of policy and lawmakers. In the context of SRH services for youth, the implications for young people's rights are significant. This is exacerbated in a climate of austerity and resource poverty, where tightening the screws on service provision increases the pressure on nurses, and constrains young people's lives, health and choices.

Austerity and Healthcare in South Africa

South Africa, classified as a middle-income country, occupies a unique position with regards to healthcare provision and fiscal austerity. South Africa's national budget does not reflect European austerity measures such as proportional cuts across the board, targeted cost containment policies or the search for productivity and efficiency gains (Ongaro et al. 2015). In fact, the national budget reflects continuous annual growth in health spending in the years 2010–2015 (National Treasury, Republic of South Africa [2010–2015]—Budget Highlights). However, due to historical inequality under apartheid, the South African public health system is severely under-resourced, and reflects many of the challenges experienced by other health systems under austerity measures, including an emphasis on outpatient and primary care, increased user charges and cut or unfilled posts, resulting in less services available to patients and longer waiting times for care (Quaglio et al. 2013). Additionally, neo-Liberalism, as an ideology that holds market exchange and economic rationalism as ethics in themselves, and as being capable of acting as a guide for all human action, has seeped into public service provision in South Africa as much as elsewhere internationally (Harvey 2005).

South Africa's health system is highly unequal: 84 % of South Africans rely on the public sector (Mayosi and Benatar 2014), which is financed through tax, government subsidy and service user fees, while only 16 % of South Africans have private health insurance and access to the private sector. Up to 25 % of uninsured people pay out of pocket for private sector care, if and when they can afford it. Patients who run out of the financial means for private care default back into the public system. The disparities in resource allocation between the parallel systems are wide. Despite catering for the large majority of the population, the public system employs some 30 % of doctors nationwide, while the remaining 70 % are employed by the private sector, as are 95 % of all medical specialists (Breier 2008). The public sector is thus in a state of crisis: struggling with a high burden of disease, higher than in most countries of comparable economic profile (Coovadia et al. 2009), and weakened by staff shortage, lack of infrastructure and resources, mismanagement and neglect (Von Holdt and Murphy 2007; Coovadia et al. 2009).

The public system and, with a less clear framework, the private system follow a healthcare approach that focuses resources at primary care level with an emphasis on health promotion and prevention (see National Health Act of 2003). Public primary care facilities in particular experience a shortage of physicians with 113,000 nurses and only 16,000 physicians at a nurse–physician ratio of 7:1 (Department of Health n.d.). In this context, nurses provide the vast majority of SRH services. Primary healthcare policy has expanded the role of nurses to include 'the promotion of health and family planning by teaching to and counselling with individuals and groups of persons' (Anon 1991). Here, nurses are perceived as an important link to the community, increasingly finding themselves with more community-oriented duties.

In 2011, the National Department of Health (DoH) introduced a large-scale reform of health systems financing under the proposal for a National Health Insurance (NHI) scheme, which aimed to decrease the disparities between public and private sector care (National Department of Health 2011). The NHI scheme provides a package of free health services, on top of which individuals can choose to take out private health insurance. The new national Adolescent SRH Framework Strategy (Department of Social Development 2015) prioritises integrated and accessible SRH services for adolescents, and suggests a number of intersectoral interventions between the Departments of Health, Social Development and Education. Crucially, at the time of writing none of the suggested initiatives have been budgeted for by National Treasury. It remains unclear how integrated adolescent SRH services will be funded, concentrating the burden of service provision on healthcare providers in already under-resourced settings.

This continues a worrying trend. Historically, access to SRH services was used as a political tool through which the apartheid government attempted to reduce the population of black South Africans while encouraging higher birth rates among whites. Government family planning clinics became politicised, such that by the late 1960s, free birth control services had become 'black birth control' and contraception labelled as a tool of white oppression (Department of Health & Reproductive Health Research Unit 2001; Hoffman-Wanderer et al. 2013). Demand for contraceptive services was often unmet, or delivered in ways that breached human rights, failed to prioritise patient needs or respect choices in relation to preferred methods of birth control. Unfortunately, as we illustrate below, this social and historical legacy endures (and is even exacerbated), and poor service delivery for the majority of patients remains entrenched.

Post-apartheid, health policies 'hollowed out' finances as budgets shrank between the mid-1990s and early 2000s but the DoH promised to expand infrastructure to address apartheid inequalities, roll out the NHI scheme and abolish user fees in the primary healthcare system (Watson et al. 2014). Despite healthcare being a key government priority, health spending from 2006 to 2012 largely went to HIV/AIDS care, and service provision (especially for women and children) suffered enormously. These trends look set to worsen, with continued shrinking of medium-term public healthcare spending, growing healthcare costs, and Parliament's reluctance, influenced by a neo-Liberal rationale, to intervene despite its ability to make budgetary recommendations and amendments (Watson et al. 2014).

The Legal and Policy Framework

South Africa's 1996 Constitution and Bill of Rights provide the basis for rights related to access to healthcare services for both adults and children, as well as reproduction-related decision-making. These constitutional rights are made accessible to children through several laws. One of the first Acts passed post-apartheid, the Choice on Termination of Pregnancy Act 92 of 1996, allows pregnant women or girls to request a termination of pregnancy up to 12 weeks of gestation. The National Health Act 61 of 2003, deals with a wide range of health-related issues, addresses healthcare providers' duties and patients' rights. It states that all information concerning a patient (of any age) is confidential—a critical aspect of SRH for adolescents. The Children's Act 38 of 2005 mandates that children from the age of 12 must be provided condoms and contraceptives, and reiterates that such services must be confidential. The Criminal Law [Sexual Offences and Related Matters] Amendment Act 32 of 2007 (the Sexual Offences Act [SOA]), and the Criminal Law [Sexual Offences and Related Matters] Amendment Act 5 of 2015 (the SOA Amendment Act) set the age of consent to sexual activity at 16 years, and define statutory offences committed with adolescents between the ages of 12 and 16 years. These provisions are summarised in Table 11.1.

Taken together, these laws not only provide SRH rights to adolescents, but also regulate access, and specify obligations and responsibilities (including, in some cases, mandatory reporting). This is a complex,

Table 11.1. Conflicting ages of consent

Issue	Age of consent	Law
General medical treatment	Children can consent to medical treatment without the consent of a parent when they are **over the age of 12**, and have sufficient maturity and the mental capacity to understand the benefits, risks and social implications.	Children's Act
HIV test	Children who are **12 years and older** can consent to an HIV test without their parents' consent. Children under 12 can consent to an HIV test without their parents if they have sufficient maturity and the mental capacity to understand the benefits, risks and social implications.	Children's Act
Condoms	Children **over the age of 12 years** may not be refused condoms by a healthcare provider or condom seller.	Children's Act
Contraceptives	Contraceptives other than condoms may be provided to a child of **12 years or older** without their parents' consent. A medical examination must be done and proper advice given to the child.	Children's Act
Sex	A person may legally consent to sexual activity (penetrative or non-penetrative) at **16 years**. Statutory offences prohibit *consensual* sexual activity where one party is 12–15 years old, and their partner is 16–17 years old with an age difference of 2 years or less. (*Consensual* sexual activity is not criminalised where both are 12–15 years old, regardless of the age gap.)	Sexual Offences Act (2007) SOA Amendment Act (2015)
Termination of pregnancy (TOP)	**Any** pregnant woman or girl can request a TOP up to 12 weeks of gestation, without consultation/approval by a doctor or nurse. There is therefore no age restriction for a TOP, and girls can consent without their parents to ensure access for any woman or girl who needs this service.	Termination of Pregnancy Act

highly moral and value-laden area of the law and service provision that is complicated by consent and confidentiality. Access to SRH services for children encourages access to professional advice and health services and prevents sexually transmitted infections and teenage pregnancy. The

Table 11.2. Confidentiality provisions in law

Confidentiality provision	Law
A child's right to confidentiality in respect of sexual reproductive health services is limited where a medical practitioner reasonably believes that the child has been abused or neglected	Children's Act
A child has the right to confidentiality in respect of information concerning her health status, treatment or stay in a health establishment except where records need to be disclosed in the best interest of the child, for a legitimate purpose or in the scope of a health practitioner's duties.	National Health Act
A child does not have the right to confidentiality in respect of sexual activity as healthcare professionals are obligated to report knowledge of a sexual offence.	Sexual Offences Act

SOA takes a much more protectionist stance, setting the legal age of consent to sex at 16 and designating certain offences between adolescents as statutory offences which require mandatory reporting (see Table 11.2). In practice, tricky choices ensue as SRH practitioners must choose between providing services, support and counselling for sexually active adolescents, on the one hand, and reporting them to social workers and the police in terms of the law, on the other.

Understanding Decision-Making: Talking to Nurses

Given these complexities, and South Africa's well-documented resource constraints, in our research we were interested in nurses' understandings of the conflicting policies and challenges, their decision-making, and how this shaped rights and access for adolescent patients in the context of healthcare under neo-Liberalism. We base this chapter on individual interviews with 28 nurses providing SRH services at rural (n = 15) and urban (n = 13) health facilities (see Hoffman-Wanderer et al. 2013), and two one-day workshops with nurses and stakeholders in adolescent SRH policy implementation in the Western Cape Province, South Africa.

The nurses were hard-working and caring professionals, concerned about teenage pregnancy, and providing the best possible care and information for patients. They had a wide array of nursing experience (ranging from 1 to 40 years), with the majority having been nurses for more than two decades. Two-thirds of participants dealt exclusively with maternity and gynaecology, family planning, reproductive healthcare and termination of pregnancies. Most viewed nursing as a desirable career and described a passion and vocation for nursing, although some noted that discriminatory apartheid policies had effectively limited the options for them as non-white South Africans to becoming 'a teacher … to go for police … to become a nurse … or to become a prison warden, that was all'. Only two respondents worked in youth-specific clinics, although all interviewees had worked with adolescents. We had aimed to sample youth-specific facilities, but at the time of the fieldwork, these facilities had been converted to general service clinics—themselves victims of the austerity budgets in public healthcare. Clinic staff reported that fewer teens used the clinics after these changes were effected.

The Impact of Austerity on Adolescent SRH Service Provision

The erosion of public healthcare funding plays out in clinics across South Africa, particularly for adolescents who often require specialised and sensitive SRH service provision. Wood and Jewkes (2006, p.113) show that young women especially experience nurses as 'rude, short-tempered and arrogant' people who ask prying questions about their relationships and behaviours, treat them judgementally and restrict choices about contraceptive options. Similarly, nurses in our sample described problems with older judgemental staff, who 'will see a youngster go into the room and they'll comment and say "ooh, this one's you know … ripe before their time"'.

The lack of resources in the public healthcare system has created a crumbling, inadequate system characterised by infrastructural and procedural shortcomings, particularly for young teens. Primary among these concerns was the lack of privacy for adolescents who were forced to wait for long periods of time in crowded, mixed-use waiting rooms. Young people feared being identified while waiting in the clinic and also worried that their visit would be reported to parents or become community gossip. Procedural rules and routines that require patients to retrieve their medical files and undergo basic tests (e.g., blood pressure) combined with space constraints to reveal patients as SRH service users and invite 'flack' from other patients. One nurse explained that '[adolescents] don't want to come to the clinic, because then everyone will know—or they think everyone will know—that they are on birth control'. Another nurse explained:

> It's a big thing to get the teenagers to come to the clinic because … the church women, the elderly women, they sit in this waiting room and they discuss everybody that's coming in. And [this is] a small community, ok not that small, but people know each other … and they will say: 'Oh I saw your child yesterday'. And teenagers don't want to hear stuff like that.

Over-burdened budgets and inadequate facilities also limit specialised services for young people as scarce resources are earmarked for services for the wider population. Adolescent-only after-school services are clearly necessary, but only two clinics allocated specific, exclusive time, one afternoon per week, for a youth clinic. Instead, most nurses reported that constrained budgets and staff shortages meant that clinics were confined to 'usual' operating hours, eight hours per day, Mondays to Fridays. Clinics that had extended opening hours had to deal with other issues characteristic of such fraught and resource-poor social contexts, for example, it was too dangerous for nurses to journey to the clinic in the dark, and public transport was both unreliable and erratic. Although the most popular time for teenagers to access services was after 2pm, most clinics routinely closed between 3.30 and 4.30pm. Only one clinic stayed open until 7pm on one night a week (although this was for 'general' reproductive health services), and one other gave teenagers priority after 2pm, in a 'fast lane', to minimise communal waiting time. Nurses recognised that the upshot of these policies was that only a minority of teenagers in need of reproductive healthcare services actually came to the clinics and hospitals (Müller et al. 2016).

Time Is Money: The Impact of Austerity on Patient Interaction

Consistent with global trends, South African health policy has expanded the role of healthcare providers to include 'the promotion of health and family planning by teaching to and counselling with individuals and groups of persons' (South African Nursing Council Regulations). Nurses are therefore perceived as an important link to the community and increasingly find themselves with more community-oriented duties. However, many nurses in our study related practical challenges to fulfilling that role, which impacted negatively on their ability to provide necessary technical, physiological information about sex and contraception. This is precisely the type of information that previous research (Wood and Jewkes 2006; Ehlers 2003) found to be lacking for teenagers. The majority (*n* = 17/28) of the study's participants emphasised the need for better sex education in schools. Half of our participants (*n* = 14) described difficulties in providing information on SRH in schools. These included a lack of available time and personnel, the closure of school clinics or removal of nurses from schools, and the reluctance of parents and school principals to have sex education taught in schools. Healthcare providers were also frustrated by restrictions on the kind of information and services they were permitted to provide (e.g., condom-use demonstrations and discussions on contraception).

Q: What do you think could be done to reduce the number of teenage pregnancies?
A: Oh I think education. In schools. You know that we're not allowed to go to the schools to talk about condom use.
Q: Are you not allowed?
A: No. You can put [condoms] down but you're not allowed to talk about it. Or do demonstrations. Especially not [at] the Afrikaans[1] schools.
Q: Oh really, not at the Afrikaans [schools]?

---

[1] Afrikaans is one of South Africa's 11 official languages, and is widely spoken in the Province in which the fieldwork was undertaken.

A: No. I think they [are] so short-sighted. No we're really not allowed, I think if you speak to any of the Sisters at the clinic they say we're allowed to go and put the condoms in the, in the toilets whatever, but we're not allowed to give a demonstration how to use a condom and why they should have condoms.

Nurses were confident that teenagers who actually came to the clinic would receive the necessary information, and told us how they seize the opportunity to provide SRH education whenever teenagers present themselves:

> For every teenage patient that comes we go through that as part of a basic integrated information that you've got to do with every patient. If they come for a coffee even, we will ask them if they are sexually active; when was their last menstruation; what are they using as family planning?

While all of the nurses reported that their clinics provided *some* verbal information about contraception to teenage patients, time constraints meant that they relied on others (such as HIV counsellors, Health Promoters or NGO-based volunteer counsellors) to supplement this. Only seven facilities had more than one of these health professionals available for teenagers. These counsellors clearly performed an important support role for time-strapped nurses who described that: 'with a busy clinic ... you'd like to give [clients] more time but that's why we have the counsellor there'.

Healthcare education takes time and resources, and these are not always available at healthcare facilities whose primary function is to provide care. Nurses need additional resources to be able to fulfil this role, and nurses who provide these services need training to do so. Better co-operation is needed between health and education authorities to make Reproductive Health Care education widely available in schools to reach teenagers who do not attend clinics. Despite nurses' motivation to tackle health promotion and community-oriented roles, the process is not always smooth and there are many complex policy challenges including high workloads, a lack of skills training, a shortage of funding, uncommitted community members, role ambiguity and unclear legal mandates (Borrow et al. 2011; Reid et al. 2006).

Austerity, Training and Its Impact on Nurses' Decision-making in a Complex Legal Environment

South Africa's legal framework gives nurses an important interventionist role, in addition to their health promotion role. They must report all cases where they suspect child abuse (defined as ill treatment or deliberately inflicted emotional or psychological harm, assault, bullying or sexual abuse) or neglect to the relevant authorities. SRH nurses are on the front line of service provision, and may therefore be the first to encounter signs that abuse is taking place. Given the endemic high levels of violence against women and children in South Africa (Abrahams et al. 2013), nurses must have the training and guidelines to enable them to intervene and/or refer patients appropriately. Yet, training on the legal aspects of SRH service provision remains critically low: nurses and facility managers reported that there is no training budget and insufficient relief staff to release those who seek training. This means that posts remain empty and waiting rooms full when training takes place. As a result, nurses 'mostly … teach ourselves'.

Only 6 of the 28 nurses in our study knew that the age of consent was 16 years. While this lack of knowledge is perhaps unsurprising, given that the law provides adolescents the right to contraception at a younger age, the confusion creates a problematic context for mandatory reporting, and blurs the line between what respondents think *is* against the law and what they think *should be* against the law, between questions of law and practice. This discretionary space fosters patient interactions that are shaped by personal values and beliefs, and which risk being moralistic and alienating for patients. With such low levels of training, it is also unsurprising that nurses are reluctant to become involved (Joyner 2009), often because they feel ill-equipped to document injuries and care for victims, or fear having to testify in court. This is highly problematic as medical evidence is often crucial to the outcomes of domestic violence, sexual offences and child abuse cases. This situation also runs entirely contrary to values of care that many of our nurses espoused.

Interdisciplinary models are widely recognised as best practices in health promotion. Yet the lack of training for health professionals on the legal aspects, the fear among medical professionals of entering into the domain of the criminal justice system, and a severe lack of resources required to foster interdisciplinary understanding and working relationships between social services, health and the police, have the effect of eroding the integrity and intent of mandatory reporting requirements and of undermining the quality and accessibility of care (Hoffman-Wanderer et al. 2013).

Nurses' Dissatisfaction with Providing Services Under Resource Constraints

Street-level bureaucracy theorists hold that real policy-making occurs at the 'coal face', in other words, from the bottom-up rather than from top-down. Day-to-day processes, workloads and the work environment shape front-line workers' decision-making and behaviour (e.g., Lipsky 1980; Maynard-Moody and Musheno 2003). In our study, understaffing, procedural processes at health facilities, lack of physical space and the socio-cultural context of the community all influenced the way that nurses provided services. The tension and friction experienced in this environment is exacerbated in a climate of austerity and resource scarcity, where 'tightening the screws' on service provision increases the pressure on nurses, and constrains young people's lives, health and choices.

While the participants in our study had virtually no impact on the high-level strategic and financial decisions that govern their service provision (e.g., setting departmental budgets and priorities), they had relatively high levels of autonomy in the clinic environment. Straddling the gap between law and policy against the service provision reality in over-burdened, under-resourced clinics, nurses used this discretionary space to mould implementation in ways that assuaged their dissatisfaction with the structural environment, and to find a better 'fit' with their own understanding of the moral context of their work (Müller et al. 2016). This policy adaptation cut both ways: sometimes serving clients' needs through adaptation, but often 'massaging' implementation to dissuade service utilisation. On the one hand, nurses told how they avoid reporting clients to social workers where doing so may invite harmful (parental) scrutiny or may bend the clinic's rules to meet service needs:

> [Teenagers] are too shy to go to the front, to sit in the front [of the clinic]. ... One day there was four of them ...and they said, one of them ... think[s she] is pregnant [and] they want me to test the urine. ... All four of them go to the toilet and then all four of them come back, so I never know [whose urine sample had been provided]. It was negative eventually; if it was positive I would have known. But that's how I want to do it.

Nurses also frequently used their discretion in negative ways: for example, providing impractical referrals to TOP clinics that are far away, providing by-the-rules service that discourages access, and by displaying pictures of foetuses taped to TOP service desks under the guise of providing so-called complete information (Müller et al. 2016). In doing so, nurses claim to have served client needs, but they did so in ways that were more aligned with their own values. The rules, norms and standards of practice—in essence, the 'what we do here' of service provision—sometimes went beyond their responsibilities, and obstructed adequate service provision and clients' rights. Nurses recognised these tensions, but did not imagine how they could effect change. Rather, they were the very end point of the service chain and there was no feedback loop that ensured that their front-line experiences shaped the upstream financial decision-making, policy articulation or law reform.

Nurses' Views on Decision-making and Participation in Policy Processes

The majority of South African nurses have had little, if any, training in the principles and pragmatics of a health promotion approach (Onya 2007). This suggests a knowledge translation gap from health policy to nursing practice. In order to be effective in their community-orientated roles, nurses require competency skills such as analytic assessment skills, therapeutic, communication, brokerage and facilitation skills. They need basic public health science knowledge and community dimensions of practice (Sistrom and Hale 2006). Nurses work in multidisciplinary teams and therefore also require networking and collaborative skills to effectively engage with other community institutions and other healthcare professionals. One might expect that this knowledge translation gap would result in nurses' strict adherence to a clinical regimen, a hesitation to delve into education, advocacy and prevention efforts. Our evidence suggests, however, that nurses *do* view these health promotion activities as their responsibility, but in the absence of formal training, their interactions with patients are often tempered by personal values and beliefs, and efforts to 'educate' swiftly devolve into moralising (Wood and Jewkes 2006).

Maynard-Moody and Musheno (2003) argue that front-line workers will often feel disdainful of 'ungrounded' directives from lawmakers and politicians who are perceived as out of touch with policy realities. Our findings echo these sentiments, as nurses felt excluded from processes that gave rise to policy shifts related to adolescent SRH. This lack of consultation with the 'experts on the ground' was seen by many as one of the reasons for the existing complex and conflicting laws:

> This is the problem of not consulting the relevant stakeholders; they don't consult the people who provide the actual services. If they had consulted the people who are involved in this, they would not have ended up with conflicting laws. Because at the end of the day, you turn a blind eye. It's just again a new thing. Those people who write up the laws need to involve the people who are involved.

The structural challenges described above were also the key obstacles to involving nurses in policy processes. Nurses felt that they did not have time for reflection on their service provision, let alone time to spend in policy meetings and drafting committees. Talking about the values and ethics of diversity in neo-Liberal contexts, Milatovic and Wånggren (2014, p.33) ask, 'So where do questions of race, equality and diversity end up in a system which privileges quick and easy answers above a dedication to social justice?' We can adapt this question to ask where questions of provider reflexivity and patient participation, both crucial to envisioning and enacting a more just and responsive health system, end up in a system that necessitates quick patient 'processing' in large numbers

according to a neo-Liberal paradigm? Nurses in our study sought opportunities to attend workshops on SRH service provision and expressed
gratitude for spaces to discuss implementation challenges. However, their
resource-limited service environments meant that participation in such
day-long workshops was either impossible because nobody could relieve
their duties, or resulted in a cancellation of patient services for the day.
As a result, nurses' voices are usually not heard in policy spaces. This is a
missed opportunity: if nurses are consulted and participate in the development of health policies, the gaps between 'top-level policy makers' and
'street-level bureaucrats' can be narrowed, resulting in policies that are
more informed by the 'realities on the ground' and accepted among the
implementers (Maynard-Moody and Musheno 2003).

Such a participatory approach is particularly useful in resource-limited
settings, and on issues that have moral content and elicit a certain level
of discretion from healthcare providers, such as SRH service provision.
For example, Fonn and Xaba (2001) employed the 'Health Workers for
Change' programme in a participatory exploration of nurses' perceptions of provision of adequate health services, and how these constraints
affected their work in general and their relationship with female patients
in particular. They found it to be a useful methodology for supporting
nurses to link policy provisions to the challenges that they experience in
their working environment, thus creating a health systems management
tool from the 'bottom up' (Vlassoff and Fonn 2001).

Conclusion

Our findings show that South African nurses who provide SRH services
to young people navigate conflicting roles as service providers, educators
and law enforcers. In trying to negotiate their conflicting obligations, a
restrictive work environment and the complex demands of their teenage
clients, these front-line workers revert to value judgements when making decisions about service implementation. Given the morally charged
nature of adolescent sexuality, and SRH service provision, this is not surprising, and results in front-line workers effectively implementing public
policy based on their moral frameworks.

In the context of austerity, service providers are important not only for potentially buffering or exacerbating the effect of austerity measures on clients, but also for acting as a feedback mechanism linking the system's resources to the people who are receiving them. We have seen all three played out in our data. While accepting that service providers fulfil the potential conflicting roles of buffering and exacerbating, they are *not* fulfilling the policy-linking third role. We argue that this is a crucial role. Where policy is made without incorporating the views of key implementing stakeholders, it should be unsurprising that service provision at the 'coal face' often bears little resemblance to the intention of policy and lawmakers. In youth sexual health services in South Africa, the implications for young people's health and rights are significant, and the public health challenges are made substantially worse in a context of resource scarcity and austerity.

References

Abrahams, N., S. Matthews, L. Martin, C. Lombard, and R. Jewkes. 2013. Intimate Partner Femicide in South Africa in 1999 and 2009. *PLoS Med* 10(4): e1001412. doi:10.1371/journal.pmed.1001412.

Anon. 1991. *Regulations Relating to the Scope of Practice of Persons Who are Registered or Enrolled under the Nursing Act*, Pretoria.

Borrow, S., A. Munns, and S. Henderson. 2011. Community-based child health nurses: An exploration of current practice. *Contemporary Nurse* 40(1): 71–86.

Breier, M. 2008. Medical Doctors. In *Skills shortage in South Africa: Case studies of key professions*, eds. J. Erasmus and M. Breier. Cape Town: HSRC Press.

Coovadia, H., et al. 2009. The health and health system of South Africa: Historical roots of current public health challenges. *Lancet* 374(9692): 817–834. Available from: http://www.ncbi.nlm.nih.gov/pubmed/19709728. Accessed 1 May 2014.

Department of Health & the Reproductive Health Research Unit (WITS). 2001. *National Contraception Policy Guidelines*. Johannesburg: University of the Witwatersrand.

Department of Social Development. 2015. *National Adolescent Sexual and Reproductive Health Rights Framework Strategy*. Pretoria: Department for Social Development.

Ehlers, V. 2003. Adolescent mothers' utilization of contraceptive services in South Africa. *International Nursing Review* 50(4): 229–241.

Fonn, S., and M. Xaba. 2001. Health Workers for Change: Developing the initiative. *Health Policy and Planning* 16(Suppl. 1): 13–18.

Harvey, D. 2005. *A Brief History of Neoliberalism*. Oxford: Oxford University Press.

Hoffman-Wanderer, Y., L. Carmody, J. Chai, and S. Röhrs. 2013. *Condoms? Yes! Sex? No! Conflicting Responsibilities for Healthcare Professionals Under South Africa's Framework on Reproductive Rights*. Cape Town: Gender, Health and Justice Research Unit, University of Cape Town. Available from http://www.ghjru.uct.ac.za/sites/default/files/image_tool/images/242/documents/Condoms_Yes_Sex_No.pdf. Accessed 13 Dec 2015.

Joyner, K. 2009. *Health Care for Intimate Partner Violence: Current Standard of Care and Development of Protocol Management*, Ph.D Dissertation. University of Stellenbosch.

Lipsky, M. 1980. *Street-level bureaucracy: Dilemmas of the Individual in Public Service*. New York: Russell Sage Foundation.

Maynard-Moody, S., and M. Musheno. 2003. *Cops, Teachers, Counsellors: Stories from the Front Lines of Public Service*. Ann Arbor: University of Michigan Press.

Mayosi, B.M., and S.R. Benatar. 2014. Health and health care in South Africa—20 years after Mandela. *The New England journal of medicine* 371(14): 1344–1353 .Available from: http://www.ncbi.nlm.nih.gov/pubmed/25265493. Accessed 19 Mar 2015.

Milatovic, M., and L. Wånggren. 2014. Spaces of possibility: Pedagogy and politics in a changing institution. In *The Para-Academic Handbook: A toolkit for making-learning-creating-acting*, eds. A. Wardrop and D.M. Withers. Bristol: HammerOn Press.

Müller, A., S. Röhrs, Y. Hoffman-Wanderer, and K. Moult. 2016. "You have to make a judgment call"—Morals, judgments and the provision of quality sexual and reproductive health services for adolescents in South Africa. *Social Science & Medicine* 148: 71–78.

National Department of Health. 2011. Policy Paper for National Health Insurance. Available from http://www.gov.za/sites/www.gov.za/files/national-healthinsurance_2.pdf. Accessed 19 Mar 2015.

Ongaro, E., F. Ferré, and G. Fattore. 2015. The fiscal crisis in the health sector: Patterns of cutback management across Europe. *Health Policy* 119: 954–963.

Onya, H. 2007. Health Promotion in South Africa. *Promotion & Education* 14(4): 233–237.

Quaglio, G., T. Karapiperis, L. van Woensel, E. Arnold, and D. Mcdaid. 2013. Austerity and Health in Europe. *Health Policy* 113(1): 13–19.

Reid, S.J., L. Mantanga, C. Nkabinde, N. Mhlongo, and N. Mankahla. 2006. The community involvement of nursing and medical practitioners in KwaZulu-Natal. *South African Family Practice* 48(8): 16–16e.

Republic of South Africa. 2015. *Budget Highlights 2015.* Pretoria: National Treasury. Available from http://www.treasury.gov.za/documents/national%20 budget/default.aspx#. Accessed 19 Aug 2015.

Sistrom, M.G., and P.J. Hale. 2006. Outbreak investigations: Community participation and role of community and public health nurses. *Public Health Nursing* 23(3): 256–263.

Von Holdt, K., and M. Murphy. 2007. Public hospitals in South Africa: stressed institutions, disempowered management. In *State of the Nation: South Africa 2007*, eds. S. Buhlungu, J. Daniel, and R. Southall. Cape Town: HSRC Press.

Vlassoff, C., and S. Fonn. 2001. Health Workers for Change as a health systems management and development tool. *Health Policy and Planning* 16(Suppl. 1): 47–52.

Watson, J., L. Vetten, P. Parenzee, T. Madonko, and S. Bornman. 2014. *Eye on the Money: Women and government priorities in South Africa.* Cape Town: Women's Legal Centre. Available from https://za.boell.org/sites/default/files/ wlc_eye_on_the_money_2014.pdf. Accessed 14 Jan 2016.

Wood, K., and R. Jewkes. 2006. Blood blockages and scolding nurses: Barriers to adolescent contraceptive use in South Africa. *Reproductive Health Matters* 14(27): 109–118. Available from http://www.ncbi.nlm.nih.gov/pubmed/ 16713885. Accessed 26 Nov 2014.

Legislation and Policy Documents

Children's Act 38 of 2005.

Criminal Law [Sexual Offences and Related Matters] Amendment Act 32 of 2007.

Criminal Law [Sexual Offences and Related Matters] Amendment Act Amendment Act 5 of 2015.

Choice on Termination of Pregnancy Act 92 of 1996.

National Health Act 61 of 2003.

The South African Nursing Council Regulations Relating to the Scope of Practice of Persons Who are Registered or Enrolled under the Nursing Act, 1978, Government Notice No. R. 2598, 30 November 1984 as amended by: No. R. 146 10 July 1987; No. R. 2676 16 November 1990; No. R. 26015 February 1991.

Part III

Young People, Welfare States and *Their* Futures

12

Pre-assembling Our Young: Points of Movement in Post-Austerity Ireland

Annelies Kamp

Introduction

The chapter offers something of a post-critical reading of youth transition through and beyond secondary school towards some form of work in the context of the Republic of Ireland (Ireland). The chapter takes material-semiotic tools, media reportage and extant research to consider what I refer to as the 'pre-assemblage' of young people moving through, and beyond, second-level school in what appears as some kind of post-austerity context. In doing this, the chapter brings into focus actors, both distant and local, human and nonhuman, who in various ways shape and form, by subtle and not-so-subtle means, and contribute, or impede, the movement of young people beyond a primary engagement with formal

A. Kamp (✉)
University of Canterbury, Christchurch, New Zealand

© The Editor(s) (if applicable) and The Author(s) 2017
P. Kelly, J. Pike (eds.), *Neoliberalism, Austerity, and the
Moral Economies of Young People's Health and Well-being*,
DOI 10.1057/978-1-137-58266-9_13

education and the consequences of this for young people's health and well-being, broadly defined.

The gathering of this chapter occurs in my current standpoint in Aotearoa, New Zealand. My approach will be, in keeping with a material-semiotic sensibility, to look very closely at one of the central techniques of transition in Ireland—colloquially referred to as 'the points race'. I will consider how points have evolved to a 'black box' status, and demonstrate their mediating role in enabling certain events to flow while others can only stutter. First, I will provide a more detailed overview of the Irish context and the pivotal role of the points system in this context. I will then introduce the tools of material semiotics that I am taking up in my exploration. Finally, I will attempt to portray the potential for some form of reassemblage of what happens between school and work and the contribution such a rethinking might make to the health and well-being of the young people of contemporary Ireland.

Beginnings in Aotearoa New Zealand

It seems to me that the best beginning of this chapter is its end. By 'end', I refer in part to where this chapter is being drawn together, in Christchurch, a very particular part of Aotearoa, New Zealand. For me, New Zealand is tūrangawaewae. A place to stand. Tūrangawaewae refers to the place where a person feels particularly strong in standing, where she is empowered and connected. I have recently returned to my home country after 15 years abroad, most recently in the Republic of Ireland.

Before leaving New Zealand in 2002, I worked for a number of years as National Advisor for the then Skill New Zealand[1]. I reference this context as a counter-point to the educational context in the Republic of Ireland, a reflection to which I will return later in the chapter. I am suggesting that New Zealand's outcomes-based qualifications strategy, operationalised through radical reform; the implementation of the National Certificate of Educational Achievement (NCEA) at levels 1, 2

---

[1] Skill New Zealand was a Crown Agency working at the interface of education and employment. Its former responsibilities are now managed by the Tertiary Education Commission.

and 3; and a transformative qualifications framework—the New Zealand Qualifications Framework (NZQF)—have made explicit the spaces that exist for productive learning and assessment assemblages that, in the context of precarious labour markets, are of even greater benefit to young people securing their initial qualifications and moving from school to some form of sustainable work and consequent well-being[2].

While a detailed review of the evolution of these institutional arrangements is beyond the limits of this chapter, a brief overview might be helpful to the reader. The implementation of outcomes-based education has the potential for 'profound impact' on the content and style of schooling systems (Lee et al. 2013). This potential was realised in the New Zealand context. The shift away from traditional, externally assessed examination-based senior school qualifications and towards the NCEA was the result of over 34 years of advocacy (Lennox 2001). From the 1960s, the existing qualifications of School Certificate and the University Entrance Examination were being challenged by employers and educational professionals (and their Union) as insufficient to the needs of the emerging technological society and a desire for a 'radical social meliorist agenda' (Lee et al. 2013). The alliance of (at times) opposing ideological stakeholders in setting the scene for such wide-ranging reform illustrates the duality of the reforms: on the one hand, meeting the needs of *all* young people in assembling qualifications that would retain relevancy in the context of a rapidly changing world; on the other hand, acting as a powerful mechanism for the measurement and accountability arrangements of neo-Liberal mentalities of government (Pierre 2000).

New Zealand's NZQF when implemented was also the most comprehensive qualifications framework in the world, a 'grand design' version that encompassed all sectors of education and training, including schools (Young 2005, 2003)[3]. With its seeds in the neo-Liberal economics that were dominant in the 1980s New Zealand (Philips 2003), the NZQF was a 'strong' framework, highly prescriptive and designed to realise the 'intrinsic logic' of such frameworks: to be transparent to its users

---

[2] This is not to suggest that a job, any job, is inherently good. That issue is canvassed elsewhere in this collection.

[3] During its early years, there was some roll-back on the form of involvement of the university sector.

in terms of what a given qualification signified; to minimise barriers to progression (both vertical and horizontal); and to maximise access, flexibility and portability between different sectors of education and employment and of different sites of learning (Young 2003). In this, both the NZQF and the NCEA, which followed it in implementation, would attempt to change the way 'positional advantage' by way of education was ordered in New Zealand (Strathdee 2003).

Developments in the Republic of Ireland

> SOME months ago I began to think I should start getting my head around the labyrinth that is the CAO application process, the points system and college courses.
>
> Not for myself, you understand, but I have two daughters currently in secondary school, the eldest of whom will be heading into fifth year in September. But it seems that events have overtaken me. Changes are apparently afoot.
>
> I read the reports with interest. I was hoping to discover that finally this 'points' madness, which has transformed our system of education into a game, was going to be addressed.
>
> But sadly, no. (Scully 2015)

As the introduction to this book attests, there is a broad body of work demonstrating the ways that a disproportionate burden of the fallout of the Global Financial Crisis (GFC) in Europe has been, and will be, carried by the youngest and future generations (Eurofound 2013; Commission 2014; Traynor 2013; Carney et al. 2014). As the crisis swept beyond the USA, the Irish economy collapsed from the extreme, precarious highs of the preceding Celtic Tiger years (see Lewis 2011 for a detailed overview). The collapse had consequence for all residents but, particularly, for children and young people in transition to first-time employment. In terms of youth unemployment, Ireland (along with Greece and Spain) was a standout statistic. Youth unemployment rates moved from a low of 6.2 per cent just before the collapse to 31.20 per cent in 2012 (Central Statistics Office 2012). Youth unemployment became something of a poster child of the economic collapse, fostering a flurry of European Union (EU)-level youth policy initiatives (European Commission 2012).

Even in 2015, with Ireland's startling recovery to 7 per cent economic growth (Beesley 2015) subsequent to five years of EU/International Monetary Fund (IMF) dictated policies of austerity, youth unemployment rates remained at around 20 per cent and concerns about long-term impacts remained. As Allen (2012) argues, the Irish people paid heavily to 'gain the prize for the model pupil of the IMF and EU'. Even if economic recovery is now underway, radically decreased unemployment does not mean that stable, decent jobs will suddenly become available for young people (UNICEF Office of Research 2014; Standing 2011). There is potential for young people to be 'scarred' by prolonged periods of joblessness they may have to endure as the economic recovery moves beyond unused capacity that remains available to employers: increased future unemployment risks and/or reduced future earnings.

Scarring can also risk a young person's future happiness, job satisfaction, wages and health (Bell and Blanchflower 2010). In Ireland more generally, the impact of the recession, the EU/IMF bailout and austerity policies are evidenced in worsening well-being indicators from 2007 to 2013: only Turkey, Cyprus and Greece fared worse (UNICEF Office of Research 2014). 'Abundant individualism' appeared to be the order of the day; the largely peaceable acceptance of 'a harsh and protracted programme of austerity' by the Irish people (Carney et al. 2014) is, for some, as concerning as the policies of austerity themselves signally, as it does the 'progressive destruction of our collective provision against risk' (Levitas 2012). In a study of solidarity between generations in austerity Ireland, Carney et al. (2014) demonstrate the role of Ireland's 'familial welfare state' in ameliorating both the individual impacts of the financial collapse and policies of austerity, and the potential for any effective collective protest. However, if the 'lifetime risks' of school to work transition in a recession (UNICEF Office of Research 2014) demand action, the role of other key actors in that transition, most particularly schools, become a central concern.

Ireland is unusual in that the vast majority of students (currently around 93 per cent) enrol in programmes focussed on eligibility for higher education (Banks and Smyth 2015). This eligibility is established by way of what is colloquially referred to as the 'points race', conducted by the Central Admissions Office (CAO). Over the years, the process of transition from school to work, training or higher education in Ireland has become increasingly dependent on academic grades, assessed by a final examination. Students are assigned points based on the subject level they enrol in and the grade achieved. In 2015, with the Irish economy once again burgeoning, the number of higher education courses requiring more points was 'higher than it has been for years' (Donnelly 2015a).

Ireland's qualifications framework is not comprehensive and does not include school qualifications. The secondary school curriculum in the Republic of Ireland currently comprises a three-year lower secondary programme followed by a two- or three-year upper secondary programme. Both the lower and upper programmes culminate in nationally standardised examination: at lower level, the Junior Certificate examination[4] influences what programmes students can access at the upper level; at the upper level, the Leaving Certificate examination decides entry to higher education. The upper-level programme is composed of an optional non-examination Transition Year which students can complete before moving to one of a number of Leaving Certificate qualifications for two years. Transition Year first appeared in 1974 during an earlier period of economic crisis in Ireland. With its focus on personal development, exploration and community engagement, Transition Year has been 'embraced and resisted simultaneously' (Jeffers 2011), even labelled at times as a 'doss year' (Walshe 2009). However, there has been consistent growth in Transition Year take-up over the years (Clerkin 2013) and acknowledgement that students who opt into it ultimately perform better in the Leaving Certificate with all the consequential benefits that high achievement in the Leaving Certificate bestows (Smyth and McCoy 2009).

International research indicates that such high-stakes testing in secondary education has a disproportionately negative effect on some groups of students, most notably those who do not come from privileged families (Au 2008; Nichols et al. 2005; Grodsky et al. 2008; McCoy et al. 2010) or dominant cultures (Au 2009; Ladson-Billings 2006). For those who seek, as is the norm in Ireland, to win in the points race and attend university in a 'quality' course that maximises their ability to compete in the

---

[4] Since 2009, there have been concerted attempts by Ministers of Education to undertake radical reform of the Junior Certificate, moving it away from a 'high-stakes' summative examination. At the time of writing, this has not been achieved MURRAY, N. 2015. Junior Cert Reform at Risk After Poll. *Irish Examiner*, 25 September 2015.

context of the risk society (Beck 1992), money matters: students from fee-paying school students dominate enrolments in high-points courses (McAuliffe 2015). High-stakes testing does not have to, but often does, have unintended consequences for classroom practices, narrowing curriculum and fragmenting knowledge (Au 2007). Research indicates that this context also has an impact on the well-being of young people; in the USA, students depicted their perceptions of high-stakes testing through images that reflected anxiety, anger, boredom and withdrawal (Triplett and Barksdale 2005); wide-ranging research in Ireland on stress, particularly for young women, of examination years and a lack of attention to personal and social development has been available since the 1980s (Hannan and Shortall 1991). Perhaps of greatest concern to the current collection is recent research that outlines how the Irish context has altered the views of young people themselves around what they value in formal education contexts:

> Their impatience with teachers who go 'off message' is in stark contrast to their critique of exam-oriented teaching 2–3 years earlier and can be seen as reflecting the high stakes involved for young people in securing access to the kinds of tertiary education which will maintain their middle-class position. (Smyth and Banks 2012)

It is the interwoven actions of human and nonhuman actors in maintaining this points race, with all its consequences in framing the opportunities for young Irish people in transition beyond school, that I will traverse in what remains of this chapter.

The Research and Conceptual Framework

In what follows, I am drawing on mixed methods research[5] undertaken by a research team from Dublin City University and the University of Ulster in Northern Ireland that explored the opportunities for meaningful

---

[5] The research was funded by the Standing Conference on Teacher Education North and South (SCoTENS).

workplace for students in the context of the senior second-level curricula on the island of Ireland (Kamp and Black 2014). For this chapter, I limit the data to findings from the Republic of Ireland. The chapter is also informed by subsequent desktop research using Nexis of media articles published in Ireland between 1 January 2015 and 31 December 2015 using the keyword 'points' with over 500 words. A total of 473 articles resulted, which were then filtered by the 'education and training' subject field. This resulted in 44 articles, which have been selectively used for illustrative purposes. In this chapter, I am considering the points race as an assemblage that mediates the opportunities afforded to young people in the Republic of Ireland as the country emerges from its entanglement with the GFC, a recession and its accompanying austerity processes. Here, I present a necessarily brief overview of my conceptual toolkit.

The broad field of material semiotics including but not limited to actor-network theory (ANT) is the name of an 'array of practices' (Fenwick and Edwards 2010) that engage with the idea of exploring—rather than either assuming or ignoring—the full range of actors that are present in a social practice such as transition from school to work. These research approaches demand the tracing of processes of assemblage of many kinds of 'actants'. The term actant refers to the *potential* agents—both human and nonhuman—involved in a given event; the actant always has the potential to become a 'performing part' (Fenwick and Edwards 2010: 10) of the network. A defining position for ANT is that there is no difference in the treatment of human and nonhuman actants: a generalised 'symmetry' prevails that dispenses with the kinds of categorical distinctions that are usually taken to be foundational (Law 2009).

Material semiotics aims to render visible this diverse range of actants—and their 'intimate nature' (Latour 2007) as intermediaries or mediators. An entity that is an intermediary 'transports meaning or force without transformation': whatever is its input will also be its output. Intermediaries are rare exceptions. However, there are endless mediators which 'transform, translate, distort, and modify the meaning of the elements they are supposed to carry'. Latour notes that no matter how complicated an intermediary is, it can be easily forgotten. A mediator, however, is complex no matter how simple it may look. This distinction is important because, to paraphrase Latour (2007: 105) if a social factor such as a policy that seeks to mediate the transition from school to work for young people in a context of austerity is transported through intermediaries, then everything important is in the policy, not in the intermediaries (be they teachers, school buildings, curriculum, parental aspirations, university admission processes, clocks, textbooks, the labour market, impending examinations, workplaces, qualifications frameworks, educational media, administrative schedules, etc.). Clearly this is not the case. A given policy plays out with immense variation to greater or lesser benefit—in terms of the possibilities for education, employment, civic engagement and long-term health and well-being—for young people.

However, the concept of mediation can, and must, be further differentiated to consider the different ways that nonhumans make us act. Latour (1993) outlines four meanings of mediation. First, mediation can relate to interference whereby each agent—human and nonhuman—interferes with, or translates, the original goal of the other. In this, it becomes clear that responsibility for action must be shared among the various actants with their diverse programmes of action.

The second meaning of mediation is composition. Here, mediation allows us to consider how, if attention is drawn to the full range of actors, the composite goal becomes the common achievement of each of the agents. Thus, the 'prime mover' of an action becomes a 'nested' series of practices, the sum of which—the outcome—can be calculated but only by being attentive to all mediating actors. Here, the focus is on how action is composed; how action is 'a property of associated entities'.

The third meaning of mediation considers the folding of time and space or 'black boxing'. Here, Latour is interested in how the production of both actors and artefacts is somehow rendered opaque: in how action is 'made invisible by its own success' (Latour 1993: 304). The argument here is that the more something succeeds, the less it can be understood as attention needs focus only on inputs and outputs rather than the complexity that inheres between input and output.

The fourth and most important meaning of mediation is crossing the boundary between signs and things or 'delegation'. Delegation here refers to the process whereby both meaning and expression are translated in nonhuman actors through whom delegation is achieved. Consider the speed bump. Whereas a law requiring drivers to slow down may be intended to make the roads safer, the speed bump achieves the 'slowing down' by delegation. What was a moral imperative now becomes a selfish imperative; the driver slows down not to protect people but rather to avoid damage to the car.

Techniques of Transition

In what remains of the chapter, I want to work with these four meanings of mediation to consider one of the prime movers present in the school to work transition of contemporary Ireland: the points race. I will then close the chapter by reflecting on some of the possibilities that have been created by introducing a different 'species' of actor in the context of Aotearoa, New Zealand: a comprehensive and strong qualifications framework that includes school qualifications.

The First Meaning of Mediation: Goal Translation

Clearly, teachers are high-level mediators with, seemingly, immense scope for goal translation. This refers to the way teachers can make other mediators—potential employers, classrooms, curriculum documents, parents of their students, examination scripts, community projects and so on—do things that would not be on the agenda without some form of interference. In an article in the *Irish Examiner*, this process of goal translation is apparent. The article speaks to a policy decision that allowed Leaving Certificate students to gain 25 extra points if they sat and passed higher maths. While the intention of the bonus points might have been 'well meaning' (although the question is posed in the article as to whether these good intentions are focussed more on the needs of the knowledge economy than on the 'ambitions and confidence of young people'), 764 students got zero for translating their original learning goals to incorporate higher maths to an effort to boost their points:

> As principals group NAPD pointed out [...] it is further evidence of just how much the points system that dictates college entry is responsible for much more as well. Young people are pinning their hopes and investing a

lot of time, stress, and perhaps even their parents money on efforts to get a good grade in honours maths; in fact any grade at all above a D may boost their CAO scores. But is it worth all that sweat and tears? (Anonymous 2015b)

This 'much more as well' is far reaching with one student interviewed by Smyth and Banks reporting 'I just hate this year because it's changing my personality and stuff' (Smyth and Banks 2012). In keeping with a material semiotic approach, any question of responsibility for this kind of negative impact is, and must be, *shared*. It is through a process of assemblage that connection influences the very particular range of individual actors and, in the process, changes the potential of the potential.

The Second Meaning of Mediation: Composition

In this perspective on mediation, the idea is that a composite goal becomes the common achievement of each of the agents by way of a 'nested' series of practices. A given outcome can be calculated but *only* by being attentive to all mediating actors with all their own, very particular, goals in a competitive, neo-Liberal environment. For example, the goal of universities who pick students based on their position in the points race; the goal of schools to maintain funding levels and avoid bad press; the goal of parents in aspiring for university as is the norm (an actor in itself) in Ireland; the goal of students to meet the expectations of their parents (or not); and the goal of the media in 'giving the public what it wants' which, in this case, is information on strategies to get points, on which schools' students secured the highest point rankings, on what points are required to get into a given course and on a detailed analysis of what was in the examination. All of these are provided to ensure wise decision-making in a context of individualisation, and with an eye to future return on investment (Bauman 2012; Beck 1999).

In the research, the data suggested that once students moved into the Leaving Certificate cycle, points become an end in themselves, assembling with aspirations, various concerned adults, CAO procedures, curriculum documents and so on, displacing study of a given subject area for the learning inherent in it with instrumental, high-stakes goals—goals laden with stress (Banks and Smyth 2015). Regardless of the richness of what might go on in the context of a school, anything that threatened time for what was deemed to be academic work was compromised, lessened, articulated as a distraction of questionable value for many stakeholders, even for some teachers:

> At the moment there is the points system, there are the points [...] I wouldn't see that [workplace learning] had any benefit at the moment because do you know as I said they don't get any recognition for it. (Teacher interview, Ireland)

The Third Meaning of Mediation: Black Boxing

Black boxing as a form of mediation draws attention to how action becomes invisible: the more something succeeds, the less can be known about it. That the points race has become a black box—made invisible by its own success—is perhaps indicated in that a recent book entitled *Education in Ireland: Challenge and Change* (Drudy 2009) appears to make only passing mention of 'points'. This 'disappearance' of nonhuman actors in particular is a central concern for material semiotics: 'objects, no matter how important, efficient, central or necessary they may be, tend to recede into the background very fast [...] and the greater their importance, the faster they disappear' (Latour 2007). Being attentive to moments of 'breakdown' is one technique that can be used to make nonhuman actors speak.

There is some kind of consensus in Ireland that the assessment regime in secondary school may be in 'breakdown', although there is no consensus regarding the question of how badly it is broken. Over recent years, there has been high-level attention to 'the worst excesses of the points race' (Anonymous 2015a). These included the 'massaging' by universities of points to maximise 'marketing signals'. This 'excess' references the 'harsh fact of Irish life' where universities have responded to the psychology around how parents and students judge the value of given courses: high points are equalled with quality; students who achieve lower point courses are deemed to be 'wasting their points'. In this context, universities set points to indicate desirability or design courses with small numbers to 'force' the courses to higher levels of competition.

The Fourth Meaning of Mediation: Delegation

Delegation refers to a process whereby the introduction of an actor results in a process of translation, drawing back into focus those actors who are no longer present, yet remain fully active. This process of mediation as delegation is well illustrated by the role of media in and of itself as a full-fledged actor in allowing points to assemble a range of allies. For example, on 14 August 2015 (Mooney 2015), *The Irish Times* offers the following:

> The question uppermost in the minds of most Leaving Cert students—and their parents—since the results came out on Wednesday is whether their results will secure them a course from their top choices.

The article then goes on to reference their *Results 2015* supplement, published earlier in the week, which included the points for all tertiary courses in 2014 as 'a guide to what they may be next Monday when the CAO makes its first round offers'. The article proceeds to detail how entry points from the previous year will of course be different, before exploring 'trends' from the 2015 data sets. This kind of detailed and constant analysis constructs a discourse of risk: the meaning of a given Leaving Certificate course, and its successful examination, ceases to be about learning. Rather, the young person, their potential and their aspiration (or lack of aspiration) becomes defined by distant actors: university administrators, the CAO office and the man in the office of *The Irish Times* who knows that this is what sells papers at this time of the year. Media connects CAO processes with teachers in schools, who connect with pressured students:

> They are making you feel it's one of the most frightening things you are ever going to do. ... Like, every subject, if you don't pass English, your Leaving Cert is gone, if you don't pass Maths, your Leaving Cert, your don't have a Leaving Cert [...] nearly every teacher is telling us the same thing. (Smyth and Banks 2012)

Reassembling Assessment Practices

There is one bright light in our secondary education system, however, and that is Transition Year.

This year did not exist in my day and provides students with opportunities to explore far outside not only of the curriculum but also themselves. It embodies what education should be—an opening of minds, an exploration of our world, a pause in which to think and debate and sing and climb and challenge.

And, of course, it is the only year out of the six spent in secondary school that you will only very rarely hear the words 'points' and 'Leaving Cert'.

We need a radical overhaul of secondary education and there would be no better start than with continuous assessment, which operates successfully in other countries.

However, the difficulty surrounding the introduction of such change is obvious, as the teachers have already gone on strike for two days over reform of the Junior cycle and they do not seem to be for turning on the issue after more than 20 years of discussions, study papers and expert groups. Resistance to change is endemic.

I cannot possibly contemplate my grandchildren (I am getting a bit ahead of myself here, I know) having to undergo the same education that I did. (Scully 2015)

It seems a strange assemblage indeed that a country such as Ireland—land of scholars and saints—and one that positions itself having 'one of the best education systems in the world and an internationally renowned reputation for academic quality' (www.educationinireland.com) can, at one and the same time, be a the subject of such concern around the consequences of its high-stakes secondary school system.

This chapter has focussed on the complicated role that the second-level school system in general, and its assessment process in particular, has to play in contributing, or not, to the possibilities for young people to engage with the world they will meet beyond school, in post-austerity Ireland. The chapter has mapped the ways 'points' have assembled a range of allies—a 'surviving-the-Leaving-Certificate' rite of passage resplendent with after-parties and media coverage, grind schools, fee-paying schools, teacher unions, tight educational budgets, third-level funding mechanisms, established forms of professional development, parental aspirations and so on—(each bringing with them their own current assemblages of interests) to aggravate this impasse, this 'black boxing' by which 'the points race' is a 'harsh fact of Irish life'. While Ireland has the potential tools—NZQF, Transition Year—and advocates for radical change of the senior school assessment system, these tools are not grasped with commitment, not even in the face of current, and anticipated future, challenges.

This event is also about how assemblages of learning and assessment that occur in various learning environments might be facilitated by radical system change, might offer possibilities for useful forms of curriculum not constrained before the event by customary structures and practice. In a context such as Ireland where the education system remains trapped in its own paradigm and does not act as a mechanism for meritocracy; where the familial welfare state acts as the primary safety for the individual (whatever their stage of life); and where it is argued that the intensification of inequality will, therefore, outlast policies of austerity, have we witnessed a shift of Ireland closer to a sub-protective youth transition regime rather than a liberal youth transition regime (Walther 2006)? It is not that there is no reform of the Leaving Certificate process: there is currently a 'quiet revolution' which involves a new grading system for the Leaving Certificate, and a new way of converting grades through to CAO points (Donnelly 2015b). For some involved in the reform process that is underway, the radical reform that is 'constantly called for' is not required. As Donnelly quotes in her article, Professor Philip Nolan—President of Maynooth University—argues that there is much about Ireland's points system that is excellent and in line with 'best international standards'.

I began this chapter by positioning myself in New Zealand where this particular battle over the form of senior school assessment was fought long ago. Reform has been both revolutionary, and evolutionary, and was enabled by a very particular, powerful, assemblage of allies. The current global emphasis on accountability in education has led to an increasing emphasis on stating and measuring learning outcomes. *How* this emphasis has been actioned makes all the difference (Edwards 2011) but in New Zealand, and in other contexts, this kind of reform has created an explicit space for learning beyond the school, for collaborative endeavours and for assessment in the service of learning rather than learning only in the service of assessment. It is my position that such reform opens spaces for citizenship, solidarity, well-being and life-wide learning. Such examples provide evocative contrast to an education system that focuses on, teaches (either implicitly or explicitly) and rewards strategies of 'abundant individualism', rule following and skills in surviving the stress of sitting external examinations. As John Walshe (2015) writes in the *Irish Independent*, the points system in Irish second-level schooling may indeed be 'brutally fair' but its 'backwash effect' is profound.

References

Allen, K. 2012. The model pupil who failed the test: Social policy in the Irish crisis. *Critical Social Policy* 32: 422–439.

Anonymous. 2015a. Briefing: How colleges inflated points to make courses more attractive. *Sunday Business Post*, August 16.

———. 2015b. Leaving Certificate results: Students being left behind in the face for CAO points. *Irish Examiner*, August 13

AU, W.W. 2007. High-stakes testing and curricular control. *Educational Researcher* 37: 258–267.

———. 2008. Devising inequality: a Bernsteinian analysis of high-stakes testing and social reproduction in education. *British Journal of Sociology of Education* 29: 639–651.

———. 2009. High-stakes testing and discursive control: The triple bind for non-standard student identities. *Multicultural Perspectives* 11: 65–71.

Banks, J., and E. Smyth. 2015. 'Your whole life depends on it': Academic stress and high-stakes testing in Ireland. *Journal of Youth Studies* 18: 598–616.

Bauman, Z. 2012. *On education*. Cambridge: Polity Press.

Beck, U. 1992. *Risk society. Towards a new modernity. Theory, culture & society.* London: Sage.

———. 1999. *Individualization*. London: Sage.

Beesley, A. 2015. Irish economic growth hits 7% as recovery outstrips targets. *The Irish Times*, December 10.

Bell, D.N.F., and D. Blanchflower. 2010. *Youth unemployment: Deja vu?* Bonn, Germany: Institute for the Study of Labor.

Carney, G.M., T. Scharf, V. Timonen, and C. Conlon. 2014. 'Blessed are the young, for they shall inherit the national debt': Solidarity between generations in the Irish crisis. *Critical Social Policy* 34: 312–332.

Central Statistics Office. 2012. *Profile 3 At work.* Dublin: Stationery Office.

Clerkin, A. 2013. Growth of the 'Transition Year' programme nationally and in schools serving disadvantaged students, 1992–2011. *Irish Educational Studies* 32: 197–215.

Commission, E. 2014. *EU measures to tackle youth unemployment.* Belgium: European Commission.

Donnelly, K. 2015a. CAO: Points race speeding up as students chasing top jobs. *Irish Independent,* August 17.

———. 2015b. Getting to the point of the new CAO scale. A quiet revolution has been going on in relation to the Leaving Certificate. *Irish Independent,* September 9.

Drudy, S., ed. 2009. *Education in Ireland. Challenge and change.* Dublin: Gill & Macmillan.

Edwards, R. 2011. Translating the prescribed into the enacted curriculum in college and school. *Educational Philosophy and Theory* 43: 38–54.

Eurofound. 2013. *Young people and temporary employment in Europe.* Brussels: European Foundation for the Improvement of Living and Working Conditions.

European Commission. 2012. *Commission staff working document accompanying the proposal for a Council recommendation on establishing a Youth Guarantee.* Brussels: European Commission.

Fenwick, T., and R. Edwards. 2010. *Actor-network theory in education.* London: Routledge.

Grodsky, E., J. Warren, and E. Felts. 2008. Testing and social stratification in American education. *Annual Review of Sociology* 34: 385–404.

Hannan, D., and S. Shortall. 1991. *The quality of their education. School leavers' views of educational objectives and outcomes.* Dublin: Economic and Social Research Institute.

Jeffers, G. 2011. The Transition Year programme in Ireland. Embracing and resisting a curriculum innovation. *The Curriculum Journal* 22: 61–76.

Kamp, A., and D. Black. 2014. *3 Ply: Exploring the potential of transformative workplace learning for and by teachers.* Armagh, NI: SCoTENS.

Ladson-Billings, G. 2006. From the achievement gap to the education debt: Understanding achievement in U.S. schools. *Educational Researcher* 35: 3–12.

Latour, B. 1993. *We have never been modern.* Harvard: Harvard University Press.

———. 2007. *Reassembling the social. An introduction to Actor-Network-Theory.* Oxford: Oxford University Press.

Law, J. 2009. Actor network theory and material semiotics. In *The new Blackwell companion to social theory*, ed. B.S. Turner. Chichester: Wiley-Blackwell.

Lee, H., G. Lee, and R. Openshaw. 2013. Radical assessment and qualification reform in New Zealand: The rocky road to National Certificate of Education Achievement. *World Studies in Education* 14: 25–45.

Lennox, B. 2001. *Where did NCEA come from?* [Online]. Wellington: New Zealand Qualifications Authority. [online]. Available from: http://www.nzqa. govt.nz/qualifications-standards/qualifications/ncea/understanding-ncea/ history-of-ncea/where-did-ncea-come-from/. Accessed 3 Mar 2016.

Levitas, R. 2012. The just's umbrella: Austerity and the Big Society in Coalition policy and beyond. *Critical Social Policy* 32: 320–342.

Lewis, M. 2011. *When Irish Eyes Are Crying. Vanity Fair.* United States: Conde Naste.

Mcauliffe, N. 2015. Fee schools dominate high-points courses. Table-topping Coláiste Eoin in Stillorgan bucks trend as one of just three non-fee-paying schools in top 10 with high progression rates. *The Irish Times*, December 3.

Mccoy, S., D. Byrne, P. O'connell, E. Kelly, and C. Doherty. 2010. *Hidden disadvantage? A study of the low participation in higher education by the non manual group.* Dublin: Higher Education Authority.

Mooney, B. 2015. Will the points go up or down for the CAO course you want? We list the courses that are likely to rise and those that are likely to fall. *The Irish Times*, August 14.

Nichols, S.L., G. Glass, and D. Berliner. 2005. *High-stakes testing and student achievement.* Arizona: Arizona State University.

Philips, D. 2003. Lessons from New Zealand's national qualifications framework. *Journal of Education & Work* 16: 289–304.

Pierre, J. 2000. *Debating governance, authority, steering, and democracy.* Oxford: Oxford University Press.

Scully, B. 2015. Our rigid education system is an unfair points game largely unchanged since 70s. *Irish Independent*, May 6.

Smyth, E., and J. Banks. 2012. High stakes testing and student perspectives on teaching and learning in the Republic of Ireland. *Educational Assessment, Evaluation and Accountability* 24: 283–306.

Smyth, E., and S. Mccoy. 2009. *Investing in education: Combating educational disadvantage.* Dublin: Economic and Social Research Institute.

Standing, G. 2011. *The Precariat: The new dangerous class.* London: Bloomsbury Academic.

Strathdee, R. 2003. The qualifications framework in New Zealand: Reproducing existing inequalities or disrupting the positional conflict for credentials. *Journal of Education & Work* 16: 147–164.

Traynor, I. 2013. EU pledges E6bn to tackle youth unemployment. *The Guardian*, June 28.

Triplett, C.F., and M.A. Barksdale. 2005. Third through sixth graders' perceptions of high-stakes testing. *Journal of Literacy Research* 37: 237–260.

UNICEF Office of Research. 2014. *Children of the Recession: The impact of the economic crisis on child well-being in rich countries*. Florence: UNICEF Office of Research.

Walshe, J. 2009. Cullen wants transition 'doss year' scrapped. *Irish Independent*, June 4.

———. 2015. Obsession with college entry points and university rankings will only intensify. *Irish Independent*, April 30.

Walther, A. 2006. Regimes of youth transitions. Choice, flexibility and security in young people's experiences across different European contexts. *Young* 14: 119–139.

Young, M. 2003. National qualifications frameworks as a global phenomenon: a comparative perspective. *Journal of Education & Work* 16: 223–237.

———. 2005. National qualifications frameworks: Their feasibility for effective implementation in developing countries. In *Focus Programme on Skills, Knowledge and Employability*. Geneva: International Labour Office.

13

Austerity and the 'Workfare State': The Remaking and Reconfiguration of Citizenship for the Young Unemployed in the Great Recession

Alan France

Introduction

Since the 1980s, the UK, Australia and New Zealand have embraced neo-Liberalism as the way to do social and economic policy (France 2016). While the 'roll out' of neo-Liberalism has varied across time and place, it is clear that even in times of more centralist or left governments the expansion of neo-Liberal practice has continued to both maintain a central place in policy making and increase its influence. This is clearly creating an environment where personal responsibility and active citizenship is the 'norm' for how the young engage with both the state and civil society (France 2007). For example, New Zealand undertook a successful (though painful) economic restructuring of all walks of life in the 1980s. Neo-Liberal ideas reshaped policies in the economy, in social policy, in

A. France (✉)
University of Auckland, Auckland, New Zealand

© The Editor(s) (if applicable) and The Author(s) 2017
P. Kelly, J. Pike (eds.), *Neoliberalism, Austerity, and the Moral Economies of Young People's Health and Well-being*,
DOI 10.1057/978-1-137-58266-9_14

education, in health and even in the political system itself. The watershed period for New Zealand was seen as 1984 when the then Labour government introduced 'Rogernomics', and even though more centralist governments have been in power since, neo-Liberalism remains of central importance (Craig and Cotterell 2007). In the UK, we also see successive Conservative and Labour governments continue to use neo-Liberal approaches first introduced by Margaret Thatcher, while in Australia the neo-Liberal agenda has its origins in the 1970s and was accelerated by the Hawke government and then by the Howard administration in 1996 (Deeming 2014). The Labour government elected in 2007 offered an alternative to this agenda; however, a number of its economic and social policy strategies were clearly strongly influenced by neo-Liberal philosophy. In 2012, the Liberal–National Party coalition was elected with a strong drive towards neo-Liberal policies and practice.

While each country has varied in its use of policy, the impact has been to shift youth policy in ways that aim to create act, self-responsible neo-Liberal citizens (France 2016). For Wacquant (2012, p.71), most analysis of neo-Liberalism concentrates on the 'thin side', that is, the economic conception of the approach, giving little attention to the 'thick side' of the 'institutional machinery involved in the establishment of market dominance and its operant impact on effective social membership'. He suggests that while there may be many forms of neo-Liberalism there remains an

> institutional core that makes it distinct and recognisable. This core consists of an articulation of *state, market and citizenship* that harnesses the first to impose the stamp of the second onto the third. So all three of these institutions must be brought into our analytical ambit. (Wacquant 2012, p.71)

In this context, young people in the neo-Liberal order are required to think of themselves as 'flexible, creative, and not to blame failure on structural conditions but to see this as a result of their own underdeveloped entrepreneurial spirit' (Woodman and Wyn 2015, p.47). As a result, what we have been seeing throughout youth policy in countries such as the UK, Australia and New Zealand is the emergence of a 'new' form of citizenship that emphasises the 'entrepreneurial self' (Kelly 2006). This requires the young to be 'rational, autonomous, responsible … and [having] dispositions of a free, prudent active subject', who are engaged in the process of 'reflexivity, continuously, endlessly for the term of [their] natural life' (Kelly 2006, p.18). We are therefore seeing a form of citizenship emerging through policy and institutional arrangements that demands a person to be responsible for themselves 'in the business of life, as an enterprise, a project or a work in progress' (Kelly 2006, p.18).

Economic Crisis and Austerity

As we are all aware, 2007 was the start of one of the most significant crises in the history of capitalism, or what Harvey called 'the mother of all crisis' (Harvey 2010, p.6). While crisis is not unusual to capitalism the Global Financial Crisis (GFC) had massive ramifications across the global landscape. For example, the impact of the GFC saw gross domestic product (GDP) across the globe adversely affected: between the first quarter of 2008 and the first quarter of 2009, GDP across the Organisation for Economic Co-operation and Development (OECD) countries dropped, on average, by 4.9 %. The initial impact was mild, but by the last quarter of 2008, it had increased rapidly. In the USA, it declined 4.3 %. In Europe, the impact was greater, with the average drop being 5.7 %, although some countries such as the UK (7.2 %) and Italy (7.2 %) suffered more. Internationally, some countries were hit even harder. In Japan, GDP dropped 9.2 % in one year. In Estonia, GDP dropped 20 % and in Ireland, where three of the largest Irish-based banks collapsed, GDP dropped 12.8 %. That said, the impact was not felt as strongly by those economies that either had access to the expanding Asian market (Australia, 0.9 %, and New Zealand, 2.6 %) or had substantial national resources (Norway 3.4 %). There was also a massive drop in consumer demand of 2.7 % on average across OECD countries, although again this hides national variations. The downturns were concentrated in manufacturing, with a fall of 16.3 % between 2007 and 2009 in Europe, and 11.5 % in the USA (Moulton 2014).

The crisis and recession that followed also brought with it high levels of youth unemployment. Between 2007 and 2009, youth unemployment increased across the OECD countries from 11.5 % (69.9 million) to 12.7 % (75.6 million). Over the following two years, it declined to 12.3 % (72.6 million) then gradually increased again until it reached 12.6 % (73.4 million) in 2013. Projections suggest that this increase is set to continue well into 2016 (ILO 2013). Young people are three times more likely to be unemployed than adults and they presently make up almost half of the world's total unemployed (43.7 %), confirming that in times of crisis young people are the hardest hit (ILO 2013). Moving into 2014, evidence from countries such as the UK, Australia and New Zealand confirmed that high levels of youth unemployment remained a major issue in the advanced economies. For example, in Australia youth unemployment remained high but the length of time a young person was unemployed had also grown from 16 weeks on average in 2008 to 29 weeks in 2014, with 18 % of all unemployed young people being classified as long-term unemployed (ABS 2014). In the UK, youth unemployment jumped quite dramatically between 2007 and 2013, but it has since started to decline and continued to fall until July 2014 when it had dropped to 15.9 %. Yet by the end of 2014, it had crept back up to 16.6 % (Office of National Statistics 2014). In New Zealand, the youth unemployment rate increased to 18.9 % in early 2013 then dropped to 16.3 % by the middle of the year; it was seeing a slow and gradual movement downward in 2014 (Statistics New Zealand 2014).

It is important to recognise that the economic crisis of 2007 was in fact a 'crisis in neo-Liberalism' and is related to problems of capital accumulation (Harvey 2010; Dumenil and Levy 2011; King et al. 2012). It is also the case that we need to talk about not one crisis but two with the second being driven by the use of austerity as a policy response to the great recession (Ortiz and Cummins 2012; Konzelmann 2014). The initial response worldwide to the crisis was to develop a number of national and international economic stimuli (Farnsworth and Irving 2012). In the first phase, a number of high-level international agreements were made that involved multibillion dollar cash injections into the banking market leading to suggestions that a new multilateralism was being formed (Farnsworth and Irving 2012). In fact, some went so far as to say that neo-Liberalism was dead (Konzelmann 2014). The growing consensus about strategy across a range of nation states was to increase spending.

It has been claimed that 'for a short period of time in 2009 and 2010, there was a 'Keynesian moment' when all governments implemented fiscal stimulus packages (Seccareccis 2012, p.64).

But by 2011, this had changed and 'austerity' had become the dominant hegemony with respect to how to respond to the crisis (King et al. 2012; Ortiz and Cummins 2012; Konzelmann 2014). A number of factors came into play. Firstly, there remained an 'ideological war' over how to tackle the growing problems created by the crisis (Clarke and Newman 2012). Neo-Liberal advocates constructed the problem as one of 'public debt'. This approach proposed cutting public spending and moving towards 'surplus budgets', rather than drawing on fiscal stimulus. This ideological position was also re-enforced by the International Monetary Fund and others such as the European Bank through loan programmes, and by the academic work of Reinhart and Rogoff (2009) who gave academic credibility to the rationale of tackling debt as a key priority. Even though the article has since been discredited (Herndon et al. 2014), its impact was to re-enforce the hegemonic positioning of 'austerity' across a number of significant economies (Theodoropoulou and Watt 2011) creating what Ortiz and Cummins (2012) claim is a second economic crisis caused by the reduction of public and consumer spending.

Austerity policies have a long history[1]; yet in reality, they have a strong association with neo-Liberal ideology and practice. The types of options open to governments under 'austerity programmes' include cutting back government spending, reducing public debt and reducing the tax burden on individuals, allowing them to have extra money for consumption (King et al. 2012). These strategies can clearly be seen as neo-Liberal and reflect the ideological positioning of 'freeing up markets' and 'tackling the excesses' of the state (Konzelmann 2014). However, the evidence for austerity as a successful measure of tackling the problem remains weak, in so far as the proposition that high levels of public debt impact on economic growth is unproven. Indeed, as Taylor et al. (2012) have shown, over the last 50 years, fiscal expansion and the use of public debt has repeatedly increased economic growth across the USA.

---

[1] See Konzelmann, 2014 for a historical perspective

A major analysis by Ortiz and Cummins (2012) on how national economies were engaging with the austerity agenda found that by 2012, 133 countries had reduced their annual expenditure: 93 of these countries were from the advanced economies and 39 countries were undergoing excessive contraction. This included 73 countries where wage bills or caps were being imposed, 55 countries that were rationalising social protection schemes including the reform of pensions and welfare benefits and another 73 countries where subsidies on food and transport were being removed. Similarly, Theodoropoulou and Watt (2011) examined the use of austerity measures in 17 European countries and found that all of them had planned programmes between 2012 and 2016. It was estimated that this would save or generate over €500 billion across the region. The types of programmes included cutting the minimum wage, a reduction in welfare programmes, the reduction in pensions and other social benefits, job losses in public administration and increased indirect taxes.

The Growth of the 'Workfare State'

One of the most significant areas of intervention by those advocating neo-Liberal strategies to policy making has been the introduction and expansion of welfare-to-work programmes. While welfare-to-work is generally credited to developments in the USA, across Europe and in a wide range of OECD countries, the development of Active Labour Market Policies (ALMP) has been a driving force for intervention into the labour market (France 2016). ALMP are defined as 'a wide-ranging set of measures designed to "actively" intervene in the labour market in order to improve its functioning' (Sunley et al. 2006). Four key areas of policy have been identified under this banner: job search assistance; labour market training or the increase of 'human capital'; private sector incentives for employing the unemployed; and finally, public sector employment (Kluve 2014). Those advocating for ALMP want to focus on the more positive aspects of this approach resisting the negative associations of the US-type schemes that appear to be strongly punitive in their nature. For example, in Sweden and Denmark, the focus on ALMP has been on developing a more social democratic model that aims to balance rights and responsibilities providing both benefits for workers and employers (Sunley et al. 2006). Torfing (1999) distinguishes between 'offensive' and 'defensive' workfare, suggesting that 'offensive' approaches rely on improving skills while 'defensive' approaches concentrate on sanctions and benefit reductions. Peck and Theodore (2012) see the distinction more between 'work first' schemes that compel individuals to take employment and 'human capital' programmes that concentrate on building skills through training. Sunley et al. (2006) suggest that in fact it is possible to distinguish between more social democratic and neo-Liberal activation policies. While both policies tend to make job search a core requirement, the social democratic model tends to concentrate on training and temporary public employment and providing qualifications. The neo-Liberal approach is more focused on lowering wages, reducing benefits and increasing work incentives. As Peck (2001, p.80) suggests, in the neo-Liberal model:

> Workfare is a creature of these political-economic circumstances mobilizing and socializing workers for jobs at the bottom of the new economy. Under conditions of wage stagflation, growing underemployment, and job casualization, workfarism maximizes (and effectively mandates) participation in contingent, low paid work by churning workers back into the bottom of the labour market.

ALMP programmes such as welfare-to-work consistently focus on 'supply side problems' such as lack of jobs skills and poor job searching skills. They also operate as a policy to attend to 'skills deficit' by increasing the role of business and industry in 'reskilling' the young. This is achieved through wage subsidies to the private sector for employing the unemployed, or by funding apprenticeships. Training and incentivising the young unemployed is now big business, with massive government subsidies and resources being targeted at employers and industry (France 2016). Welfare-to-work programmes are also now being provided mainly by the private sector through payment by results. In Australia, public sector employment services were abolished in the mid-1990s and replaced with a system of private and non-profit providers. Currently, there are over 100 providers who compete for contracts at over 2300 sites across Australia (Martin 2014). Similar models have been developed in the UK and New Zealand. At the same time, individuals are consistently 'encouraged' or required to undertake training or further education which for many carries high financial costs and burdens (France 2016). This attention to supply problems not only benefits capital but also operates to locate the problem of unemployment with the unemployed, by increasing personal (and financial) responsibility of the individual for their failure to get work (France 2016).

In the UK, Australia and New Zealand, the type of approaches that have dominated are those defined as 'defensive' (Peak and Theodore 2001), with, largely, a focus on sanctions and penalties for 'non-compliance'. In this context, welfare-to-work tends to 'churn' the most vulnerable and poor into 'poor work' (Peck 2001). This acts not only to socialise and discipline participants but also to shift poverty from 'out-of-work poverty' to 'in-work poverty' helping to reduce the welfare budget of national economies. Such an approach brings the unemployed closer to the labour market but also creates a 'reserve army' of labour that can be drawn on when required (Peck 2001). Such welfare-to-work programmes have emerged unevenly and in different shapes and sizes across time (and place), although this form of practice

> has become the institutional codification of work-oriented welfare reform and as such it must be understood as *both* a reactive, reform strategy *and* a would be successor to the welfare state. (Peck 2001, p.81)

In this context, it is 'fit for purpose' for the new political and economic context driven by neo-Liberal ideals and principles (Wacquant 2012). But such regimes also have a strong role in contributing to the 'moral economy' of neo-Liberalism. Not only does it locate the problem in the individual but also it introduces and normalises a discourse on welfare reform that rejects 'entitlement' as a right, and moves to one that emphasises the 'new social contract of "personal responsibility"' (Hamilton 2014). Such discourses are moralising and powerful in shaping public opinion and perspectives of what is right and wrong in the welfare system (Humpage 2014).

Welfare-to-work programmes can also have a significant role in 'policing' and 'monitoring' the poor. Such programmes are embedded in forms of surveillance that can de-humanise or ignore human rights, especially of the powerless (Maki 2011). For example, in the UK, Work Programme surveillance is a central part of monitoring conditionality and participation (O'Hara 2014). Such approaches tend to reassert the notion that the poor are untrustworthy, feckless and immoral and need to be continually under surveillance (Gazso and McDaniel 2010). Regulating and policing of the poor and of young people in particular are central to the ways these programmes are organised (Wacquant 2009). Such approaches also gained substantial traction in the UK, Australia and New Zealand (France 2016). For example, in Australia, the move to welfare-to-work programmes was introduced in the 1980s under the Hawke Labour government, in the 'New Start' programme which encouraged 'active job searching' for the unemployed. This approach was further expanded by the Keating Labour government who introduced the 'Job Compact' that guaranteed the long-term unemployed a job, but in return claimants had to accept any 'reasonable' offer of work. Non-compliance brought harsher penalties (Hamilton 2014).

By 2000, welfare-to-work programmes gained a stronger foothold across the UK, Australia and New Zealand. With the introduction of so-called Third Way policies, 'welfare-to-work' was seen as having a major role to play in tackling 'the dependency culture' of the young unemployed (France 2016). In Australia, the 1996 Howard Conservative coalition government introduced the 'Work for Dole' (WfD) programme. Under this scheme, all unemployed 18–24-year-olds who had been on a benefit for six months were forced to participate in a range of 'job preparedness' programmes as a condition of receiving benefits. Conditionality was also continually strengthened (Hamilton 2014). In the UK, during this period, we saw the introduction of the 'New Deal' programme that aimed to end a welfare system that 'chains people to passive dependency instead of helping them to realise their full potential' (Department of Social Security 1998, p.9). Funded by a large tax on the profits of privatised utilities, it introduced a range of programmes aimed at young people aged 18–24 and required them to actively participate in order to receive benefits. It was proposed in the New Labour election manifesto as a 'new' deal or settlement between the individual and the state and created the first-ever compulsory scheme in the UK (France 2016).

In the late 1990s, in New Zealand, the National (conservative) government campaigned on the question of 'welfare dependency' and advocated a number of critical reforms that saw the introduction of reduced benefit rates, increased conditionality and sanctions for claimants who left work voluntarily. The newly elected Labour government in 2000 introduced the 'work first' approach, which initially saw them soften many of the welfare-to-work initiatives. However, over the early part of the time in office, it set up a new Jobseeker agreement that increased claimant obligations, increased case management systems, introduced work testing and created a new pre-benefit requirement (Humpage 2014).

As we entered the great recession, all of the national governments in the UK, Australia and New Zealand expanded their welfare-to-work programmes. For example, in the UK, the newly elected Conservative government abandoned New Deal and replaced it with the Work Programme, which increased the welfare-to-work approach by requiring those receiving a Jobseekers' allowance to be part of the programme. It has a strong focus on 18–24-year-olds, and those not in employment, education or training (NEET) aged 16 and 17. Non-compliance by young people at various stages of the Work Programme brings a wide range of sanctions including the loss of benefits. In 2014, the UK government increased restrictions on young people getting access to Jobseeker's allowances and introduced the 'Help to Work' programme for those who have been out of work for over two years. Before they get any benefits, they have to attend the jobcentre every day and either work for free or undertake training.

In Australia, while the 2008–2012 Labor government explored ways of reducing any negative impacts of the 'WfD' programme, it was extended in 2011, giving substantial new powers to providers to suspend payment to job seekers for failure to attend interviews or agree to go onto the programme. This development saw the use of sanctions increase once again with eight-week suspensions increasing substantially (OECD 2012). This continued and was expanded by the incoming Liberal coalition government in 2012. In his first budget in 2013, the newly elected Prime Minister Tony Abbott revealed that job seekers applying for a New Start or Youth Allowance, who had not been previously employed, would face a six-month waiting period before they were eligible for payments. They would also need to undertake 25 hours a week in the WfD programme. Once they had spent six months on the programme, they would lose income support altogether for another six months unless they undertook further training or study after completion.

In New Zealand, the National government have had an extended period of increasing and 'tightening up' on the rules applying to getting benefits (Humpage 2014). For example, the unemployed are now required to actively look for work, accept any suitable job offered and undergo work experience. Sanctions have been increased and for the first breach of the work obligations contract, the main benefit of claimants will be reduced by 50 %. For a second breach, all benefits will be suspended and for a third, the claimant's benefit will be cancelled. Other initiatives have seen the introduction of policies that act to 'quarantine' behaviour (France 2016). For example, the New Zealand government has introduced the Youth Payment for 16–17-year-olds which can only be claimed in exceptional circumstances. Payments will only be distributed through redirections (for accommodation and utility costs), a payment card (for food and groceries) and an in-hand allowance. Beneficiaries must be in full-time education, training or work-based learning,[2] and they must undertake an approved budgeting programme.

While welfare-to-work programmes have been expanded in the UK, Australia and New Zealand, there remains limited reliable evidence that they are successful in meeting their core aims of getting the young into work (Crisp and Fletcher 2008; Martin 2014; Watts et al. 2014; France 2016). Where they are most effective tends to be in removing the young from receiving benefits. For example, a recent UK report based on a five-year evaluation into the effectiveness of sanctions concluded that

- Those under 25 are hit hardest by the sanctions.
- Vulnerable people and those with multiple and complex needs, such as lone parents, disabled people or homeless people, have been

---

[2]Training or work-based learning leading includes undertaking an National Certificate of Educational Achievement level 2 qualification, or an equivalent or higher qualification

disproportionately affected by the recent expansion of welfare conditionality and sanctions.

- This policy has a number of unintended consequences that include distancing people from social support; creating hardship; and displacing rather than solving issues such as long-term worklessness and substance misuse (Watts et al. 2014).

Evidence in New Zealand also shows that sanctions and penalties for those who are seen not to comply continue to grow although much remains unknown about who is sanctioned and why they are sanctioned (Wynd 2013). Yet international evidence on the effectiveness of sanctions suggests they tend to increase exit from benefits but do little for long-term employment prospects. Based on a systematic review of international evidence, Griggs and Evans (2010, p.5) conclude that

> sanctions for employment-related conditions (full-family sanctions in the case of US welfare systems) strongly reduce benefit use and raise exits from benefits, but have generally unfavourable effects on longer-term outcomes (earnings over time, child welfare, job quality) and spill-over effects (i.e. crime rates).

What is interesting to note here then is that even though the welfare-to-work programmes have showed little positive effect on getting people into work, policy makers still see this policy as the primary way of tackling the 'problem' of youth unemployment.

Welfare-to-Work Programmes, and Young People's Health and Well-being

One of the most important points to make when considering the impact of welfare-to-work programmes on young people's health is that health questions remain of little concern to politicians and evaluators. Most assessments of such programmes concentrate on exploring the 'successes' of the programme in terms of employment rates, job readiness, attitudinal change and engagement levels. Very few evaluations give much attention to the impacts of such programmes on participant's health and well-being. For example, in a recent evaluation of the Work Programme in the UK that drew on participant's experiences, health got eight pages of focus in the evaluation report out of 196. But even then its main interest was on health as a barrier to employment. The only time the UK government mentioned possible negative impacts on health in the programme was to deny that changes in health conditions could be attributed directly to involvement in the programme and that contradictory evidence existed:

> In other cases, participants with health conditions reported deterioration in their health, including worsened depression, increased levels of stress and anxiety, and loss of confidence. Such changes were attributed to difficult personal circumstances, an extended period without work, increased indebtedness. These factors could not be directly attributed to Work Programme experiences. However, some reported concerns about pressure from advisers or stress from a perceived threat of sanctioning. Their fears, however, were not always borne out—many participants who had missed appointments with advisers through ill-health said if they phoned in straight away to explain what happened, advisers had been 'fine' about this. (Meager et al. 2014, p.170)

This lack of interest in health impacts of being sanctioned was also missing in New Zealand where the government do not even keep regular detailed records of how many people are sanctioned and what the impacts these experiences might have on a person's or families' financial position, or on the health consequences of being sanctioned and punished by the programme (Wynd 2013). A recent debate in the UK also highlights the lack of state knowledge about the personal consequences of sanctioning on participants' well-being. The Conservative government initially refused to release figures on suicide rates of those participants had been sanctioned on the Work Programme. After sustained pressure from the press and the public, it did release mortality statistics that showed that between December 2011 and February 2014, more than 80 people a month were dying after being declared 'fit for work'. The report also showed that 7200 claimants died after being put onto the programme. The report clearly distanced the programme from these effects stating that: 'Any causal effect between benefits and mortality cannot be assumed from these statistics' (Department of Work and Pensions 2015, p.2). The report also suggested that higher rates of mortality among benefit claimants than the population at large was inevitable due to the fact that a higher number of people on benefits had illnesses than the general population. While there remained growing anecdotal evidence, and individual cases that make the news linking suicides to sanctioning, governments are always able to refute the claims arguing that there remains no clear causal evidence (while also not trying to gather the evidence).

However, there is a growing body of evidence that suggests a link can be made, and does exist. Hale (2015), who researched the experiences of 500 disabled claimants who entered the Work Related Activity Group (WRAG), claimed this programme not only failed to get people back into work but also failed to either understand their health needs or put in adequate forms of support for individuals. Added to this was a practice of conditionality and sanctions that 'left participants in the WRAG fearful, demoralised, and further away from achieving their work-related goals or participating in society than when they started' (Hale 2015, p.5). As a result, many participants expressed high levels of anxiety and increased health problems. In a similar vein, Philip and Mallan (2015, p.8) argued that there is substantial international literature that shows a clear linkage between unemployment and high levels of mental illness: 'Recent meta-analyses have aggregated several hundred studies finding compelling evidence that unemployment is associated with poor mental health.' Finally, O'Hara (2014), in her investigation on austerity, also identified individuals who felt trapped and vulnerable by the way they were treated in the sanctioning process. She also found those responsible for implementing such programmes had grave concerns and worries that they were adding to participant's health issues.

Conclusion

Over the past 30 year's welfare-to-work programmes in countries such as the UK, Australia, New Zealand and the USA have become a 'normal' part of how social welfare for the young unemployed is constructed. The 'workfare state' is at the heart of the neo-Liberal project and makes significant contributions to our understanding of citizenship for the young. As a response to the austerity agenda that has developed in the Great Recession, welfare-to-work has continued to expand its influence and has been used as a way of not only getting people back to work but to reduce the social benefit budget. Having to earn your benefits by being active is now accepted across most liberal nation states as the best way to tackle the 'problem' of dependency and worklessness among the young unemployed. Yet, little evidence exists to suggest that such programmes are effective in getting young people into the labour market. In fact, evidence suggests that most of these strategies are targeted at disciplining, regulating and controlling the poor and operate to show that the state is doing something about the 'feckless', the 'work shy', and the undeserving. The real consequences of these types of programmes remain unknown. Questions over how people manage financially when sanctioned or what impact of living under the stresses that such programmes promote remain of little concern to those who advocate such programmes. For those who have been most affected by the GFC welfare-to-work policies create a form of citizenship that is significantly different from those who are working or managing to cope. Young people who are required to be on welfare-to-work programmes find themselves having few benefits and rewards, but significant responsibilities and obligations. If they are seen to fail these, they are sanctioned, punished and further stigmatised and problematised.

What we are therefore seeing, especially in the liberal economies of countries such as the UK, Australia and New Zealand, is the embedding, through the use of welfare-to-work policies and practices, of a moral economy of unemployment that re-enforces individual responsibility and self-blame while also punishing those who are unable to access work (regardless of its quality and value). Yet, little is known about the impacts and consequences of this experience for the young unemployed. There remains a serious need for a more critical engagement with these policies and for more research on the impacts for those who are being 'churned' consistently through the system.

References

Australian Bureau of Statistics. 2014. Unemployment by Age 15–24. Available from www.abs.gov.au. Accessed 25 Nov 2014.

Clarke, J., and J. Newman. 2012. The alchemy of austerity. *Critical Social Policy* 32(3): 299–319.

Craig, D., and G. Cotterell. 2007. Periodising neo-Liberalism? *Policy & Politics* 35(3): 497–514.

Crisp, R., and R. Fletcher. 2008. *A comparative review of workfare programmes in the United States, Canada and Australia. Report No. 533.* London: Department of Work and Pensions.

Deeming, C. 2014. Social Democracy and social policy in neo-Liberal times. *Journal of Sociology* 50(4): 577–600.

Department of Social Security. 1998. *New Ambition for Our Country: A New Contract for Welfare.* London: HMSO Stationary Office.

Department of Work and Pensions. 2015. *Mortality Statistics: Employment and Support Allowance, Incapacity Benefit or Severe Disablement Allowance.* Sheffield: Department of Work and Pensions.

Duménil, G., and D. Lévy. 2011. *The Crisis of Neo-Liberalism.* Cambridge, MA: Harvard University Press.

Farnsworth, K., and Z. Irving. 2012. Varieties of crisis, varieties of austerity: social policy in challenging times. *Journal of Poverty and Social Justice* 20(2): 133–147.

France, A. 2016. *Understanding Youth in the Global Economic Crisis.* Bristol: Policy Press.

———. 2007. *Understanding Youth in Late Modernity.* Buckingham: Open University Press.

Gazso, A., and S. Mcdaniel. 2010. The 'Great West' Experiment: Neo-Liberal Convergence and Transforming Citizenship in Canada. *Canadian Review of Social Policy* 63: 15–35.

Griggs, J., and M. Evans. 2010. *Sanctions within conditional benefit systems: A review of evidence.* York: Joseph Rowntree Foundation.

Hale, C. 2015. *Fulfilling Potential? ESA and the fate of Work-Related Activity Group.* London: Mind.

Hamilton, M. 2014. The 'new social contract' and the individualisation of risk in policy. *Journal of Risk Research* 17(4): 453–467.

Harvey, D. 2010. *The Enigma of Capitalism and the Crises of Capitalism.* New York: Oxford Press.

Herndon, T., M. Ash, and R. Pollin. 2014. Does high public debt consistently stifle economic growth? A critique of Reinhart and Rogoff. *Cambridge Journal of Economics* 38(2): 257–279.

Humpage, L. 2014. *Policy Change, Public Attitudes and Social Citizenship*. Bristol: Policy Press.

International Labour Office. 2013. *Global Trends for Youth: A Generation at Risk*. Geneva: International Labour Organization.

Kelly, P. 2006. The entrepreneurial self and 'youth at risk': Exploring the horizons of identity in the twenty-first century. *Journal of Youth Studies* 9(1): 17–32.

King, L., M. Kitson, S. Konzelmann, and F. Wilkinson. 2012. Making the same mistake again—or is this time different? *Cambridge Journal of Economics* 36(1): 1–15.

Kluve, J. 2014. *Active Labour Market policies with a focus on youth*. Turin: European Training Foundation.

Konzelmann, S. 2014. The Political Economics of Austerity. *Cambridge Journal of Economics* 38(4): 701–741.

Maki, K. 2011. Neoliberal Deviants and Surveillance: Welfare Recipients Under the Watchful Eye of Ontario Works. *Surveillance & Society* 9(1/2): 47–63.

Martin, J. 2014. *Activation and Active Labour Market Policies in OECD Countries: Stylized Facts and Evidence on their Effectiveness*. Bonn: Institute for the Study of Labor.

Meager, N., B. Newton, R. Sainsbury, A. Corden, and A. Irvine. 2014. *Work Programme Evaluation: the participant experience report. Report No. 892*. Sheffield: Department for Work and Pensions.

Moulton, B. 2014. The 2007–2009 Financial Crisis and Recession: Reflections in the National Accounts. In *Eurostat Conference The Accounts of Society National Accounts at the Service of Economic and Monetary Policy Making*, ed. Eurostat. Luxembourg, Alvisse Parc Hotel: Eurostat.

OECD. 2012. *Activating Jobseekers: How does Australia do it?* Paris: OECD.

Office of National Statistics. 2014. Unemployment by age 15–24 year olds. Available from www.ons.gov.uk. Accessed 25 Nov 2014.

O'hara, M. 2014. *Austerity bites: A journey to the sharp end of cuts in the UK*. Bristol: Policy Press.

Ortiz, I., and M. Cummins (eds.). 2012. *A Recovery for All: Rethinking Socio-Economic Policies for Children and Poor Households*. New York: UNICEF Division of Policy and Practice.

Peck, J. 2001. *Workfare States*. New York: Guilford Press.

Peak, J., and N. Theodore. 2012. Reanimating neo-Liberalism: process geographies of neo-Liberalisation. *Social Anthropology* 20(2): 177–185.

Philip, T., and K. Mallan. 2015. *A New Start? Implications of Work for Dole on Mental Health of the Unemployed*. Brisbane: Queensland University of Technology, Children and Youth Research Centre.

Reinhart, C., and K. Rogoff. 2009. *This Time is Different: Eight Centuries of Financial Folly*. Princeton: Princeton University Press.

Seccareccia, M. 2012. The role of public investment as principle macroeconomic tool to promote long-term growth: Keynes's legacy. *International Journal of Political Economy* 40(4): 62–82.

Statistics New Zealand. 2014. *Youth employment 16–24*. Available from www.stats.govt.nz. Accessed 25 Nov 2014.

Sunley, P., R. Martin, and C. Nativel. 2006. *Putting Workfare in Place*. Oxford: Blackwell Publishing.

Taylor, L., C.R. Proaño, L. de Carvalho, and N. Barbosa. 2012. Fiscal deficits, economic growth and government debt in the USA. *Cambridge Journal of Economics* 36(1): 189–204.

Theodaropoulou, S., and A. Watt. 2011. *Withdrawal Symptoms: An assessment of the austerity packages in Europe*. Brussels: European Trade Union.

Torfing, J. 1999. Workfare with Welfare: Recent Reforms of the Danish Welfare State. *Journal of European Social Policy* 4: 485–510.

Wacquant, L. 2012. Three steps to a historical anthropology of actually existing neo-Liberalism. *Social Anthropology* 20(1): 66–79.

———. 2009. *Punishing the Poor: The neo-Liberal government of social insecurity*. Durham NC: Duke University Press.

Watts, B., S. Fitzpatrick, G. Bramley, and D. Watkins. 2014. *Welfare sanctions and conditionality in the UK*. Joseph Rowntree Foundation, Available at https://www.jrf.org.uk/report/welfare-sanctions-and-conditionality-uk.

Woodman, D., and J. Wyn. 2015. *Youth and Generation: Rethinking change and inequality in the lives of young people*, Sage: London.

Wynd, D. 2013. *Benefit Sanctions: Children not seen, not heard*. Auckland: Child Poverty Action Group.

14

Bush Kinder: Thinking Differently About Privileged Spaces Through/With/In Children's Geographies

Barbara Chancellor and Marg Sellers

Opening the Conversation

From the outset, we saw this chapter as an opportunity to consider children's geographies within the context of a Melbourne (Australia) Bush Kinder early childhood setting. We wanted to explore how young children's health and well-being might be configured differently in this alternative early childhood setting, and how the children negotiate and engage with different attempts to shape their experience and learning in that space. Essentially, we were interested in exploring, 'how geographical context is significant to moral practice, and how ethical deliberation is incomplete without recognition of the geographical dimension of human existence' (Smith 2000 p. viii). This sits well with how we position Bush Kinder as a place of children's well-being and learning. Then, in a conversationally inspired moment, we considered the notion that Bush Kinder is a privileged

B. Chancellor • M. Sellers (✉)
RMIT University, Melbourne, Victoria, Australia

© The Editor(s) (if applicable) and The Author(s) 2017   **277**
P. Kelly, J. Pike (eds.), *Neoliberalism, Austerity, and the Moral Economies of Young People's Health and Well-being*,
DOI 10.1057/978-1-137-58266-9_15

space, but what then followed was a Deleuzo-Guattarian 'and ... and ... and' (Deleuze and Guattari 1987, p. 25) 'moment ... and ... ongoing moments'. Was the Bush Kinder a privileged space? If so, in what ways? What did the notion of privilege mean for this space? Could it be understood as not being a privileged space?

These questions gnawed away; we were not sure whether the Bush Kinder was entirely a place of privilege given that such spaces are accessible to the general public. In terms of lived experience, the availability and choice of Bush Kinder is not widespread in Melbourne, but children's play/learning opportunities in such open, natural places are not restricted only to early childhood education provision. Those nature spaces can be accessed publicly at almost any time as Melbourne has many green spaces scattered through all parts of the city. But in the first instance, we thought that how any given family accesses those green spaces that likely reflects how they value play and recreational opportunities. Also, how difficult it may be for some families to get to those spaces without their own transport or money for public transport is not to be overlooked.

Other questions then emerged, ideological in nature: Is privilege a notion of the privileged, conjured up to sustain privilege? Does the notion of privilege or establishing what is or is not privileged territory set a benchmark for those who can access whatever is deemed to be privileged territory to maintain some distance from those who cannot; for those above the line to be able to keep out those below it? Is privilege the flip side of the coin of centres and peripheries? Is it like 'morality'? Who decides what is good or right or bad and wrong in terms of differentiation of decisions, actions and intentions as a code of conduct for socially regulating lives?[1]

Marg Reflects on Privilege

I guess I was thinking about privilege in relation to my childhood. I grew up believing I was privileged in that we lived in a new house in a working-class suburb. I didn't know suburbs were subject to class differentiation. I

---

[1] From various dictionary definitions of 'morality'.

had good food to eat, didn't ever have to wear hand-me-downs; we had school shoes and going-out shoes; Mum didn't have to work—in my family that was a sign of financial well-being; we went on camping holidays; and so on. But as I grew older, I saw at high school that a few kids went off on American Field Scholarships to the USA and beyond, they lived in prestigious houses and their Dads drove upmarket cars. But even then, I never felt underprivileged. Relatively speaking to other working-class kids in the area I was privileged but compared to those from higher socio-economic demographical areas, not having the same economic position was not in my perception a disadvantage. That my cultural capital did not always work to my advantage eluded me. So I'm thinking that it depends where you are looking from as much as where you might be positioned (by others?) in society as to whether one is or is not privileged; similarly, thinking about how Bush Kinder experiences fit into a discourse of privilege. As soon as something like Bush Kinder is treated as privileged space, I'm wondering who has what agenda?

Barb Responds

Yes, I agree that a discourse of privilege is always problematic and likely to be seized upon by groups with different agendas. I view my childhood as privileged from the perspective of being outdoors, playing freely with my friends, on a daily basis. I was able to provide the same opportunities for my own children and they reflect on their childhoods as I do my own; fun in the outdoors, playing with friends; privileged. Contrary to many, I don't believe that a privileged upbringing is connected with schools or money. My views sit in a Deleuzo-Guattarian imagining of smooth and striated spaces, smooth being the creative and flowing aspects, striated the rigid and structured. While I acknowledge both as important, I believe today's children have little opportunity to operate within the smooth spaces and that is why I view Bush Kinder as a privileged space.

Like Horton and Kraftl (2006a, p.260) mulling over memories that tugged at them as they attended to children's geographies, we too felt that:

somehow, [our] attention to the deeply banal and affective stuff of everyday lives might give us yet more reason to critically ponder some long and deeply taken-for-granted understandings.

About, in this instance, notions of privilege alongside/through/with/in the Bush Kinder space that children territorialise as unique individuals, working/playing in concert with other unique individuals, both children and adults, and as an attempt to perhaps understand more of what matters to young children.

Inspired to think differently in this moment by Deleuze (2004) and Guattari (1995), our thinking resonates initially with the Deleuzean 'image of thought' (Deleuze 2004, p. 185). A notion that is open to possibilities for thinking thought not yet conceived of, through/with/in happenings of previously unthought questions, practices and knowledge which may emerge from/with/in various ways in various contexts. Opening to such an apparently repetitive and complexly chaotic processual multiplicity is likely a disrupting and disruptive process for writers and readers alike. Massumi (2002, p.8) alludes to how we might 'think open a space for change in a grid-locked positional system'. With this in mind, our response is to (re)turn to earlier discussions (Elliott and Chancellor 2014; Chancellor et al. 2017) and flow through similar yet always changing spaces of children's geographies.

In engaging with this thought experiment, what follows resists conventional analysis and instead flows with an aesthetics of expression which involves 'creative uncertainty' (Guattari 1995, p. 134), 'chang[ing] mentalities' and 'reinvent[ing] social practices' (Guattari 1995, p. 119). This goes beyond focussing on interpretation and meaning towards a consideration of what matters for the moral geographies of young children in the Bush Kinder space explored here. In this, we acknowledge from the outset that we are 'at risk of encountering incomprehension and of being isolated' (Guattari 1995, p. 132) by many others, albeit from what we would consider parallel fields and perspectives. However, what matters to us is to 'open the field up to a different deployment of aesthetic components' (Guattari 1995, p. 132) always/already opening (to) possibilities (Sellers 2013).

Bush Kinder: A Space of Self and Social Transformation

In Australia, there is a range of early childhood service models, which facilitate the provision of government-subsidised preschool for all four-year-old children. Many preschool providers offer unsubsidised programmes for three-year-olds as a way of providing service and gaining income. The national early childhood curriculum document, the *Early Years Learning Framework*, suggests that children learn best through play (DEEWR 2009). However, understandings and facilitation of children's play by adults working in early childhood settings in Australia are at best, questionable. Prior to the emergence of a childcare industry in Australia in the 1970s, all kindergartens were run by degree-qualified teachers, largely using a play-based approach. This remains a credible approach: Valentine and McKendrick (1997, p.223) argue that, 'the geographical literature on children [emphasises] the importance of play to children's quality of life and to their geographical and social development'. In Australia, it becomes harder to be confident in interpretations of play-based curriculum due to the bourgeoning of a childcare industry run for profit, and the subsequent lowering of education requirements for the adults employed therein. Employing a business model, the marketisation of early childhood education is pervasive (Kilderry 2006; Duhn 2010). In such a neo-Liberal environment, adult-imposed learning outcomes are seldom queried (Press and Woodrow 2005). Adult-directed activities and routine-driven learning programmes have become de rigueur, bringing into question children's quality of life in early childhood settings and, particularly, their geographical and social development—or their moral and social geographies.

As Rustin (2013, p.27) points out, neo-Liberalism imposes a 'universal model' for the social provision of services in the (mis)belief that such services become effective and efficient only when there are financial incentives for providers. It is his belief that children should be considered as primary stakeholders, and that education should have a genuine human welfare agenda, one that is not governed by economic means or ends. Rustin (2013, p.25) states:

> When children first enter the world, they already bring with them complex material and relational needs, whose satisfaction or otherwise by their primary carers will always have lasting consequences for their later development and well-being. A child's entry into the world beyond his or her family, and into the different stages of education and the challenges which this brings, carries with it another cluster of needs, for the provision of which children and their families depend on others, in schools and other supportive social agencies.

An example of the tension between social and economic agenda is the Australian Government's politically driven, universal access directive to provide 15 hours per week of sessional time in an early childhood educational setting for all four-year-old children by 2013. Arguably, this time frame was largely impossible within the early childhood services operating at the time. Not only did it put pressure on providers in terms of being able to meet the new requirement but it also opened the way for more private providers to enter the market-oriented business of early childhood education. So, while on the surface this government initiative appeared to benefit children, it came at a high cost as early childhood settings tried to find solutions to manage this new directive. As Pike and Kelly (2014) point out, 'government is always a moral project' (p. 9), the question here being, whose moral geographies was this politically charged, essentially economic agenda likely to compromise? They argue that in such

> ongoing debates this moral project of the self should be a central concern because it tells us much about how, at the start of the 21st century, we imagine ourselves, who we are, what we should become ... these hopes and aspirations are most often invested and embodied in the young people, that we parent, that we school, that we govern. (Pike and Kelly 2014, p. 191)

However, whatever the political agenda of the government, the Westgarth Kindergarten parent–teacher body sidestepped and opened a different way through.

Westgarth Kindergarten parent–teacher body responded to the universal access directive in an unexpected and innovative way. They conceived an idea and created something new and different, namely, a Bush Kinder.[2] Going against the grain of conventional compliance, rather than reducing sessions for three-year-olds, to enable them to meet the directive of increasing the number of sessions for four-year-olds, they devised an innovative way to maintain the three-year-old sessions and increase available sessions for four-year-olds. The parent–teacher body

---

[2]It should be noted that since the emergence of the Westgarth Bush Kinder (in Melbourne, Victoria), the first of its kind in Australia, other bush and beach kinder have started up, mostly in the state of Victoria.

of this community Kindergarten opted to establish a Bush Kinder as part of the Westgarth Kindergarten programme. In this innovative Bush Kinder space, notions of childhood play-as-learning, relations with and within the space of the local parkland setting and the play of power relations become visible. Moral geographies of this early childhood setting are significant as they disrupt traditional hierarchical power relations and spatial and moral dimensions of practices, and responses by children, teachers and the wider community to these different kinds of geographies emerge. Geographies of/with/in this localised Bush Kinder space open up the vision of the parent committee who forged this initiative, the subsequent engagement of children in the space and a further rippling of ideas about young children's well-being and learning in outdoor, open spaces into the wider community.

Disturbing Unequal Power Relations: Transforming Self in the Social

In this setting, power relations are turned upside down and inside out as children drive the play and the learning, creating new geographies of/with/in the Bush Kinder space. Pike (2008) talks of Foucauldian notions of power, which are not always coercive and negative but circulatory, contextual, fluid in nature. In this real-time contextual space, in circulating fluidly through/with/in the natural setting the children's moral geographies emerge as contours; contours (re)formed through/by children responding to the natural features of the space and responding within relations with each other. This is different to the power relations, spatial and moral dimensions of practices and responses of children and teachers more commonly played out in early childhood settings where, in a similar way to Pike and Kelly's description of children in schools, children are cajoled, directed, encouraged and rewarded to behave in certain ways, ways that sustain unequal power relations (Pike and Kelly 2014, p. 9). Fielding (cited in Hemming 2007, p. 364) describes the school as a hot bed of moral geographies—of moral codes dictating when and where children ought to learn and behave; this is also true in many kindergartens and childcare centres in Australia. However, within Bush Kinder type settings, possibilities open for operating otherwise and in other ways.

Bush Kinder is arguably one kind of children's place and spaces thereof where unequal power relations are more readily disrupted, being outside of dominating structures—of buildings, fenced property and programme routines designed to work within the physical space rather than serve the social and learning well-being of the children involved. As Rasmussen (2004, p. 171) explains,

> The many meanings and kinds of 'children's places' should make us aware of children as social and cultural actors who create places that are physical and symbolic and call attention to 'the interfaces' between adults' understanding of what one can and should do in a place for children and children's understanding of this matter.

Children operating in these kinds of spaces are leading the way for optimising their socialising and learning experiences, primarily among themselves, but also in more equitable relations with the adults in the setting and also in corporeal relations with the natural resources surrounding them. Horton and Kraftl (2006b, pp.80–82) suggest the need for reflection on 'the moral, affective and material work involved in doing education, in a variety of contexts'—such as with/in/through the highly charged, child-initiated human–nonhuman relations in a Bush Kinder setting involving interrelationships of the people there and relations with the materiality of the natural world—in order to avoid merely viewing childhood as a condition, image, category or signifier. Turning the story over to children and opening up spaces for their voices and actions to be heard and seen, that is, centralising their perspectives is all too frequently not achieved. However, we have attempted to redress this here in our ongoing explorations around/of Bush Kinder, to ensure children proceed as power-full players, figuratively and physically. We also value the quiet(ened) voices of the teachers who, humbly respectful of the children as power-full players in their well-being and learning, describe their roles as relatively subordinate to the children, opening up spaces for equitable and complementary interrelationships. This reversal of this binary opens spaces for more equitable operations (St. Pierre 2011).

Bush Kinder: A Space of/for (the) Privilege(d)?

It could be argued that Westgarth Kindergarten established the Bush Kinder by virtue of a position of privilege, in terms of cultural, economic and educational capital. From having a parent body with knowledge and expertise relative to policy writing, and time for negotiating regulatory requirements, through developing the proposal to establish the Bush Kinder, and for managing its operations. Ostensibly, this privileged position enabled the development of an innovative response to the government directive—most commonly, centres envisaged discontinuing the three-year-old sessions as a quick and easy fix for complying with the regulation. However, while the Westgarth Kindergarten agenda of establishing the Bush Kinder was not from the economically driven position associated with privilege but from within a socially responsible aim of continuing to provide an educational programme for 3-year-olds, the notion of privilege is relationally complex in these apparently binarial discourses.

Admittedly, this 'privileged' Westgarth Kindergarten parent body had the nous and expertise, which likely included a network of professionally useful contacts. But the underpinning philosophical foundation upon which the parents based the plan and their stated aspirations and ideals for establishing a Bush Kinder suggests a socially relational rationale. Their website says that Bush Kinder Vision aims to promote a community with a closer connection with nature; a community that values and participates in nature-based activities more regularly; a healthier and more environmentally aware community; a well-connected and cohesive community; and creative, independent and resilient children (www.wgkg.vic. edu.au). Yet, while this reflects a critical agenda of social responsibility, the ideological notion of neo-Liberal 'privilege' is still not entirely dismissible given the relatively higher socio-economic demographics of the early childhood centres operating Bush and Beach kinder programmes around Melbourne.

This complexity continues. It is apparent that the parent–teacher body simultaneously worked with and challenged the newly instigated government policy, in itself part of a neo-Liberal political agenda. In doing so, Westgarth Kindergarten was providing early childhood education for the maximum number of young children in their catchment area. Internationally, economies are recognising the worth of participation in early childhood education as contributing to successful outcomes in the adult workforce.[3] Such prospective adults are, as young children, purported to have need of attending an early childhood setting for a significant number of hours per week from an early age. So maximising potential participation in the Westgarth Kindergarten programmes becomes a mechanism for ensuring these children, as future adults, are well positioned to function as ideal economy boosters; for working with and in a neo-Liberal agenda. At the same time, it allows greater participation by their parents in the labour market. But, the emergence of the Bush Kinder simultaneously provides challenges to this dominant neo-Liberal ideological framework. In refusing to cut the sessional hours for the three-year-olds, the Westgarth Kindergarten parent–teacher body were, at least in part, refusing a singularly economic-focussed, political agenda by concurrently prioritising social aspects of growth, learning and development for these younger children through maintaining their access to the kindergarten programme.

Moreover, conventional ideological discourses of notions of privilege generally favour proponents of an economic agenda in regard to who benefits, whose interests are being served and why. For example, early childhood centres operating primarily as business ventures are bound to return a profit. These corporate priorities secure their directors and shareholders as the main beneficiaries of the early childhood setting. But such a critique of privilege collapses around this bunch of three-year-olds at Westgarth Kindergarten. There is no economic benefit or advantage to the kindergarten beyond the given functionality of financially 'breaking

---

[3] See, for example:

- National Economic Review 2014, Australian Department of Education. http://www.globalaccesspartners.org/National-Economic-Review-2014-Report.pdf
- Calman, L.J. and L. Tarr-Whelan. 2005. *Early childhood education for all: a wise investment.* New York: Legal Momentum. http://web.mit.edu/workplacecenter/docs/Full%20Report.pdf
- Bartik, T.J. 2014. *From preschool to prosperity: the economic payoff to early childhood education.* Kalamazoo, MI: W.E. Upjohn Institute for Employment Research. http://www.upjohn.org/publications/upjohn-institute-press/preschool-prosperity-economic-payoff-early-childhood-education

even' in their operations. As well, there is no disadvantage that adversely impacts the three-year-olds as the primary stakeholders. Rather, the children become the main beneficiaries as their programme is saved from being phased out, and the four-year-olds benefit from having the extra hours (required by the government policy) as a Bush Kinder experience. Something they may not have otherwise had. All this circulating around, and through, an apparently neutral Bush Kinder space. Ironically, it was from within the shadows of the political economy that the Bush Kinder emerged yet there is no revenue-gathering opportunity associated with operating in this publicly owned parkland. No monetary gains to be had from land ownership, from capital investment in the property or from rental contractual agreements. The geography of the space has been irreducible in terms of contributing to the 'production of saleable products' (Rustin 2013, p. 33).

The extent to which any of this matters is, then, arbitrary. Ideological notions of privilege are complex and in this instance seem to dissolve into a non-hierarchical horizontal plane where things are not pitched in binary opposition one against the other, but where commingling relations of coexistence flow more freely. Where disrupting the primacy claimed by ideals attributed to economic growth and development enables 'a relational society' in which the quality of social institutions and education, for example, 'depends substantially on what qualities of human relationship they facilitate' (Rustin 2013, p. 24), including relationships between people and the nonhuman material world of nature in particular. What better place to enable this kind of well-being to emerge and grow than in spaces like the Westgarth Bush Kinder? What better place for this to happen than in this kind of play-as-learning space that in its operations outside human-made, manufactured structures and resources (e.g., buildings, fences, playground equipment, plastic, wood, concrete, steel, artificial grass, safety matting, sandpits, diggers) by default disrupts governing systems in favour of personal interrelations? With oneself, with others and with forces and affects of nonhuman material/natural worlds? This distances us from an essentially individualistic, economically oriented position that neo-Liberalism presupposes in its focus on profit-seeking and market imperatives (Rustin 2013). In Rustin's (2013, p.35) view, the world of individualist, acquisitive capitalism has become unsustainable, for many reasons [including how the] ideology of individual self-interest violates human needs for connectedness and mutual care.

Similarly, connectedness with one another and/in the Parklands setting is generated through Bush Kinder type spaces. The experiences of the children in those spaces override a purely market-dominated, business-oriented, neo-Liberal agenda.

Children Complexly Engaging with/in/Through Geographies

Westgarth Bush Kinder is located within the Darebin Parklands and offers relatively open native bushy areas, large rocks, trees for climbing on and swinging from and a long boomerang-shaped mound, all in an area the size of about two tennis courts. As such, Westgarth Bush Kinder is an ephemeral space, a complex system, 'open, recursive, organic, non-linear and emergent' (Gough 2012, p.42). With no visible boundaries such as fences or lines marked on the ground, boundaries at Bush Kinder are neither constructed nor managed through foundations of power relations. Instead relations move fluidly within negotiated territories where the players are children, teachers, families and the wider community. Smith (2010) comments that the more adult structuring of play there is, the more authentic play is disrupted with more scope for manipulating activities in the interests of adults. That is, the more governance of children's well-being and learning the more children's moral geographies are played out to adult agenda. Valentine and McKendrick (1997) discuss the common mismatch between adult-directed play provision and what children actually want. They claim that children often prefer to play in 'flexible' landscapes, such as waste grounds and open spaces, rather than playgrounds and other formally designated play sites. For the children at Bush Kinder, play choices are largely theirs alone. The ebb and flow of their play moves with and through the contours of the land, always already emerging as something different. Sutton-Smith (1997) notes that play can involve active, participatory forms of energetic engagement as well as passive or vicarious forms, such as daydreaming or just being in the moment, the latter easily attainable in the unstructured, open, natural setting of the parkland.

In relation to the operations of the Bush Kinder and to the children territorialising the space, play is central to the study of children's environments (Valentine and McKendrick 1997), and by extension to their moral geographies, as it is the primary mechanism for becoming acquainted with their environment and shaping the relations therein. For example, Blaut and Stea (cited in Valentine and McKendrick 1997) consider the opportunity to move and play freely in the environment as moving beyond developmental discourses that valorise the individual engaged solely in human interactions, and (re)focuses our thinking towards children's broader, collective geographies. Consequently, possibilities open for understanding children as 'emergent in a *relational* field, where *nonhuman* forces are equally at play in constituting children's becomings' (Hultman and Taguchi 2010, p. 525, original emphasis)—of their moral geographies, for example.

In an evaluation of the Bush Kinder pilot, Elliott and Chancellor (2014) noted that children become adept at climbing high up into the trees, and in so doing learn the 'language of the tree'. Connecting and being with the tree through feeling the bark, experiencing uneven surfaces, negotiating unexpected shapes of branches and discovering footholds and places for hands to grab onto is arguably more helpful to transformation of self—emergent through/with/in a relational field of human and nonhuman forces—than the constructed climbing frames common in many outdoor play spaces where dimensions are mathematically regular and predictable, and surfaces are smooth and even. The manufactured climbing frame 'gives information' to the climber in a differently ordered and structured way from the relational field of children's interactions and interconnections with natural features and contours of the land in the Bush Kinder space.

Affrica Taylor (2011, p.425) interrogates not only the essentialised nature of childhood but also the essentialised nature of 'nature'. Drawing on social studies of childhood and human geography, Taylor describes the impossibility of disentangling the social and the natural and so employs the term, 'socionature'. The pedagogical approaches used by the teachers at the Bush Kinder demonstrate a willingness to let go of possible nostalgic notions of childhood and nature by allowing the child and the natural space to interact in 'authentic' ways through play (Taylor 2011, p.429). Teachers recall that initially Bush Kinder was a 'blank canvas' and was about 'being in the moment' (Elliott and Chancellor 2014). In this, children's becomings are understood in terms of children becoming something different—not more than or better than—through complex systems of activity of human–human and human–nonhuman relations.

The openness of the unstructured programme of the Bush Kinder and the freely flowing activity of the children's play generates possibilities for different encounters in our thinking through young children's moral geographies, considering ways in which children engage with the natural spaces, with the space of the open Bush Kinder programme and with the relational spaces emerging between each other and the adults in the space. Possibilities arise for transformation of self of all those participating the Bush Kinder setting. Observations at Bush Kinder show the complexity of the performativity of being in the moment, always already in a(n) (un) timely manner that suggests a sense that these children are rarely interrupted by adult-imposed agendas for learning. There thus appears little if any space for power and control to exist within these open(ed) spaces, although perhaps it manifests in different ways and is then perceived less rigidly organised along generational lines (see e.g. Pike 2012).

The notion of 'power-fullness' as a way of problematising conventional notions of power, being powerful and empowerment (Sellers and Honan 2007) is also useful:

> When power is perceived as complex and non-linear in ongoing operations of relations with/in a multiplicity of forces rather than a singular force acting on specific bodies, different possibilities for conceiving power-fullness emerge around/ with/in/through encounters of relationships. (Sellers 2013, p. 147)

This is a response to Deleuze's (1988, p.71) incitement to ask not what power is and where it comes from, but to ask, 'How is it practiced?' If we open up to thinking of children as power-full human beings engaging with adults in the Bush Kinder, we perturb disabling modernist understandings of unequal power relationships through recognising that anybody is embodied in any other body's expressions of power-fullness. In this way of thinking, 'children are (re)conceived in operations of always already becoming-power-full' (Sellers 2013, p. 148). This became increasingly apparent in the evaluation data (Elliott and Chancellor 2014), elaborated in the following discussion.

Teachers commented how children set their own pattern of activity, spending periods of time sitting, reflecting and participating in philosophical discussions, among themselves and with teachers. One of the teachers reported that there was a 'softening of the louder, bigger voices and the lifting of the quieter voices for some children'; the teachers suggested that the bush environment seemed to have a 'calming and levelling' effect on group dynamics. We might also infer that the setting promoted conditions for unfettered expressions of power-fullness and that this affected how the children operated as individuals, and with/in the group. This reflects Smith's (2000, p.viii) proposal outlined in our opening comments that 'geographical context [is] significant to moral practice, and how ethical deliberation is incomplete without recognition of the geographical dimension of human existence'. Not only were the children engaged in relations with each other—anybody is embodied in any other body's expressions of power-fullness (Sellers 2013)—they were also engaging with nonhuman bodies. Bush Kinder is a place in which children, teachers and community are social actors in their own right in the present (Horton and Kraftl 2006b, p. 83), a space for opening up (to) children's moral and social geographies.

not Concluding Thoughts. Continuing Thinking Differently

In this chapter, we have attempted to show that Bush Kinder is a setting where young children's play is power-fully arranged through their moral geographies, perturbing more common power relations and spatial and moral dimensions of practices and responses of conventionally structured early childhood settings. All this, by thinking open possibilities (opening up possibilities through/with/in our thinking) for the children to initiate and distribute what matters for their learning through play as learning, and learning as play in an open, natural space. The benefits perceived by teachers and the community (Elliott and Chancellor 2012) reveal Bush Kinder as a space which could be easily described as privileged in terms of its establishment—an innovation that required particular knowledge, expertise, networks and time. However, for us it remains debatable as to whether the Bush Kinder can be considered a privileged space in term of its operations alongside the Westgarth kindergarten and the children's participation through (simply) engaging and interacting with other children, adults and the natural resources of the space itself. All the while, this involved a complex array of relational activity among non/human bodies, opening possibilities for a space of self and social transformation. The moral project of the self in human and nonhuman relations becomes apparent in the Westgarth Bush Kinder, opening a collective assemblage, a Deleuzean image of thought for thinking differently about how we see and make the world of young children's well-being and learning in this differently privileged geographical space.

References

Chancellor, B., A. Gough, and M. Sellers. 2017. Moving with the contours of the land: open(ing) transformative spaces of play, natural environments and environmental sustainability in an early childhood setting. *Children's Geographies*.

Deleuze, G. 1988. *Foucault*. London: Athlone Press.

———. 2004. *Difference and Repetition*. London: Continuum Press.

Deleuze, G., and F. Guattari. 1987. *A thousand plateaus: capitalism and schizophrenia*. Minneapolis: University of Minnesota Press.

Duhn, I. 2010. 'The centre is my business': Neo-liberal politics, privatisation and discourses of professionalism in New Zealand. *Contemporary Issues in Early Childhood* 11(1): 49–60.

DEEWR. 2009. *(EYLF) Early Years Learning Framework*. Australia: Australian Government Department of Education, Employment and Workplace Relations. Available from: http://www.ag.gov.au/cca. Accessed 11 Nov 2015.

Elliott, S., and B. Chancellor. 2014. From forest preschool to bush kinder: An inspirational approach to preschool provision in Australia. *Australasian Journal of Early Childhood, Early Childhood Australia* 39(4): 45–53.

———. 2012. *Westgarth Kindergarten Bush Kindergarten website* [online]. Available from: http://e-publications.une.edu.au/1959.11/14412. Accessed 11 Sept 2015.

Guattari, F. 1995. *Chaosophy*. In , ed. S. Lotringer. New York, NY: Semiotext(e).

Gough, N. 2012. Complexity, Complexity Reduction, and 'Methodological Borrowing' in Educational Inquiry. *Complicity: An International Journal of Complexity and Education* 9(1): 41–56.

Hemmng, P.J. 2007. Renegotiating the primary school: children's emotional geographies of sport, exercise and active play. *Children's Geographies* 5(4): 353–371.

Horton, J., and P. Kraftl. 2006a. Not just growing up, but going on: Materials, spacings, bodies, situations. *Children's Geographies* 4(3): 259–276.

———. 2006b. What else? Some more ways of thinking and doing 'Children's Geographies'. *Children's Geographies* 4(1): 69–95.

Hultman, K., and H. Lenz Taguchi. 2010. Challenging anthropocentric analysis of visual data: A relational materialist methodological approach to educational research. *International Journal of Qualitative Studies in Education* 23(5): 525–542.

Kilderry, A. 2006. Early childhood education and care as a community service or big business? *Contemporary Issues in Early Childhood* 7(1): 80–83.

Massumi, B. 2002. *A shock to thought: Expression after Deleuze and Guattari*. London: Routledge.

Pike, J. 2008. Foucault, Space and Primary School Dining Rooms. *Children's Geographies* 6(4): 413–422.

Pike, J. 2012. 'I don't have to listen to you! You're just a dinner lady!': Power and resistance at lunchtimes in primary schools. *Children's Geographies* 8(3): 275–287.

Pike, J., and P. Kelly. 2014. *The moral geographies of children, young people and food: Beyond Jamie's school dinners*. Hampshire, United Kingdom: Palgrave Macmillan.

Press, F., and C. Woodrow. 2005. Commodification, corporatisation and children's spaces. *Australian Journal of Education* 49(30): 278–291.

Rasmussen, K. 2004. Places for children—Children's places. *Childhood* 11(2): 155–173.

Rustin, M. 2013. A relational society. *Soundings: A journal of politics and culture* 54: 23–36.

Sellers, M. 2013. *Young children becoming curriculum: Deleuze, Te Whāriki and curricular understandings*. London: Routledge.

Sellers, M., and E. Honan. 2007. Putting rhizomes to work: (e)merging methodologies. *International Journal of Qualitative Studies in Education* 20(5): 531–546.

Smith, D. 2000. *Moral geographies: Ethics in a world of difference.* Edinburgh: Edinburgh University Press.

Smith, P.K. 2010. *Children and play.* London: Wiley-Blackwell.

St. Pierre, E.A. 2011. Post qualitative research: The critique and the coming after. In *The Sage Handbook of Qualitative Research*, eds. N. Denzin and Y. Lincoln, 611–625. Thousand Oaks CA: SAGE Publications.

Sutton-Smith, B. 1997. *The ambiguity of play.* Cambridge, MA: Harvard University Press.

Taylor, A. 2011. Reconceptualizing the 'nature' of childhood. *Childhood* 18(4): 420–433.

Valentine, G., and J. Mckendrick. 1997. Children's outdoor play: Exploring parental concerns about children's safety and the changing nature of childhood. *Geoforum* 28(2): 219–235.

15

From Health to Hard Times: Fairness and Entitlement in Free School Meals *After Neo-Liberalism*

Jo Pike

Introduction

Following the election of the Conservative–Liberal Democrat Coalition Government in the UK elections of 2010, the then Education Secretary Michael Gove announced that plans to extend a pilot scheme to provide free school meals for children in primary school would be abandoned. The previous Labour Government's pilot scheme was implemented between 2009 and 2011 and extended free school meals entitlement in Wolverhampton (UK) and provided universal free school meals for all primary school children in Newham and Durham (UK). These pilot schemes replaced previous eligibility criteria, where pupils were entitled to free school meals if their parents claimed 'means-tested out-of-work benefits (such as Income Support) or Child Tax Credit (and not Working Tax Credit) with an annual income of no more than £16,190' (Kitchen et al. 2013, p.1).

J. Pike (✉)
Leeds Beckett University, Leeds, West Yorkshire, UK

© The Editor(s) (if applicable) and The Author(s) 2017
P. Kelly, J. Pike (eds.), *Neoliberalism, Austerity, and the Moral Economies of Young People's Health and Well-being*,
DOI 10.1057/978-1-137-58266-9_16

Extending these pilot projects would have meant that school meals would be available, free of charge, for a limited period of time to all primary school children living in other areas of deprivation including Bradford, Nottingham and Islington (UK). The Coalition Government's decision to abandon the extension of the scheme was justified on the basis of cost. If school meals were provided to children free of charge, other services would have to be cut—it was simple economics. In a parliamentary debate, the newly appointed Minister for Children, Tim Loughton (HC Deb, 30th June 2010) responded to criticism of this decision by asking

> If hon. Members are now talking about a universal free school meal programme, where will that money come from? Which programmes would they cut? They cannot have it both ways.

The money saved by abandoning the extension of the free school meals pilots was estimated to be around £160 million (Loughton, HC Deb, 30 June 2010). This was one of the first of many cuts to public services that characterised the economic policy of not only the Coalition Government in 2010–2015 but also the subsequent Conservative Government elected in 2015. The extent of the cuts to public services during this time was unprecedented. Hastings et al. (2015, p.3) suggest that

> Local authorities in England lost 27 per cent of their spending power between 2010/11 and 2015/16 in real terms. Some services, such as planning and 'supporting people' (discretionary social care with a preventative or enabling focus) have seen cumulative cuts to the order of 45 per cent.

These cuts led to widespread dissent and public and political protests as welfare budgets bore the brunt of the austerity measures, and low income families, people with disabilities, the unemployed and young people were adversely, and arguably, disproportionately affected. So it came as something of a surprise when only three years later in September 2013 the then Deputy Prime Minister, and leader of the Liberal Democrats, Nick Clegg announced that '[e]very child in reception, year 1 and year 2 in state-funded schools will receive a free school lunch from September 2014' (DPMO 2013). The estimated cost of this was over £1bn (£450 million in 2014–2015, and £635 million in 2015–2016). Questions were raised about how this would be paid for, and how a scheme which, when limited to a number of specific geographic locations was regarded as unaffordable, could now be rolled out nationally. The official narrative used to explain this decision was that the austerity measures had worked so efficiently that the government could now afford Universal Infant Free School Meals (UIFSM). The less official narrative according to statements made to *The Independent* Newspaper, UK, by Department of Education advisor Dominic Cummings was that 'The DfE wasn't told until about an hour or so before the announcement. No policy work was done in advance', and that the free school meals scheme was a policy 'gimmick' devised 'on the back of a fag [cigarette] packet' in exchange for other policy concessions (Morris 2014).

Perplexing as this decision was, it is difficult, and perhaps not particularly fruitful, to speculate on the motivations behind it. It is certainly not the aim of this chapter to do so. Rather, what I wish to explore here are the ways in which policy decisions related to school meals and more specifically, free school meals, are justified to the public, and how these debates are morally framed within public discourse. In doing this work, I want to follow Stuart Hall and Alan O'Shea's (2013) lead in *After Neoliberalism? The Kilburn Manifesto* to focus on the concept of 'fairness' and how 'fairness' is differently configured in public and policy discourse. Particularly when concepts of 'fairness' are deployed in response to questions regarding the relative obligations of the state and the family with respect to the well-being of children and young people. Thinking about 'fairness' in these contexts and in these ways can 'help to clarify our obligations concerning public goods' (Cullity 2008, p. 2) and vice versa. My intention here is to extend Hall and O'Shea's (2013) work to explore the moral dimensions of 'fairness' and how particular moralities are mobilised to support or oppose the UIFSM scheme.

Initially, I suggest that the ways in which public and policy discourses operate are dependent upon how the aims of the UIFSM scheme are presented. When UIFSM is framed as a health or education intervention, 'common sense' thinking dominates both public and policy commentary. In line with Hall and O'Shea (2013), I suggest that 'common sense' thinking requires little evidence to support the efficacy of such interventions.

I attempt to illustrate how the 'common sense' assumptions about the health and educational benefits of school meals become sedimented in popular thinking. The second half of the chapter discusses how the meanings of UIFSM are shifted when the scheme is presented as a 'welfare intervention'. This work involves detailed consideration of the different moralities that are implicated in both justifications for and opposition to the UIFSM policy. Opposition to the UIFSM scheme came from across the political spectrum, and in some cases, commentators appeared to frame their opposition using similar vocabulary, albeit with slightly different emphases. In seeking to explore the more common and pervasive moralities featured in such discourses I aim to discover how concepts of fairness and entitlement are configured in both the policy justifications for the UIFSM programme, and in the opposition to it. Following Hall and O'Shea (2013), I argue that moral concepts such as fairness have become 'monetarised' in the context of neo-Liberalism and have replaced more welfarist perspectives premised on notions of 'public good'. I conclude the chapter by considering whether school meals can be classified as a 'public good' and, whether this might consequently reshape the ways in which young people are positioned in neo-Liberal policy discussions and developments. This chapter does not attempt to discuss whether the UIFSM scheme should or should not be implemented. Rather, what I am interested in here are the particular moralities that shape and are constructed in these debates about certain dimensions of young people's health and well-being in the moral economies of neo-Liberalism and austerity in the UK during the last half decade.

School Meals Policy Rationale

As I have argued elsewhere (Pike and Kelly 2014; Pike 2010) discourses surrounding school meals policy in the UK have historically been linked to achieving three outcomes for children and young people: improving health, improving educational attainment and alleviating the effects of poverty. According to a Department for Education (DfE 2013, p.1) memorandum, the UIFSM policy is designed to

- improve educational attainment and children's social skills and behaviour;
- ensure that children have access to at least one healthy meal each day, and support the development of long term healthy eating habits;
- help families with the cost of living, and remove disincentives to work.

These aims have, historically, been interwoven in different and complex ways since the inception of the school meals service (Gelbier and Randall 1982; Welshman 1997; Gustafsson 2002; Passmore and Harris 2004; Morgan 2006; Sibley 2004). The school meals service in the UK was initially implemented as a solution to young men's poor state of nutrition during the Boer War where between 40 % and 60 % of potential army recruits were declared physically unfit for service. The resulting Education Act (1906) further stated that the provision of state education was only beneficial if children were sufficiently nourished to be able to 'benefit fully from their education' (Passmore and Harris 2004, p. 221). Subsequently, school meals policies have been used as a mechanism to ameliorate a range of public health concerns including under-nutrition, obesity and type II diabetes (Blair 2006). However, I want to suggest that the ways in which school meals policies have been justified to the public have varied according to the nature of their aims. Policies which purport to achieve education and health outcomes tend to require very little justification since it is difficult to argue *against* improving young people's health and educational attainment. Consequently, it is relatively straightforward, politically speaking, to generate public support on these grounds. In *After Neoliberalism?* Stuart Hall and Alan O'Shea (2013, p.1) argue that what is happening in this context is a form of 'common sense' thinking. This 'common sense' suggests the reasonableness of policies because they draw on 'what everybody knows, takes for granted and agrees with'. Common sense, they suggest

> is a form of 'everyday thinking' which offers us frameworks of meaning with which to make sense of the world. It is a form of popular, easily-available knowledge which contains no complicated ideas, requires no sophisticated argument and does not depend on deep thought or wide reading. It works intuitively, without forethought or reflection. It is pragmatic and

empirical, giving the illusion of arising directly from experience, reflecting only the realities of daily life and answering the needs of 'the common people' for practical guidance and advice. (Hall and O'Shea 2013, p.1)

What everybody knows is that school meals are healthy, healthy food creates healthy children and healthy children do better in school. The benefits are obvious, taken for granted, and require little explanation. At these times popular consensus is achieved so that, as Richard Adams writes in *The Guardian* newspaper, 'few doubt the benefits of free lunches for reception, year-one and year-two pupils' (Adams 2013). Such comments not only invoke popular opinion but also play a key role in shaping and influencing it: 'By asserting that popular opinion *already agrees*, they hope to produce agreement *as an effect*. This is the circular strategy of the self-fulfilling prophecy' (Hall and O'Shea 2013, p. 1). The following exchange between Comment is Free (CiF) contributors, *Rochdalelass* and *Pixie Frou frou*, in *The Guardian* newspaper in the UK illustrate how these common sense notions are taken up in public debates about the apparent health and well-being benefits for young people that flow from the provision of free school meals:

Pixie Froufrou—You are absolutely correct about this. Ensuring that all children get two nutritious meals every school day would go a long way towards (a) improving their learning capabilities because they are not hungry or hyped up on junk food, and (b) improving their health by ensuring that they eat well, and get used to eating healthy meals.

Rochdale Lass—I think so. But then what do I know having spent years on the chalkface with children who were much too pale and inches shorter than those of the same age in other parts of the city, suffering from behavioural and attention deficit problems.[1]

---

[1] CiF sections in web-based newspapers allow members of the public, anonymously or through the use of pseudonyms, to post comments about stories, opinions or the contributions of others. As I have argued elsewhere (Pike and Kelly 2014), these CiF sections provide insights into what some people are thinking about (often in the moment) in relation to a variety of issues. They are, in this sense, interesting spaces in which to do social science (all spellings, grammar and punctuation from CiF contributions reproduced here are as they appear in the original).

Here, the common sense discourse is rooted in everyday experience at 'the chalkface' and supported by empirical evidence witnessed first-hand by *Rochdale lass*. In this sense, it appears fair and right that children are given a free nutritious school meal because not doing so would be to condone child hunger, malnutrition and various cognitive impairments. It is very difficult to argue against this sentiment, this logic.

However, there is by no means consensus that providing healthy, free school meals does in fact deliver these benefits. While it is noted that school meals tend to be more nutritionally sound than packed lunches brought from home (Evans et al. 2010a, b, Rees et al. 2008), there are both methodological and ethical issues involved with demonstrating the efficacy of whole population nutritional interventions; particularly in populations that are relatively well nourished (Verheijden and Kok 2005). It is perhaps unsurprising then that results from the evaluation of the free school meals pilots (2009–2011) suggest there was 'there was no evidence that the FSM pilot led to significant health benefits during the two year pilot period' (Kitchen et al. 2013, p.3). Furthermore, despite children making between four and eight weeks' more educational progress than pupils in control areas, the report's authors concluded that

> the evaluation findings thus provide some suggestive, but not conclusive, evidence that rolling out the universal pilot, including all pilot-related activities, might help to reduce educational inequalities. (Kitchen et al. 2013, p.10)

However, the lack of evidence and consensus regarding the benefits of UIFSM is not reflected in political discourse where the link between free school meal programmes and consequent improvements to young people's health and educational attainment is taken as axiomatic and presented, in a press release from the Deputy Prime Minister's Office on 2 September 2014, in the seemingly unassailable language of clear cut evidence:

> The evidence is clear. Providing children with nutritious and delicious meals gives them the fuel they need to excel both inside and outside the classroom, while making them more likely to opt for fruit and vegetables at lunchtime rather than junk food such as crisps. (Laws 2014) (Schools Minister)

> All the evidence, including the pilots in Durham and Newham, shows
> that free school meals will not only help ease the pressure on household
> budgets and encourage positive eating, but will also help improve concen-
> tration and raise educational performance. (Clegg 2014) (Deputy Prime
> Minister)

Because the claimed health and education benefits of free school meals
are based on common sense thinking, arguing *against* UIFSM in terms of
health and education outcomes becomes problematic since to do so is to
argue outside of common sense and to appear irrational. However, this
apparent consensus dissolves or disappears when the UIFSM is presented
as a 'welfare intervention' designed to address economic inequality. In
this case, reactions are more complex, and concepts of fairness feature
more prominently in public and policy debates. In general, opposition to
free school meals as welfare interventions run along the following three
lines: first, feeding children is the responsibility of parents and not the
State (Welshman 1997); second, providing welfare to poor families sub-
sidises their lifestyle 'choices' (see below); and third, UIFSM is an unnecessary subsidy for affluent families and therefore a waste of money (see
below). All three of these arguments draw on moral concepts of fairness
to frame their opposition to the scheme. In the remainder of this chapter,
I review how moral concepts of fairness and entitlement are mobilised
within discourses surrounding the UIFSM scheme, and how these moral
concepts are configured within the context of neo-Liberal austerity programmes in the UK.

A Moral Economy of Fairness?

Hall and O'Shea (2013, p.8) suggest that in the context of neo-
Liberalism, the concept of fairness has become 'a quasi-market relation, a
reward for personal effort'. While broadly supporting this assertion (I will
return to this later), it does tend to obscure some of the complex ways in
which the concept of fairness is deployed in public and policy discourse,
and the different moral judgements that accompany such discussions.
For Cullity (2008, p.5), an action is regarded as fair when 'something

ought, all things considered, to be done' and 'doing it as it ought to be done requires a form of impartiality'. The kind of impartiality required varies according to different contexts. In June 2010, following the UK Coalition Government's decision not to extend the free school meals pilot scheme, Roberta Blackman-Woods MP accused the government of acting unfairly because of their failure to implement cuts to services impartially:

> The coalition promised to prioritise fairness when implementing cuts and to meet the 2020 target of eradicating child poverty, but deeds speak louder than words and it is appalling that one of the first acts of the coalition Government has been to attack the poorest in our society by cancelling the extension of the free school meals programme. (Blackman-Woods, HC Deb 30th June 2010)

The thrust of her argument relates to a distributive notion of fairness where the scaling back of publicly funded goods and services *ought to* begin with those that have the greatest ability to privately fund such goods and services, and/or those who are otherwise able to absorb such cuts without it adversely affecting their access to goods and services. In this way, fairness would be achieved as an *outcome* of some action, since the effects of the cuts would be felt equitably. The goal of fairness as an outcome of particular policies was also alluded to in a press release from the Deputy Prime Minister's Office (2013). Announcing the launch of the scheme Nick Clegg suggested that

> Every child deserves the best possible start in life, and at the same time we are doing all we can to help ease the pressure on household budgets. ... Providing universal free school meals will help give every child the future they deserve, building a stronger economy and a fairer society.

In this instance, Clegg explicitly appeals to the public's sense of fairness, and to concepts of children's deservingness, to mobilise support for the policy. In the same press release, he refers explicitly to ideas of fairness and justice by suggesting that critics of the policy 'won't cloud my goal to create a level playing field for all of our children so their success will be determined by their talents and efforts alone and not by their parents' bank balance' (DPMO 2013). Clegg's suggestion appears to be that all children need to be treated equally in terms of distributing public goods. However, we might question the impartiality of such an approach since different children may have different levels of need. Providing school meals to *all* children irrespective of need may be regarded as a fair process, but it may be considered unfair in relation to the outcome since it would not create a level playing field as Clegg suggests. Rather, it would simply move the playing field further up the hill. Using Cullity's model (2008), distributing goods equally may be a form of impartiality, but it would not be considered an *appropriate* form of impartiality in this instance, if the aim of the policy is to create a fairer outcome. This argument is illustrated in comments from CiF discussion on *The Guardian* where *Polhotpot* argues, vehemently, that

> This is a waste of money. Why the hell should middle class parents (and I speak as one) get free school meals? Much better to increase the income threshold for the existing programme. Maybe make it so that anyone whose parents currently receive income-linked benefits gets free meals?

Indeed, commentators on the left, who might ordinarily be assumed to support a universal benefit, mobilise moral concepts of fairness to oppose UIFSM 'for reasons of profligacy' (Williams 2014). Zoe Williams, a traditionally left-leaning journalist at *The Guardian* newspaper argues that UIFSM is a waste of money at a time when the country can least afford it. She alludes to some of the moral judgements made about the poorest families as she describes the welfare cuts imposed by the Coalition Government suggesting that in the context of the austerity agenda

> a new universal benefit looks like an active insult, a deliberated punch in the face: apparently the nation can afford substantial sums, for the betterment of its citizens' lives. Just not for scumbags. (Williams 2014)

What is suggested in both cases is that creating a fair outcome for children necessarily involves treating them differently. If this view is accepted, achieving fairness involves identifying those children and young people for whom the present system of allocating free meals on a means tested basis is unfair. It is in these discussions that moral judgements regarding the deservingness and entitlement of young people and their families become most evident. *Paddyme*, from Yorkshire, puts it this way in a CiF contribution in *The Daily Mail*:

> What do we do with dogs and cats, we neuter. If the parents of the kids in the school can't afford to feed them then they shouldn't breed them. And we live in a bleeding heart welfare state which allows people to live off welfare as a life choice (though not all). If said feckless parents quit smoking, drinking, fancy iphones, takaways etc then no child WOULD (or should) be hungry. No its not the childs fault, but until something is done about the 'entitled' culture then the cycle will continue. I am SICK of hearing the words 'entitled' 'human rights'—what about the poor taxpayer who is funding these lazy 'entitled's'. Which is why I am voting UKIP—I voted Conservative for almost 30 years, but I have had enough!

In this rather extreme example, it is not difficult to see that moral judgements are being made about the sort of people that receive welfare benefits from the State, the people that make poor choices putting their own interests above those of their children. The kinds of choices that are alluded to include purchasing what *Paddyme* considers to be frivolous and unnecessary items. These sorts of comments are inflected with both explicit and implicit moral judgements about the types of choices that 'feckless' parents make. It is not only 'feckless' parents that are subject to moral judgement. In the debates about the fairness of UIFSM, more affluent parents also became subject to accusations of laziness and abdication of parental responsibility. For *Umopapsidn* in *The Guardian*,

> No offence but ... the argument that parents who are wealthy enough to provide decent food for their kids but can't be arsed to either prepare it themselves or buy in healthy stuff is letting them off the hook. To say that the well-off are not responsible for the quality of food they offer their children—ignoring what they choose to feed themselves—is senseless. You are, in essences allowing them to passively abdicate their parental responsibilities. And that's before the unlevel playing field comes into it.

For Mitchell Dean (2010, p. 19), these kinds of moral judgements are a fundamental part of governing the behaviour of individuals, since government 'presumes to know with varying degrees of explicitness and using specific forms of knowledge, what constitutes good, virtuous, appropriate, responsible conduct of individuals'. Consequently, morality can be understood not only as 'the attempt to make oneself accountable for one's own actions' but also to make others accountable.

The idea that people should be held responsible for their actions and choices even when they result in inequality is a familiar argument in moral philosophy (Wolff 1998). If inequality exists because people have voluntarily made different choices, or followed different paths, it is suggested there should be no moral compunction to redistribute resources for the purposes of equity. However, as Wolff (1998) also suggests, these debates very often utilise examples which are over-simplified (Wolff uses the example of the tennis player and the gardener where the former pursues a career she enjoys and remains poor, while the latter works hard and makes a good living). They take little account of Dworkin's (1981, cited in Wolff 1998) suggestion that we must consider the extent to which individuals have the same opportunities to acquire resources. Indeed, there can be circumstances in which it is 'fair' to redistribute resources to individuals who have suffered because of the choices they have made, since we do not all face the same kinds of choices under the same kinds of circumstances. When *Paddyme* takes issue with the *attitude* of 'feckless parents', he is suggesting that poor choices are not the result of accident or bad luck but are part of an entitlement culture. However, in both instances, it is not 'entitlement' that is being debated, since entitlement can be regarded in a relatively straightforward way in that it involves having a legitimate claim to something, according to given criteria. Rather, the issue is whether these people *should* be entitled to claim free school meals and whether they deserve to.

Here 'entitlement' is framed in moral terms which suggest that to 'be entitled' is to be 'lazy', is to expect 'something for nothing' and is to 'shirk' one's responsibilities. It is in this sense that Hall and O'Shea (2013, p.8) argue that the concept of fairness has become 'a quasi-market relation, a reward for personal effort'. As a 'quasi-market relation', or as a 'reward for personal effort', entitlement can only be enjoyed if you are deemed to have contributed to the public good, through hard work, effort or more usually, economically through taxation. In relation to debates about 'welfare scroungers', Hall and O'Shea (2013, p.9) suggest that

The debate has been conducted within a neoliberal framing of the agenda across most of the political spectrum and media output. This frame takes for granted that the market relation is central (you can only have what you pay for), the deficit is the problem, and cutting public expenditure is the only solution; and, within this, cutting welfare benefits is the priority—and it's all a result of 'Labour's mess'.

From this perspective, it is regarded as unfair to draw against the public purse without first contributing to it. As Cullity (2008, p.2) suggests, it 'is widely accepted that "free riding" by actively taking collectively produced goods without paying can be wrong'. However, this is not as straightforward as imagined since there are instances where people inadvertently receive public goods, and where doing so does not diminish others' access or enjoyment of those goods. For example, many of us may benefit from public street lighting or improved air quality without directly contributing to any costs associated with their provision. In some senses, we might argue that children and young people cannot be accused of 'free riding' since there is no expectation that children will have contributed to the public purse, or that they should be held accountable for the choices that their parents make. In which case, it could be seen as fair and impartial that all children receive school meals free of charge. The fact that their parents derive different levels of benefit from such a scheme could be regarded as irrelevant since this does not interfere with children's ability to access the meals, and they themselves are not drawing from a collective pot.

In terms of the neo-Liberal shaping of 'fairness' as a market relation, public and policy discourses often justify expenditure on particular policy initiatives, not on the grounds of existing contributions towards the public good but on future contributions. Brown (2015) suggests that under neo-Liberalism everything is 'economised' and in a very specific way: human beings become market actors and neo-Liberalism re-casts people as different forms of 'human capital' who must 'constantly tend to their own present and future value'. In this sense, it is considered 'fair' and 'right' for the taxpayer to invest in the UIFSM scheme if we are likely to see a reasonable future return on this investment. Investing in free school meals is deemed to be worthwhile in terms of the cost to the State of treating diet-related diseases, or in educational terms:

At a cost of around £223 per pupil per year, this suggests that it has cost £100 to £120 to obtain a 1 percentage point increase in attainment at Key Stage 1 and £40 to £60 to obtain a 1 percentage point increase in attainment at Key Stage 2. (Kitchen et al. 2013, p. 121)

Indeed, the evaluation report for the free school meals pilot project devoted some 26 pages to a cost–benefit analysis suggesting that

> academic performance in primary school is strongly linked to attainment in secondary school and to subsequent education and labour market choices, suggesting a credible route through which the pilot might affect longer-term outcomes. (Kitchen et al. 2013, p. 140)

In this sense, future generations of children and young people may be held morally responsible for making good on the State's investment.

Conclusion

Debates over free school meals reveal complex and often contradictory 'common sense' discourses that have been utilised by diverse commentators and politicians since the inception of the school meals service in the early twentieth century. As Hall and O'Shea (2013) suggest, common sense thinking is used to garner support and sediment certain beliefs about free school meals within popular thinking. Such discourses make certain lines of argument regarding the efficacy of UIFSM in terms of health and education outcomes problematic. However, as a welfare intervention, no such consensus is achieved since the idea of welfare is bound up with concepts of fairness and entitlement, moral concepts which have been reframed and 'economised' in the context of neo-Liberalism. Ideas of fairness are subject to debate since fair processes do not always produce fair outcomes and what is fair for children and young people may not be regarded as fair for their parents or the taxpayer. In this sense, fairness is used both to justify and to oppose the UIFSM scheme.

In considering the kinds of moralities that accompany public and policy discourses of free school meals, notions of entitlement and deservingness often play out in rather extreme ways that attempt to render parents accountable for their 'choices'. Children and young people are regarded as deserving or otherwise on the basis of these 'choices' in ways that suggest that parents are morally deficient 'free riders' for claiming free school meals. As Hall and O'Shea (2013, p. 8) suggest, such a view of welfare provision seems to be 'a long way from the collectivism of the 1940s'. What appears to be missing from these debates is any discussion of our collective moral responsibility to ensure that children and young people, *all* children and young people, are adequately fed and nourished, irrespective of their parents' actions or 'choices'. While the health and education benefits of free school meals are not fully understood or agreed upon and are methodologically challenging to demonstrate, what is not in doubt is that those children who receive an inadequate diet can suffer health problems as a result. If diet-related diseases are classified as a public health issue, then the provision of school meals can be regarded as a public good. This way of thinking, of collective responsibility towards our children and young people, could prove potentially fruitful in opening up a space through which we might challenge what Massey (2013) describes as the vocabularies of neo-Liberalism; vocabularies which fundamentally change not only our relationship to the world but also our relationship with young people.

References

Adams, R. 2013. Free school meals policy gets lukewarm reception from educationalists. *The Guardian*, September 18. Available from http://www.theguardian.com/education/2013/sep/18/free-school-meals-lukewarm-reception. Accessed 2 Apr 2016.

Blackman-Woods, R. 2010. *HC Deb* 30 June 2010. vol 512, cols 230 WH. Available from http://hansard.parliament.uk/Commons/2010-06-30/debates/10063026000001/FreeSchoolMeals#contribution-10063026000118. Accessed 2 Apr 2016.

Blair, T. 2006. Our Nation's Future, Healthy Living. Speech given in Nottingham UK, July 26. Available from http://webarchive.nationalarchives.gov.uk/+/http:/www.number10.gov.uk/Page9921. Accessed 2 Apr 2016.

Brown, W. 2015. Booked#3 What exactly is Neoliberalism? *Dissent*. Available from https://www.dissentmagazine.org/blog/booked-3-what-exactly-is-neoliberalism-wendy-brown-undoing-the-demos. Accessed 2 Apr 2016

Cullity, G. 2008. Public Goods and Fairness. *Australasian Journal of Philosophy* 86(1): 1–21.

Dean, M. 2010. *Governmentality: Power and rule in modern society*. London: Sage.

Department for Education. 2013. 'Evidence check' memorandum Universal infant free school meals (UIFSM). Available from https://www.parliament. uk/documents/commons-committees/Education/evidence-check-forum/ Universal-infant-free-school-meals.pdf. Accessed 2 Apr 2016.

Deputy Prime Minister's Office. 2013. Free school lunch for every child in infant school. September 17. Available from https://www.gov.uk/govern-ment/news/free-school-lunch-for-every-child-in-infant-school. Accessed 2 Apr 2016.

———. 2014. Deputy Prime Minister launches free school meals. September 2. Available from https://www.gov.uk/government/news/deputy-prime-minister-launches-free-school-meals. Accessed 2 April 2016.

Education (Provision of Meals) Act. 1906. Available from http://www.legisla-tion.gov.uk/ukpga/1906/57/enacted. Accessed 2 Apr 2016.

Evans, C.E.L., D.C. Greenwood, and J.E. Cade. 2010a. *A comparison of the nutrient intakes of British primary school children: A systematic review and meta-analysis*. UK: Nutritional Epidemiology Group, Centre of Epidemiology and Biostatistics, University of Leeds.

Evans, C.E.L., D.C. Greenwood, J.D. Thomas, and J.E. Cade. 2010b. A cross-sectional survey of children's packed lunches in the UK: Food- and nutrient-based results. *Journal of Epidemiology & Community Health* 64: 977–983.

Gelbier, S., and S. Randall. 1982. Charles Edward Wallis and the rise of London's school dental service. *Medical History* 26: 395–404.

Gustafsson, U. 2002. School meals policy: The problem with governing chil-dren. *Social Policy and Administration* 36: 685–697.

Hall, S., and A. O'Shea. 2013. Common-sense neoliberalism. In *After neoliber-alism? The Kilburn manifesto*, eds. S. Hall, D. Massey, and M. Rustin. Soundings.

Hastings, A, N. Bailey, G. Bramley, M. Gannon, and D. Watkins. 2015. The Cost of the Cuts: The Impact on Local Government and Poorer Communities. York: Joseph Rowntree Foundation. Available from http://socialwelfare. bl.uk/subject-areas/government-issues/welfare-state/josephrowntreefoundati on/173775Cost_Cuts_Summary-Final.pdf. Accessed 2 Apr 2016.

Loughton, T. 2010. HC Deb 30 June 2010. vol 512, cols 243 WH. Available from http://hansard.parliament.uk/Commons/2010-06-30/debates/10063026000001/ FreeSchoolMeals#contribution-10063026000118. Accessed 2 Apr 2016.

Kitchen, S., V. Brown, C. Crawford, L. Dearden, E. Greaves, C. Payne, S. Purdon, and E. Tanner. 2013. Evaluation of the Free School Meals Pilot Impact Report. Available from https://www.gov.uk/government/uploads/system/uploads/attachment_data/file/184047/DFE-RR227.pdf. Accessed 2 Apr 2016.

Massey, D. 2013. Vocabularies of the economy. In *After neoliberalism? The Kilburn manifesto*, eds. S. Hall, D. Massey, and M. Rustin. London, UK: Soundings.

Morgan, K. 2006. School food and the public domain: The politics of the public plate. *Political Quarterly* 77(3): 379–387.

Morris, N. 2014. David Laws vs Dominic Cummings: Education Department goes to war with itself over free school meals. *The Independent*, March 11. Available from http://www.independent.co.uk/news/education/education-news/david-laws-vs-dominic-cummings-education-department-goes-to-war-with-itself-over-free-school-meals-9185048.html. Accessed 2 Apr 2016.

Passmore, S., and G. Harris. 2004. Education, health and school meals: A review of policy changes in England and Wales over the last century. *Nutrition Bulletin* 29(3): 221–227.

Pike, J. 2010. An Ethnographic Study of Lunchtime Experiences in Primary School Dining Rooms, Unpublished Ph.D. Thesis, University of Hull.

Pike, J., and P. Kelly. 2014. *The Moral Geographies of Children, Young People and Food: Beyond Jamie's School Dinners*. London: Palgrave.

Rees, G.A., Richards C.J, and J. Gregory. 2008. Food and nutrient intakes of primary school children: A comparison of school meals and packed lunches. *Journal of Human Nutrition and Dietetics* 21: 420–427.

Sibley, D. 2004. Bodies and cultures collide: Enlistment, the medical exam and the British Working Class, 1914-1916. *Social History of Medicine* 17(1): 61–76.

Verheijden, M.W., and F.J. Kok. 2005. Public health impact of community-based nutrition and lifestyle interventions. *European Journal of Clinical Nutrition* 59(1): 66–76.

Welshman, J. 1997. School meals and milk in England and Wales, 1906–45. *Medical History* 41: 6–29.

Wolff, J. 1998. Fairness, Respect, and the Egalitarian Ethos. *Philosophy & Public Affairs* 27(2): 97–122.

Williams, Z. 2014. Free school meals should be for those who need them, not those who don't. *The Guardian*, September 2. Available from http://www.theguardian.com/commentisfree/2014/sep/02/free-school-meals-need-1bn-universal-benefit. Accessed 2 Apr 2016.

16

'Generation in Waiting' or 'Precarious Generation'? Conceptual Reflections on the Biographical Trajectories of Unemployed Graduates Activists in Morocco

Christoph H. Schwarz

Introduction

At the start of the twenty-first century the population demographics of many of the Middle East and North Africa (MENA) countries are characterized by a 'youth bulge'[1], that is, a large cohort of young people. Until the uprisings of 2011, these young people and young adults were hardly present in Western media. If considered at all, they tended to be discussed as a potential threat—associated with debates on

---

[1] The term was originally coined by Gary Fuller (1995, p. 154), who defined a youth bulge as a large cohort of people aged 15–24, that is, exceeding 20% of the overall population.

C.H. Schwarz (✉)
University of Marburg, Marburg, Germany

© The Editor(s) (if applicable) and The Author(s) 2017
P. Kelly, J. Pike (eds.), *Neoliberalism, Austerity, and the Moral Economies of Young People's Health and Well-being*,
DOI 10.1057/978-1-137-58266-9_17

terrorism[2], especially after 9/11. Here, the United Nations Arab Human Development Report (2002) represents an important intervention as it problematized the unemployment rates and general social situation of the young in the MENA region. However, this Report also perceives young people and young adults mainly as statistical data and as objects of policies that had to change. The Report did not take into account their less visible forms of agency and protest. Nor did it apply an open qualitative approach that would have asked how young adults themselves perceive and make sense of their situation. Accordingly, young people tended to be seen as politically lethargic victims of failed policies of authoritarian regimes and a 'traditional Islamic culture' that somehow lacked 'development'.

Against this background, researchers such as Asef Bayat (2000, 2010) pointed to what he called 'non-movements' and the 'quiet encroachment of the ordinary', describing, for example, the sometimes contradictory strategies with which young adults negotiate their freedoms in everyday life, even in highly repressive settings like Iran or Egypt.

Other important contributions to the policy discourse[3] include publications from the Middle East Youth Initiative (MEYI), a joint project by the Wolfensohn Center for Development at Brookings and the Dubai School of Government. Between 2006 and 2012, MEYI 'engaged an active, international network of researchers working together to improve

---

[2] Most prominently in Samuel Huntington's thesis of a 'Clash of Civilizations', that actually stated the demographic development in 'Muslim societies' as the most important 'reason for the aggressiveness of 'Islamic culture': 'Finally, and most important, the demographic explosion in Muslim societies and the availability of large numbers of often unemployed males between the ages of fifteen and thirty is a natural source of instability and violence both within Islam and against non-Muslims. Whatever other causes may be at work, this factor alone would go a long way to explaining Muslim violence in the 1980s and 1990s. The aging of this pig-in-the-python generation by the third decade of the twenty-first century and economic development in Muslim societies, if and as that occurs, could consequently lead to a significant reduction in Muslim violence propensities and hence to a general decline in the frequency and intensity of fault line wars.' Huntington 1996, p. 265)

[3] I distinguish this discourse from a scientific debate that is mostly confined to academic settings and journals that are not easily accessible for the general public and often do not translate into the media discourse. In the social sciences and area studies discourse, a variety of authors like Mounia Bennani-Chraibi (1994, 2000), Linda Herrera (2006) or Asef Bayat (2010), or Herrera and Bayat (2010) have shed light on the situation of youth in different contexts in the MENA region.

outcomes for the region's youth'. MEYI offers a selection of often qualitative cross-country research and policy papers on the situation of young people in the region, problematizing their social exclusion. Diane Singerman's (2007) concept of *waithood* can be considered the project's most important conceptual contribution in this regard. Waithood describes a particular form of social exclusion of the young through a particular 'political economy of marriage' that for many results in a stalled transition to adulthood.

In this chapter, I aim to critically discuss the concept of waithood and defend it against possible neo-Liberal readings that would shift the focus away from the central problem of unemployment and precarious labor. I argue that on the one hand, the term does address central problems of young biographies in the region, while on the other hand, it can easily be used to cater to stereotypes of an economically passive, politically lethargic 'victim youth' that is to be 'mobilised' into entrepreneurship by pedagogic, institutional and economic policies.

In the following section, I will first outline and discuss the concept of waithood and its neo-Liberal readings. I will then take the Moroccan unemployed graduates movement as an example of how young adults have addressed their economic situation and have 'apolitically' protested in an authoritarian regime for over a decade before the 'Arab Spring', largely unnoticed by the Western public. I will then illustrate the psychosocial situation behind these protests, based on in-depth interviews with activists. In the conclusion, I will discuss the advantages and dangers of the concept of waithood against the background of these interviews, and elaborate on open questions for further research on young people in the region.

Waithood, Marriage and Youth Unemployment

Based on her research in Egypt, Diane Singerman (2007, pp. 9–10) describes a particular 'political economy of marriage' and emphasizes that 'adulthood equals marriage in the Middle East'. As a general rule, especially for women, it is a prerequisite for moving out and forming one's own family. But given the predominant cultural definitions, marriage comes at a certain financial price that Singerman calculates as the sum of six basic component costs: housing; furniture and appliances; gifts of gold to the bride (*shabka*); dower (*mahr*); celebrations; and the bride's trousseau, including clothing, less expensive furnishings and smaller household items. By her calculations, this is a sum that, in Egypt, amounts to four and a half times the gross national product per capita and eleven times the average annual household expenditure per capita. Taking into account the high youth unemployment, it becomes obvious that accumulating this amount of capital is next to impossible for many young adults, and that it takes them far longer than the previous generations to make this transition to adulthood. In the meantime, and often well into their late 30s, they continue to live with their parents and depend on the income of the older generation. Thus, waithood describes a particular form of social exclusion of the young generation that

> places young people in an adolescent, liminal world where they are neither children nor adults. In this liminal state, young people remain financially dependent on their families (who, in large part, finance the costs of marriage) for far longer than previous generations and they must live by the rules and morality of their parents and the dominant values of society which frown on unchaperoned fraternization and unmarried relationships. (Singerman 2007, p. 6)[4]

Singerman points to other studies that highlight the urgency of this problem for the interviewees, for example, the research by Brian Katulis (2004). In his study for Freedom House, Katulis found that the Egyptian interviewees interpreted women's rights—and human rights in general—mainly in economic terms, as the following quotations illustrate:

> '[Human rights means] the essentials—food at a suitable price, housing, and security.' (Urban man, 20–29, college graduate, Cairo)

---

[4] For a further discussion on waithood, see Silver 2007; Salehi-Isfahani 2008; Dhillon and Yousef 2009; Singerman 2011; Honwana 2014; Mulderig 2013.

'My right as a human being is to work.' (Rural man, 20–29, high school graduate)

'[Human rights mean] financial rights, because the country is deteriorating. Things are becoming more and more expensive, and in general there is an economic slump. I'm getting married, and I can't get everything I need.' (Newly urban woman, 20–29, literate) (Katulis 2004)

However, these interviewees' demand for human rights as economic rights—guaranteed by the state—is contrasted with a general neo-Liberal tendency of MEYI whose authors often encourage a further roll-back of the state as an employer. Dhillon, Dyer and Yousef (2009), for example, explicitly promote a 'post-welfare life course' in their analysis of young people's lives in the MENA region. They distinguish three ideal types of life courses: a traditional life course, in which individuals tend to pass directly from childhood to adulthood, a transition organized by family and community: this life course still prevails in some of the more rural regions, and it presents young people, especially women, with few economic opportunities. In the last 50 years, this life course was by and by replaced by a welfare life course: in parallel with the development of rent-based economies it was state institutions that organized the transitions to adulthood by providing public education for an increasing number of children and young people, and by later offering them public sector jobs. However, in the wake of the oil-price-crash in the 1980s, state institutions retracted while birth rates continued to grow, resulting in the increasing incapacity of governments to sustain the welfare life course. After describing these two life courses, the authors switch into the mode of future prognostics, when they describe a 'post-welfare life course':

In the post-welfare life course, young people's transitions are based on choice, better information, and the right signals from institutions. The education transition is built on acquiring a broad range of skills as opposed to simply the degrees necessary for public sector work. Work transitions are flexible and provide productive careers in the private sector rather than government jobs. Access to capital allows young people to build credit reputations that can be leveraged toward marriage and family formation. These critical transitions are mediated by well-functioning markets, the

private sector and governments. Because the Middle East is still transitioning from state-run to market economies, this new life course has yet fully
to emerge. (Dhillon et al. 2009, pp. 15–16)

Here, 'access to capital', mentioned as an empowering instrument toward
personal independence, marriage and family formation, apparently refers
to access to easy credit and loans, without any mention of the risk of 'lend-
ing to the poor' and the severe consequences if debtors due to economic
crisis cannot pay back, as has happened in Spain since 2007 (Colau and
Alemany 2012), or many other contexts (Soederberg 2014). Apparently,
in this political project, credit is supposed to replace the revenue that
before was provided by state-run rent economies.

The analytic approach and policy recommendations applied here
juxtapose rigid state institutions and a forlorn 'traditional' culture
with a dynamic market—a market that is associated with the dynamic
of youth and promises to mobilize their innovative potential. Thus, a
vague stereotype of 'youthful dynamic' is employed to promote a particular neo-Liberal agenda (Sukarieh 2012; Sukarieh and Tannock 2015).
Emblematic of this vision is Hillary Clinton's address to Tunisian young
people at a town hall meeting in 2012:

> Young people are at the heart of today's great strategic opportunities and
> challenges, from rebuilding the global economy to combating violent
> extremism to building sustainable democracies. … I hear sometimes from
> leaders in this region that there is a certain fear about opening their econo-
> mies, but I think that does a great disservice to the people of these coun-
> tries that have so much energy, and especially to young people. Opening
> the economies will particularly advantage the young people of Tunisia and
> other places. (Clinton 2012, February 25)

In the wake of the 2011 uprisings, to the two stereotypes of MENA
youth as a potential terrorist threat or as politically lethargic victims, a
third was added: youth is addressed as a source of valuable human capital
and young people are imagined as the future entrepreneurs who will overcome the current economic crisis, a potential that policy makers seem
eager to mobilize.

The case of the unemployed university graduates movement in Morocco offers an interesting example, precisely because it contradicts all three of these stereotypes, as we will see in the next section.

The Moroccan Unemployed Graduates Movement and Its Historical Context

The Moroccan *diplômés chômeurs*—or unemployed graduates—movement is the first of its kind in the world. It developed against the background of two related developments in Morocco: the creation of a large public sector and the expansion of public education in the 1970s and the subsequent roll-back of the public sector as a consequence of structural adjustment programs (SAPs) imposed by the International Monetary Fund (IMF) and World Bank since the early 1980s.

In contrast to states like Algeria or Egypt, where after independence one-party governments heavily centralized the economy around the state, the Moroccan monarchy opted for a multiparty political system and a 'controlled liberal economic system' (Bogaert and Emperador 2011). The monarchy has been using a semiformal network of patronage to wield influence, grant favors and exercise control and repression. Relying on and extending this network, commonly referred to as the *makhzen*[5], the state in the 1960s and 1970s brought many economic activities under its control and allotted resources to its supporters, a process that was referred to as 'Moroccanization' (White 2001). Where co-optation did not suffice to silence the opposition—left-wing, democratic or Berber activists, or student activists like the National Moroccan Student Union (Union National des Étudiants Marocains)—political violence was employed. Indeed, the phase after independence under Mohamed V. in 1956, of Hassans II's accession to throne in 1961, until the end of the Cold War is commonly referred to as the 'Years of Lead', due to the general repressive climate, in which the regime arbitrarily detained, tortured or 'disappeared' thousands of citizens.

---

[5] The respective Arabic term has been imported to European languages over the centuries and, in the English case, has been adopted to the word 'magazine'. In the Moroccan context, it can be understood as 'property of the king'.

Most importantly during the phase of 'Moroccanization', Hassan II had secured his control of Morocco's most important sector at that time, phosphate exports, which henceforth have been handled by the monopoly of the Sherifian Office of Phosphates (OCP, Office Chérifien des Phosphates). Morocco has since been the world's most important phosphate exporter, and due to a world market rise in phosphate export prices, the OCP revenues allowed the government to expand the public sector as well as the educational sector in the 1970s. According to Koen Bogaert and Montserrat Emperador (2011, p.245), between 1970 and 1977, university enrollment tripled and the number of public servants grew at an annual average rate of 5.5 so that graduates 'were practically guaranteed a job in the public sector. This formed part of a social contract between the authorities and the new urban middle class'.

However, with the fall of the Franco regime in Spain in 1975 and the subsequent decolonization processes, the Moroccan monarchy seized the territory of the Western Sahara in 1975, thus engaging in an armed conflict with the *Polisario* movement, which resulted in further public expenditures for military campaigns as well as for investing in the infrastructure of this territory. Due to these and other factors, the Moroccan semi-rentier model of economic policy and the respective social pact could not be sustained at this level. By the end of the 1970s, Morocco faced fiscal instabilities and sharply reduced public spending, which resulted in an increase in unemployment rates. Due to dropping phosphate prices in the early 1980s, government revenues declined further. At that time, major 'bread riots' broke out in Casablanca in 1981. In 1983, Morocco adopted an IMF and World Bank SAP. This SAP included a devaluation of the Moroccan currency, the *dirham*, liberalization of trade and further public budget cuts (White 2001, p. 32).

As a consequence, the unemployment rate among university graduates rose from 6.5 % in 1982 to 26 % in 1991 and 40 % in 2002 (Bogaert and Emperador 2011). This rate tended to be higher among those with higher degrees (Cohen, Jaidi 2006, p. 139). In this situation, Mounia Bennani-Chraïbi (2000, p. 143) considered the integration of the educated urban young 'the most pressing problem in Morocco today'.

In 1991, Morocco witnessed the first protests of unemployed university graduate activists, who soon would found a syndicate-like organization, the National Association of Moroccan Unemployed Graduates (ANDCM, Association Nationale de Diplômés Chômeurs du Maroc), the first of its kind in the world (Sater 2007, p. 97). The unemployed graduates movement developed out of Moroccan university students' unions. Although the first activists shared a left-wing or pan-Arab *ba'athist* ideology, the new movement arose out of the frustration with 'traditional ideological politics'. Their own and the previous generations' experiences of the 'Years of Lead' had made them cautious to avoid repression by the state forces and they opted for a form of 'apolitical mobilization' (Emperador 2011). The new-born movement centered around one subject: the right to work and the protest against employment through nepotist and patronage networks. The 'moral economy' (Thompson 1971; Pripstein Posusney 1993) of these protests can be described, in the words of Abdelrahman Rachik (2010), in terms of not being granted the social position one actually deserves after long years of effort and high investment in study. Central references were to articles 12 and 13 of the 1996 constitution, which state that all citizens 'have equally right to education and to work' (13) and that they 'can accede, in the same conditions, to positions within the public sector' (12); furthermore, they refer to two ministerial decrees that guarantee the direct employment into public service to graduates of the third degree (those holding a master's degree) (Cohen and Jaidi 2006; Bogaert and Emperador 2011).

Demanding jobs from the government was a rather open approach that from the very beginning also allowed Islamists, Amazigh[6] activists, and nonpartisan graduates to participate. However, the activists' repertoire of collective action (Tilly 1986; McAdam et al. 2001) was undoubtedly inherited from the movement of the Moroccan left. At first, activists confined themselves to sit-ins and hunger strikes in the relatively protected environments of the offices of supportive labor unions. However,

---

[6] The Amazigh—or Berber, a term that some reject—consider themselves the indigenous population of the Maghrib, those who inhabited the region before the invasion of Arab tribes. Tamazigh, a language of the Afro-Asian family that is present in Morocco in three regional varieties, is often referred to as the strongest marker of difference against Arab cultural identity. The Moroccan Amazigh movement, which has developed along social and cultural cleavages in the last decades, is a cultural and political, nationalist movement that opposes the projects of a pan-Arab or Islamist hegemony, and the concomitant social exclusion and marginalization of the Amazigh population (Maddy-Weitzman 2011).

after some years of consolidation and organizational expansion into more remote regions, the ANDCM adopted more public tactics, culminating, in 1995, in a nine and a half months sit-in—the longest in Moroccan history—in front of the Ministry of Education. Ever since, their actions have been mainly street based: demonstrations and sit-ins in front of the parliament in the country's capital, Rabat, demanding negotiations with the Minister of Works, or in case of repression with the Minister of the Interior (Sater 2007, p. 94; Rachik 2010, p. 26; Emperador 2011).

Within a couple of years a certain political ritual evolved: when protests grew stronger, the government, drawing on repression as well as co-optation, would regularly negotiate with the protesters and directly employ some of them in the public sector. The coordinators of the protests would in turn monitor their members, using lists of participation, in order to make sure that only those who regularly and actively participated in the protests were given a job. Activists would be given tokens they had to return to their local coordinator after the demonstrations (Emperador 2007, 2009; Bogaert and Emperador 2011; Emperador 2011). In some committees, those activists who exposed themselves more to police violence during sit-ins, for example, by forming the front row, would be given a higher ranking on the list of the coordinators.[7]

After successful negotiations and ensuing employment, the respective protest groups would dissolve, only to be soon replaced by new cohorts of fresh graduates who could not find a public sector job. In the course of this process, the structure of the ANDCM would more and more be sidelined and replaced by decentralized local coordinations that in recent years have organized not only based on region but also based on degree level.

At the time of conducting interviews, in autumn 2014, the activists would gather in groups (according to their local coordination) up to three days every week in a park that is situated 250 meters from the Moroccan parliament in Rabat. Usually they would gather in circles and discuss organizational and strategic questions. When they decided they were enough activists for a significant protest, they would form a disciplined demonstration, many of them dressed with vests bearing the

---

[7] Personal communication by one activist to the author, November 2014.

logos of their committees, and take to the streets. Organizers wearing special vests would walk at the side of the demonstration. In front of the parliament, the demonstration would usually be dissolved by the antiriot brigades of the police. The activists would run from the police, but return in smaller groups, mingle with tourists or passers-by in front of the parliament, where they would again take out their banners and start to shout and sing slogans until the police would run toward them again.

Exploring the Lives of Unemployed Graduate Activists

The data material that is the focus of this section consists of four in-depth narrative-biographical interviews with activists in the *diplômés chômeurs* movement, four of them individual interviews with male activists and one interview with two female activists.[8]

Educational Trajectories, Financial Situation and Family Dependency

The two female interviewees, Karima, who writes her PhD in philosophy, and Latifa, a PhD candidate in informatics, do currently not work for wage; instead, they contribute to the household of their families. They also commute weekly from their families' houses in the Middle Atlas in order to join the protests with their committee, and they stay with friends or relatives in the suburbs of Rabat.

All of the four male interviewees work, albeit all in precarious conditions: Shafik, for example, is a 32-year-old man who describes himself as the 'son of a nomad'. He has six sisters and two brothers. His grandparents, parents and older siblings are illiterate. He was the first of the family to attend school. Two of his younger sisters and his younger brother are

---

[8] These interviews were conducted in the course of three one-month-long fieldtrips to Morocco in 2014 and 2015; interview languages were French and English. The context of the fieldtrips was a general study on the biographies of political protesters and the moral economy of their protests in Morocco.

currently attending school, living in the house of their maternal grandparents in the Middle Atlas, while his parents continue to 'live in the desert', as he says. Shafik is the first and so far only member of his nuclear family to attend university. He graduated with a BA and MA in mathematics and is now writing his PhD in the same discipline. Currently, he has a PhD scholarship from the government of 1000 *dirham* (around 90€) a month, and he is working in the informal private sector, giving classes as a freelance tutor for pupils, in order to cover for his living costs in Rabat. He frequently describes his strategy to pay for his living as a sequence of precarious jobs: to 'do some bricolage' as he calls it. At the time of the interview, he was living in a room of approximately 16m² on the top of an apartment building in a poor neighborhood at the outskirts of Rabat, a room he was renting with three other PhD students for the cost of 250 *dirham* (approximately 20€) each. His family apparently cannot support him, and in any case he would refuse support by them, because he does not consider it appropriate for his age.

One of his flatmates, Hassan, lives under similar conditions. His father is a farmer, he holds a BA and an MA in biology, and he is currently pursuing his PhD. He too gives private lessons for high school pupils and undergraduate students, also doing 'bricolage'.

In contrast to Hassan and Shafik, who live in Rabat, where the protests take place, in November 2014, the rest of the interviewees commuted to the protests from cities like Meknès or Fès every week, up to four-hour train ride away.[9]

Omar, 31, who grew up in small village in the Rif mountains, shared a room with 11 other activists in Rabat and another flat with 7 other people in Fès, where he studied. His father, a tailor, died when Omar was 12 years old. He emphasizes that this was not only psychologically very hard but also socioeconomically. His oldest brother had to step in and earn the money for the family. He highlights that most of his friends and colleagues continue to financially depend on their fathers. He described his first experiences on the labor market after finishing his BA in English Literature as follows:

---

[9] Another female activist I talked to regularly commuted from Oujda, the easternmost city at the Algerian border, a twelve-hour train ride away.

I tried the private sector. I worked as a teacher for primary school students from 2007 to 2010 so it was three years in the private sector, in a private school. I would work for fifteen hours per week and I would be payed 1500 *dirhams* [around 135€] each month. So later on I just made up my mind and I realized that continuing in that position wouldn't help me to establish a family, because with 1500 *dirhams* it is simply impossible.

In this context, and in Hassan's and Shafik's mentioning of their 'bricolage' employment, it becomes salient that unemployed graduates actually do work, but their precarious wages simply do not provide for founding a family, realizing a middle-class life course, or for a living that would come close to the promise of social upward mobility associated with higher education (Bogaert and Emperador 2011). The definition of employment then becomes 'being given the job that one actually deserves', according to one's education. Accordingly, Omar explained that he continued his studies, hoping to later find a better job, and pursued an MA in Gender Studies, the subject in which he is currently writing his PhD thesis.

Marriage Prospects and Broken Relationships

In comparison to other countries in the MENA region, urban Morocco is often described as holding relatively tolerant views regarding courtship and premarital relations (Bennani-Chraïbi 1994; Cheikh 2014). Omar and another interviewee, his colleague Driss, actually had relationships with fellow students. For Omar, marriage has obviously a high relevance when it comes to career choices and to the decision to continue his studies. However, Omar and Driss both recount that their girlfriends broke up with them, and they see their 'unemployment'—or rather, their precarious employment—as the reason for this. They wanted to marry their girlfriends but they kept hoping that their protests for a public sector employment would soon pay off. So they put off their partners in order to propose later on. Omar relates that his partner was under a lot of pressure from her family to marry soon, and that she finally broke up with him and cut the contact with him. In Driss's case, his girlfriend's father married her to another man, against her will.

Hassan, however, had actually married a divorced woman with a son of a different father, and his wife was expecting his child at the time of the first interview. She lived with his parents in his village of origin in the Southern Atlas, around seven hours by public transport. Under current circumstances, due to the costs of travel and the time lost during the long trip, Hassan could only see his wife and his parents every two to three months.

For Shafik, however, marriage does not seem relevant for his idea of a transition to adulthood, and he does not have a relationship. When directly asked about his plans to form a family, he answers that this was of rather low priority: 'maybe after four years after obtaining a public sector job'. When asked what he would do if he was given the public sector job, he is currently protesting for, he first mentions that he wants to provide for his family of origin, to make up for all they have given to him, and especially to provide for his younger brothers and sisters. In addition, he would dedicate himself more to the struggle of the Amazigh movement. But then he returns to the question of providing for his family and mentions that he bought books for his younger siblings 'so they don't feel inferior'. He later remarks that his younger brother currently has problems in school, 'because he considers himself inferior. I'm trying to help him, but I don't know exactly what he is currently going through'. Apparently, his idea of providing for the next generation—a central step in the transitions to adulthood in many theories of youth and adolescence (Erikson 1959; King 2010)—first and foremost implies generationality within his family of origin, instead of founding a family of his own, as the concept of waithood would suggest.

Karima and Latifa, the two female interviewees, mentioned that some of their female colleagues were actively looking for marriage partners, but they emphasized that they themselves do not have a spouse and are not looking for one, 'because God has already decided for us'. In emphasizing this passive position, they seemed to confine to a hegemonic norm of female chastity before marriage.

Perspectives on the Moroccan 'Arab Spring'

All of the interviewees held rather negative views of the mass protests organized by the 20th of February Movement (M20F) that formed in 2011 in the wake of the uprisings in Tunisia and Egypt and can be considered the Moroccan brand of the so-called Arab Spring. According to Omar, the so-called Arab Spring 'was a curse for the unemployed graduates movement'. He relates how the *diplômés chômeurs* at first tried to exploit the volatile situation; they threatened to join the M20F-protests, and the government, then headed by the Istiqlal party, reacted with promising public sector jobs to 4.403 protesters, if the unemployed graduates did not join the M20F protests. Hassan also cited this number; however, at least half of the jobs that were actually created were then given to people that were not on the lists of the unemployed graduates coordinators: 'sons-of-someone', as he conjectured. Moreover, the subsequent parliamentary elections brought the Islamist Justice and Development Party (Parti de Justice et Development) to power, whose leaders constantly refused to stick to the written agreement signed with the former government. Thus, according to Shafik, the prospects of this current cohort of unemployed graduates of being employed in the public sector are rather dim. Shafik highlights that the M20F has 'a different agenda', and in fact interrupted the negotiation processes with the government.

These statements show that the spectacular revolts of 2011, so often hailed by the Western public that actually coined the term 'Arab Spring', also had negative side effects, at least for some of the young activists and social movements in the region. The scholarly debate still lacks a systematic comparison of both movements, and a discussion of how far the experiences of the unemployed graduates movement contributed to the repertoire of contention of M20F, or the character of collective action, or how the new modes of organization that M20F experimented with (horizontal and open assemblies) differed from the Unemployed Graduates' closed-shop model.

Conclusion

The term *waithood* marks an important contribution to research on the situation of young people in the MENA region, particularly because, in earlier public and policy discourse, youth tended to be perceived mainly as a demographic problem, while their social situation and psycho-social suffering was often ignored. Nevertheless, the concept should be used with caution as it might contribute, at least semantically, to the stereotype of a political lethargic or economically passive young adult. But a case like that of the unemployed graduates activists shows that this does not hold true. The contradictory character of their somewhat particularistic and 'apolitical mobilization' can be explained against the background of the Moroccan 'Years of Lead', a phase of significant repression and state violence against any oppositional movement that would campaign for radical change or dare to speak in the name of a general interest. Equally, when it comes to economic activity, it is significant that none of these activists are actually '*hiyateen*' ('those who lean on walls', as they are called in Cairo to describe young unemployed men who spend their day loitering in the streets) (Gregg 2005: 270). To the contrary, at least all of the young male activists are actually quite busy, and they can be described as 'working poor': the jobs they take in the private sector do not offer any long-term prospects. Their working days instead seem to be characterized by an often hectic and forcedly spontaneous improvisation under precarious conditions, as the frequently used term 'bricolage' suggests. It is also no surprise that marriage is highly relevant for them. The cases of Omar and Driss show that they are suffering from not being able to form a family, just like the cases of Latifa and Karima. However, despite the central patriarchal role of the family, these cases also show that Moroccan society offers a certain leeway when it comes to premarital relations and courtship. In addition, Shafik's case indicates that for some young adults, marriage does not have a central relevance because they feel more responsible to support their family of origin. Instead of being dependent on them, Shafik's first priority is to 'give something back' and to assume the role of a responsible older brother. It seems no coincidence that this case represents the most extraordinary educational career of the sample: a son of an illiterate nomad family who is now about to pursue a PhD in mathematics.

Diane Singerman's (2007) original discussion of waithood included open questions that are instructive for discussions of globally declining wages in some sectors of the economy. For example, her reference to Marxist-feminist discussions on how unpaid reproductive labor, usually carried out by women, is a necessary contribution in order to keep wages low for capital, points to important questions in the debate. Her critique of a 'political economy of marriage' rightly emphasizes that we are dealing with highly political questions here, instead of mere market dynamics or demographic development. A critique in this vain will take into account the role of the state, that is, the problematic nexus between the authoritarianism of a regime and its patronage politics. The objections raised in this paper should be read as directed against depoliticizing, neo-Liberal readings of the term 'waithood' that would result in simply proposing a better educational preparation of the young to 'take the initiative', to be 'active' in becoming small entrepreneurs, therefore further individualizing the risks regarding their transitions to adulthood, as it is defined in this socio-political context.

To sum up, the movement of unemployed graduates shows that, at least in the Moroccan case, the concept of *waithood* cannot be applied without discussing precarious work conditions and the lack of employment rights in the private sector; the absence of long-term prospects that this 'waiting' describes can nevertheless imply a very mobile, hectic and stressful day-to-day routine. Furthermore, the cases presented here highlight that 'unemployment' is a flexible and political category that can be reinterpreted for social struggles, and that negotiations with authoritarian regimes sometimes take on forms that are considered 'apolitical' and thus escape the views of the Western public. It is evident that the movement's practice of protesting against nepotism and patronage regarding employment, while at the same time negotiating the activists' own incorporation into these very networks, is contradictory. Unlike many of the 'Arab Spring' protesters, this movement does not offer a case for easy identification and idealization to the Western audience; instead, the movement illustrates the complex context and constraints of long-term social mobilization under authoritarianism in a postcolonial context. As it furthermore contradicts the three stereotypes of young people in the MENA region, outlined above, this largely ignored movement exemplifies the need for a critical revision of public and scientific discourses, and for more reflexive approaches when doing research on youth, in this context and elsewhere. Finally, the movement once more illustrates that the transition to adulthood, its intersection with the reproduction of social inequality and social exclusion and the potential spaces societies offer (or refuse) to pass this transition are very political issues, and that they should be discussed as such.

References

Bayat, A. 2000. From 'Dangerous Classes' to 'Quiet Rebels': Politics of the Urban Subaltern in the Global South. *International Sociology* 15(3): 533–557.

——— 2010. *Life as Politics: How Ordinary People change the Middle East.* Amsterdam: Amsterdam University Press.

Bennani-Chraïbi, M. 1994. *Soumis et rebelles: Les jeunes au Maroc.* Paris: Centre national de la recherche scientifique.

——— 2000. Youth in Morocco: An Indicator of a Changing Society. In *Alienation or integration of Arab youth: Between family state and street*, ed. R. Meijer, 143–160. Curzon: Richmond.

Bogaert, K., and M. Emperador. 2011. Imagining the State through Social Protest: State Reformation and the Mobilizations of Unemployed Graduates in Morocco. *Mediterranean Politics* 16: 241–259.

Cheikh, M. 2014. *L'économie intime: de la prostitution à une nouvelle éthique sexuelle au Maroc du XXi ème siècle* [online]. Available from: http://www.farzyat.org/leconomie-intime-de-la-prostitution-a-une-nouvelle-ethique-sexuelle-au-maroc-du-xxie-siecle. Accessed 15 Nov 2015.

Clinton, H. 2012. *Town Hall with Tunisian Youth* [online], February 25. Available from: http://www.state.gov/secretary/20092013clinton/rm/2012/02/184656.htm. Accessed 26 Jan 2015.

Cohen, S., and L. Jaidi. 2006. *Morocco: Globalization and its consequences.* New York: Routledge.

Colau, A., and A. Alemany. 2012. *Mortgaged Lives. From the Housing Bubble to the Right to Housing*, vol 2014. Los Angeles: The Journal of Aesthetics and Protest.

Dhillon, N., and T. Yousef, eds. (2009). *Generation in waiting: The unfulfilled promise of young people in the Middle East.* Washington DC: Brookings Institution Press.

Dhillon, N., P. Dyer, and T. Yousef. 2009. Generation in Waiting: An Overview of School to Work and Family Formation Transitions. In *Generation in waiting: The unfulfilled promise of young people in the Middle East*, eds. N. Dhillon and T. Yousef, 12–38. Washington, DC: Brookings Institution Press.

Emperador, M. 2007. Diplômés chômeurs au Maroc : dynamiques de pérennisation d'une action collective plurielle. *L'Année du Maghreb* III: 297–311.

——— 2009. Les manifestations des diplômés chômeurs au Maroc: la rue comme espace de négociation du tolérable. *Genèses* 3(77): 30–50.

————— 2011. Unemployed Moroccan University Graduates and Strategies for 'Apolitical' Mobilization. In *Social Movements, Mobilization, and Contestation in the Middle East and North Africa*, eds. J. Beinin and F. Vairel, 217–235. Stanford: Stanford University Press.

Erikson, E.H. 1959. *Identity and the life cycle*, vol 1980. New York: Norton.

Fuller, G. 1995. The Demographic Backdrop to Ethnic Conflict: A Geographic Overview. In *The Challenge of Ethnic Conflict to National and International Order in the 1990s*, ed. Gewin Edward, 151–154. Washington, DC: Central Intelligence Agency.

Gregg, G.S. 2005. *The Middle East: A cultural psychology*. Oxford: Oxford University Press.

Herrera, L. 2006. When does Life begin? Youth Perspectives from Egypt. *DevIssues [online]* 8(2): 7–9. Available from: http://www.iss.nl/fileadmin/ASSETS/iss/Documents/DevISSues/DevISSues_Volume_8__number_2__Dec_2006.pdf. Accessed 29 June 2015.

Herrera, L., and A. Bayat. 2010. *Being young and Muslim: New cultural politics in the global south and north*. New York: Oxford University Press.

Honwana, A. 2014. "Waithood": Youth transitions and social change. In *Development and Equity: An Interdisciplinary Exploration by Ten Scholars from Africa, Asia and Latin America*, ed. D. Foeken, 19–27. Leiden: Brill.

Huntington, S.P. 1996. *The Clash of Civilizations and the Remaking of World Order*. New York: Simon & Schuster.

Katulis, B. 2004. *Women's Rights in Focus: Egypt. Findings from June 2004 focus groups with Egyptian citizens on women's rights* [online]. Available from: https://freedomhouse.org/sites/default/files/inline_images/Women's%20Rights%20in%20Focus-%20Egypt%20.pdf. Accessed 10 Nov 2015

King, V. 2010. The Generational Rivalry for Time. *Time & Society* 19(1): 54–71.

Maddy-Weitzman, B. 2011. *The Berber identity movement and the challenge to North African states*. Austin: University of Texas Press.

Mcadam, D.G., S.G. Tarrow, and C. Tilly. 2001. *Dynamics of Contention*. Cambridge: Cambridge University Press.

Mulderig, M.C. 2013. *An Uncertain Future: Youth Frustration and the Arab Spring* [online]. Boston, Boston University. Available from: http://www.bu.edu/pardee/files/2013/04/Pardee-Paper-16.pdf?PDF=pardee-papers-16-arab-spring. Accessed 18 Oct 2016.

Pripstein Posusney, M. 1993. Irrational Workers: The Moral Economy of Labor Protest in Egypt. *World Politics* 46(1): 83–120.

Rachik, A. 2010. *Nouveaux mouvements sociaux et protestations au Maroc* [online]. Maroc: IRES—Institut royal des études stratégiques. Available from: http://www.ires.ma/sites/default/files/nouveaux_mouvements_sociaux_et_protestations_au_maroc.pdf?access=1. Accessed 14 Feb 2014.

Salehi-Isfahani, D. 2008. Stalled Youth Transitions in the Middle East: A Framework for Policy Reform. *Middle East Youth Initiative Working Paper* 8.

Sater, J.N. 2007. *Civil society and political change in Morocco*. London, New York: Routledge.

Silver, H. 2007. Social Exclusion: Comparative Analysis of Europe and Middle East Youth [online], Middle East Youth Initiative.

Singerman, D. 2007. The Economic Imperatives of Marriage: Emerging Practices and Identities among Youth in the Middle East. *Middle East Youth Initiative Working Paper* 6.

Singerman, D. 2011. The Negotiation of Waithood. The Political Economy of Delayed Marriage in Egypt. In *Arab youth: Social mobilization in times of risk*, eds. S. Khalaf and R.S. Khalaf, 67–78. London: Saqi Books.

Soederberg, S. 2014. *Debtfare states and the poverty industry: Money, discipline and the surplus population*. London: Routledge.

Sukarieh, M. 2012. From terrorists to revolutionaries: the emergence of "youth" in the Arab world and the discourse of globalization. *Interface: A Journal for and about Social Movements* 4(2): 424–437.

Sukarieh, M., and S. Tannock. 2015. *Youth Rising?: The Politics of Youth in the Global Economy*. London: Routledge.

Thompson, E.P. 1971. The Moral Economy of the English Crowd in the Eighteenth Century. *Past & Present* 50(1): 76–136.

Tilly, C. 1986. *The Contentious French*. Cambridge, MA: Harvard University Press.

White, G. 2001. *A Comparative Political Economy of Tunisia and Morocco. On the Outside of Europe looking in*. New York: State University of New York Press.

Index

Note: Page number followed by 'n' denotes notes

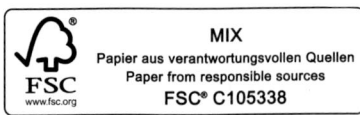

Printed by Books on Demand, Germany